OXFORD MEDICAL PUBLICATIONS

Paediatric Dentistry

Paediatric Dentistry

Third Edition

Edited by

Richard Welbury

Professor of Paediatric Dentistry
University of Glasgow

Monty Duggal
Professor of Child Dental Health
Leeds Dental Institute

and

Marie Thérèse Hosey
Department of Child Dental Care
University of Glasgow

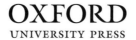
OXFORD
UNIVERSITY PRESS

OXFORD

UNIVERSITY PRESS

Great Clarendon Street, Oxford OX2 6DP

Oxford University Press is a department of the University of Oxford.
It furthers the University's objective of excellence in research, scholarship,
and education by publishing worldwide in

Oxford New York

Auckland Cape Town Dar es Salaam Hong Kong Karachi
Kuala Lumpur Madrid Melbourne Mexico City Nairobi
New Delhi Shanghai Taipei Toronto

With offices in

Argentina Austria Brazil Chile Czech Republic France Greece
Guatemala Hungary Italy Japan Poland Portugal Singapore
South Korea Switzerland Thailand Turkey Ukraine Vietnam

Oxford is a registered trade mark of Oxford University Press
in the UK and in certain other countries

Published in the United States
by Oxford University Press Inc., New York

First edition published 1997
Reprinted 1999
Second edition published 2001
Reprinted 2003, 2004

Third edition published 2005
Reprinted 2006

British Library Cataloguing in Publication Data

Data available

Library of Congress Cataloging in Publication Data

Data available

Typeset by Newgen Imaging Systems (P) Ltd., Chennai, India
Printed by CPI Bath
on acid-free paper

ISBN 0 19 8565836   978 0 19 856583 3

3 5 7 9 10 8 6 4 2

Contents

Contributors

M. J. Aldred   Department of Dentistry
Royal Childrens' Hospital Melbourne

A. S. Blinkhorn   Professor of Oral Health
University of Manchester

N. E. Carter   Department of Child Dental Health
Dental Hospital, Newcastle upon Tyne

P. J. M. Crawford   Department of Child Dental Health
University of Bristol

P. F. Day   Department of Child Dental Health
Leeds Dental Institute

C. Deery   Department of Paediatric Dentistry
Edinburgh Dental Institute

M. S. Duggal   Professor of Child Dental Health
Leeds Dental Institute

S. A. Fayle   Department of Child Dental Health
Leeds Dental Institute

P. H. Gordon   Department of Child Dental Health
University of Newcastle upon Tyne

N. M. Kilpatrick   Department of Dentistry
Royal Children's Hospital Melbourne

P. A. Heasman   Department of Restorative Dentistry
University of Newcastle upon Tyne

M. T. Hosey   Department of Child Dental Care
University of Glasgow

M. L. Hunter   Department of Child Dental Health
University of Cardiff

J. G. Meechan   Department of Oral Surgery
University of Newcastle upon Tyne

J. H. Nunn   Professor of Special Needs Dentistry
Trinity College Dublin

G. J. Roberts   Department of Children's Dentistry
Eastman Dental Institute London

H. D. Rodd   Department of Child Dental Health
University of Sheffield

J. A. Smallridge   Department of Child Dental Health
                     Guys and St Thomas' Trust London

K. J. Toumba   Professor of Preventive and Paediatric Dentistry
                     Leeds Dental Institute

P. J. Waterhouse   Department of Child Dental Health
                     University of Newcastle upon Tyne

R. R. Welbury   Professor of Paediatric Dentistry
                     University of Glasgow

J. M. Whitworth   Department of Restorative Dentistry
                     University of Newcastle upon Tyne

B. Williams   General Dental Practitioner
                     Ipswich, Suffolk

Preface to the third edition

I was very pleased when my younger colleagues Marie Thérèse Hosey and Monty Duggal accepted my offer to join me in editing this third edition. Our book has now sold four and a half thousand copies since its launch in 1997 and it is essential that we maintain a contemporary outlook and publish changes in techniques and philosophies as soon as they have an evidence base.

Since 2001 and the second edition, there have been a significant number of changes of authorship, as well as a change of chapters for some existing authors.

Gerry Winter died in December 2002. He was a wise colleague and friend who was a mentor to many of us. I continue to miss his expertise and availability for consultation, by post or telephone, which he freely gave even after his retirement.

John Murray, Andrew Rugg-Gunn, and Linda Shaw have now retired from clinical practice. I am indebted to them all for their support, both in my own personal career and in the production of out textbook. I am grateful to them for allowing the new chapter authors to use their texts and figures.

The restorative section of the book has been remodelled. The endodontics chapter in the previous editions has now been incorporated into either chapters 8 or 12, and there are separate chapters relating to the operative care of the primary and the permanent dentitions. Without the help and friendship of Jim Page the original 'Operative care of dental caries' chapter would not have been possible. I am grateful to Jim for allowing us to continue to use his original illustrations from that chapter.

Although designed for the undergraduate we hope the new edition will continue to be used by undergraduate, postgraduate, and general dental practitioner alike, and that their practice of paediatric dentistry will be both fulfilling and enjoyable.

Glasgow
January 2005

R. R. W

Abbreviations

ABC	Airways, Breathing, Circulation (for basic life support)
ADHD	attention deficit and hyperactivity disorder
ADJ	amelodentinal junction
AI	amelogenesis imperfecta
ALL	acute lymphocytic leukaemia
ALP	alkaline phosphatase
AMG	Amelogenin gene
AML	acute myeloid leukaemia
ANUG	acute necrotizing ulcerative gingivitis
APF	acidulated phosphate-fluoride
ASA	American Society of Anesthesiologists
ASD	atrial septal defects
BNF	*British national formulary*
BP	*British pharmacopoiea*
BPA	bis-phenol A
BSPD	British Society of Paediatric Dentistry
CEJ	cementoenamel junction
CLD	certainly lethal dose
DDAVP	1 desamino-8, D-arginine vasopressin (also known as desmopressin)
DIC	disseminated intravascular coagulation
DMFT	decayed, missing, filled teeth
EACA	epsilon (ε)-aminocaproic acid
EADT	extra-alveolar dry time
EAT	extra-alveolar time
ECC	early childhood caries
EIR	external inflammatory resorption
ENT	ear, nose, and throat
e.p.t	electric pulp tester
ERM	electrical resistance methods
FOTI	fibre-optic transillumination
G-6-PD	glucose 6-phosphate dehydrogenase
GJP	generalized juvenile periodontitis
GMA	glycidylmethacrylate
GORD	gastro-oesophageal reflux disease
GPP	generalized prepubertal periodontitis
HEA	Health Education Authority
HF	hydrogen fluoride
HIV	human immunodeficiency virus
HLA	human leucocyte antigens
IDDM	insulin-dependent diabetes mellitus
IHS	inhalation sedation
IM	intramuscular

INR	international normalized ratio (blood-clotting time)
IOTN	Index of Orthodontic Treatment Need
IRM	intermediate restorative material
ITP	idiopathic thromobocytopenic purpura
IV	intravenous
JP	juvenile periodontitis
JRA	juvenile rheumatoid arthritis
KG	keratinized gingiva
LAD	leucocyte-adhesion deficiency
LCH	Langerhans' cell histiocytosis
LJP	localized juvenile periodontitis
MHC	major histocompatibility complex
MIH	molar-incisor hypomineralization
MRI	magnetic resonance imaging
MTA	mineral trioxide aggregate
NAI	non-accidental injury
NME	non-milk extrinsic (sugars)
NSAIDs	non-steroidal, anti-inflammatory drugs
OCA	Operative Care is Advised
OFG	orofacial granulomatosis
OPT	orthopantomogram
p-a	posteroanterior
p.p.m.	Parts Per Million
PCA	patient-controlled analgesia
PCA	Preventive Care is Advised
p.l	periodontal ligament
PJC	porcelain jacket crown
PLD	potentially lethal dose
PLS	Papillon Lefèvre syndrome
PP	prepubertal periodontitis
PRR	preventive resin restoration
PVAC–PE	polyvinylacetate–polyethylene
RA	relative analgesia
Sp./Spp.	species
STD	safely tolerated dose
TAB	'transient apical breakdown'
TENS	transcutaneous electrical nerve stimulation
TMJ	temporomandibular joint
TTP	tender to percussion
TWI	Tooth Wear Index
VSD	ventricular septal defects
WHO	World Health Organization

1

Craniofacial growth and development

1 Craniofacial growth and development

P. H. Gordon

1.1 INTRODUCTION

This chapter describes, in general terms, the postnatal growth of the craniofacial skeleton and the occlusal development of the primary and permanent dentitions. There is a great deal of individual variation in the process of growth and in the final form of the craniofacial structures; this chapter presents a simplified, or rather idealized, account of craniofacial growth and occlusal development, then goes on to discuss the effect of individual variation in producing departures from this idealized pattern.

Figure 1.1 illustrates the typical changes that take place in the stature of an individual during growth and the extent of normal variation. A chart such as this will present an overall view of the process of growth and will help to detect instances in which growth is not proceeding in the usual manner, but it disguises the fact that the various tissues of the body grow at different rates at different ages, which is illustrated in Fig. 1.2. Neural tissues reach their maximum growth rate at a relatively early age, while the maximum rate for general skeletal growth occurs later. The maximum growth rate for lymphoid tissue occupies an intermediate position.

1.2 GENERAL PRINCIPLES OF CRANIOFACIAL GROWTH

One way of assessing the changes that take place during craniofacial growth is to superimpose tracings of two lateral skull radiographs, taken of the same person, but at different ages. The two radiographs can be compared, as shown in Fig. 1.3, and the changes that have taken place during growth can be examined. One potential difficulty with this approach is that the various bones of the skull grow at different rates at different ages, and there is no single central point about which growth occurs in a radial fashion—that is to say, there is no valid, fixed radiographic landmark on which to superimpose the films. One convention is to superimpose the tracings of the radiographs on the outline of the sella turcica, using the line from the sella to the frontonasal suture to orientate the films. If this method of superimposition is used, it appears that the cranium expands in a more-or-less radial fashion to accommodate the brain and the facial skeleton then grows downwards and forwards, away from the cranial base.

The growth of the cranium is linked to the growth of the brain, and so the calvarial bones increase in size at an earlier age than the bones of the face—the growth of which is linked to that of the musculoskeletal system. Of course, the centre of the sella turcica and the frontonasal suture are not fixed points and are themselves subject to changes in the course of growth. However, the growth of the bones in the anterior cranial fossa is largely complete by the age of 5 years and, while there is a certain amount of remodelling, the area between the sella and the frontonasal suture provides relatively stable landmarks for super-imposition from that age onwards.

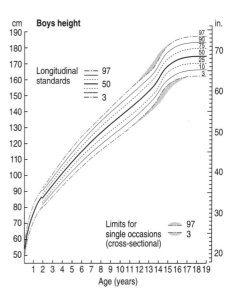

Fig. 1.1 Growth and development record.

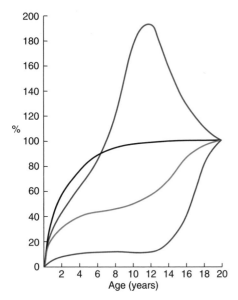

Fig. 1.2 Postnatal growth of various tissues expressed as a percentage of total gain from birth to maturity. Lymphoid type:green; neural type: black; general type: red; genital type: blue. (Redrawn from Scammon, R. E. (1930). The measurements of the body in childhood. In *Measurement of man* (ed. J. A. Harris, C. M. Jackson, D. G. Paterson, and R. E. Scammon). University of Minnesota Press, Minneapolis.)

Bones grow at their edges. Unlike soft tissues, for example the liver, the calcified structure of bone prevents growth by means of the generalized division of cells producing expansion of the organ as a whole. Alteration in the size and shape of bones takes place by deposition and resorption of material on the external and internal surfaces of the bone, by proliferation of cartilage and its replacement by bone, and by growth at the sutures. These different mechanisms all come into play at various stages in the growth of different regions of the craniofacial skeleton.

A long bone, such as the femur, increases in length by proliferation of cartilage at the epiphyses and its replacement by bone. The head of the femur and its shaft are pushed apart by the expanding cartilage, which is then replaced with bone; this process is sufficiently forceful to counteract the compressive force exerted by the owner's weight. There are not many sites in the craniofacial skeleton at which growth proceeds by this mechanism. Proliferation of cartilage in the nasal septum may be responsible, in part, for the downward and forward translation of the maxilla, and the spheno-occipital synchondrosis in the floor of the middle cranial fossa provides a mechanism for some increase in anteroposterior length of the cranial base. These epiphyses and synchondroses are capable of pushing bones apart and acting as primary growth centres rather than providing a mechanism whereby bones can respond or react to growth in other areas.

Sutures, on the other hand, form bone when subjected to traction. In the case of the calvarial bones, the suture systems form new bone and enable the bones to stay in contact with each other when the expansion of the growing brain would otherwise move the bones apart. The suture systems allow the bones to respond to growth in neighbouring soft tissue; the suture systems that lie between the maxilla and the cranial base allow the downward and forward translation of the maxilla in response to growth of the soft tissues of the face. It is not proliferation of the vascular connective tissue in the sutures that pushes the bones apart, the whole arrangement of the connective tissue in a suture seems designed to enable the suture to respond to a tensile force.

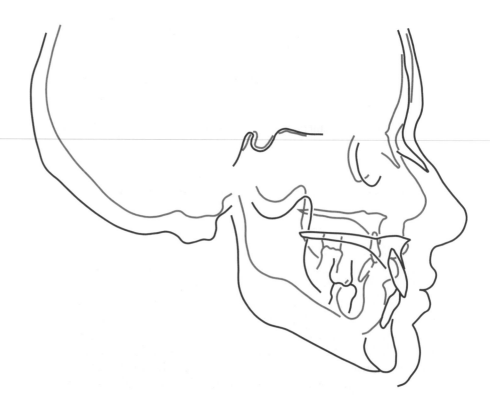

Fig. 1.3 Lateral skull radiographs of the same subject, taken at ages 6 and 18 years, superimposed on the sella–nasion line, registered on sella.

Surface deposition and resorption are very important mechanisms that allow for the translation and remodelling of bone. Deposition and resorption go hand in hand, seldom does one occur without the other. Deposition of bone on one aspect of a cortical plate of bone, accompanied by resorption on the other aspect allows for translation of bones—that is to say, a change in their relative positions—and resorption and deposition occurring on the same aspect of a bone allow for changes in shape. Change in the size of a bone will involve both mechanisms. Surface deposition and resorption of bone are functions of the periosteum or 'osteogenic membrane' that covers its surface.

The mechanisms that control the process of facial growth are not completely understood. It is likely that there is a genetic component in the control mechanism; after all, children tend to resemble their parents in facial appearance. Apart from that, the growth of the bony skeleton is influenced by signals received from its growing soft tissue integument and, probably, vice versa.

1.2.1 Cranial growth

At birth, the cranium has reached some 60–65% of its adult longitudinal dimension and about 90% by the age of 5 years. The calvarial bones are carried away from each other by the expanding brain, and respond by forming new bone in the sutures that separate the bones of the vault of the skull. The six fontanelles that are present at birth reduce in size, the largest—the anterior fontanelle—closes at about 1 year of age and the last to close—the posterolateral fontanelle—closes at about 18 months. The calvarial bones undergo a process of remodelling, with areas of bone deposition and resorption altering the contour of the bones as the volume of the brain cavity increases.

The cranial base also grows to accommodate the changes in the size and shape of the brain, but the process is different to that seen in the calvarial bones. There is considerable lateral growth of the cranial base as the cerebral hemispheres expand, but less increase in the anteroposterior dimension. No sutures are present to allow for expansion of the deeper compartments of the cranial base, a process that takes place by surface deposition and extensive remodelling. In addition, there are three synchondroses in the mid-ventral floor of the cranial base that allow for increases in the anteroposterior dimension. These are the spheno-occipital synchondrosis (the most important of the three), the intersphenoid synchondrosis, and the sphenoethmoidal synchondrosis. Growth in the spheno-occipital synchondrosis does not cease until about the age of 15 years in boys, rather earlier in girls, and it closes at about the age of 20. The pattern and the timing of growth in the cranial base is intermediate between the neural type of growth that characterizes the growth of the calvarial bones and the musculoskeletal pattern of growth exhibited by the facial skeleton.

The shape of the cranial fossae is much more complex than the relatively smooth form of the bones of the vault of the skull. The partitions which separate the cranial fossae are formed by surface deposition and subsequent remodelling, the final size and shape of the compartments being determined by the size of the lobes of the brain.

1.2.2 Nasomaxillary growth

The nasomaxillary complex grows downwards and forwards relative to the cranial base. Unlike the growth of the cranium, which occurs in conjunction with the growth of the brain at a relatively early age, being almost complete by the age of 5 years, the nasomaxillary complex grows fastest at about the time of the pubertal growth spurt, in conjunction with the general growth of the musculoskeletal system. There are two mechanisms which might account for the downward and forward growth of the maxilla. One is the proliferation of cartilage in the nasal septum, which could provide a force to actively push the maxilla in this direction. Another factor is the 'functional matrix' of the soft tissue environment of the maxilla. As the soft tissue grows, the maxilla is translated downwards and forwards. In any event, the sutures positioned between the maxilla and the cranial base respond by producing new bone, which is formed both on the maxillary and the cranial aspects of the suture system.

As the maxilla moves downwards and forwards, new bone is created by surface deposition in the area of the maxillary tuberosity, while the anterior aspect of the maxilla is remodelled not by surface apposition, as might be expected in a bone that is growing forwards, but by a process of resorption. The downward and forward movement of the maxilla is effected by a translation of the bone accompanied by surface deposition on the posterior aspect of the maxilla, rather than by surface apposition on the anterior aspect of the bone.

As bone is deposited on the external aspect of the maxilla in the region of the tuberosity, it is also resorbed from the internal aspect of the bone in this area, thereby enlarging the maxillary sinus. As the bone is translated downwards, the nasal cavities and the maxillary sinus expand by a process of bone resorption at the floor of the nose and the sinus, together with bone deposition on the palatal aspect of the maxilla.

1.2.3 Mandibular growth

Growth of the mandible, like that of the maxilla, is co-ordinated with the pattern of general musculoskeletal growth, growing at its fastest rate at about the time of the pubertal growth spurt. Growth of the mandible has to be co-ordinated with the downward and forward growth of the maxilla. This task is made more complicated by the fact that the mandibular condyles articulate in the glenoid fossa, which lies behind the spheno-occipital synchondrosis, while the maxilla lies in front of it; therefore, growth of the mandible has to keep pace not just with the translation of the maxilla, but also with growth in the cranial base.

Taking the anterior cranial fossa as a stable reference area it appears that the mandible, like the maxilla, grows downwards and forwards. As is the case with the maxilla, this downward and forward growth is not achieved by deposition of bone on the anterior aspect of the mandible; it is achieved by translation of the bone, accompanied by growth in the region of the ramus and the mandibular condyle, as illustrated in Fig. 1.4. Bone is deposited on the posterior aspects of the ramus and the coronoid processes and resorbed from the anterior aspect of the ramus. At the same time the condylar cartilage contributes to growth of the mandibular condyle. Although there are similarities between the condylar cartilage and the epiphysis of a long bone—both grow by proliferation of cartilage and its replacement by bone—it is likely that the condylar cartilage operates as a reactive growth site, responding to translation of the mandible rather than causing it. It is not proliferation of the condylar cartilage that pushes the mandible downwards and forwards.

As the ramus of the mandible grows upwards and backwards, the anterior aspect of the ramus undergoes resorption and becomes remodelled into the body of the mandible. This process involves resorption on the lateral aspect of the bone and deposition on the lingual aspect, which forms new bone in correct alignment with the body of the mandible and helps maintain an appropriate intercondylar width. Growth of the mandibular ramus and condyle has to keep pace with changes in the position of the maxilla, in both vertical and horizontal directions, and with growth in the middle cranial fossa. It is easy for a small discrepancy to arise, for example, in the amount of vertical growth of the mandibular ramus, resulting in a rotation of the body of the mandible and a corresponding tilt of the occlusal plane.

1.2.4 Regulation of craniofacial growth

It is generally accepted that musculoskeletal growth proceeds at least partly under genetic control, but there is still some uncertainty as to how this control is exercised. If it was exercised at the level of the bone itself, if the final size and shape were

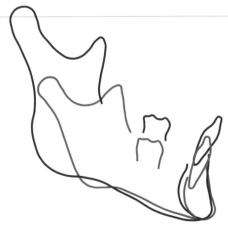

Fig. 1.4 Growth of the mandible occurs mainly in the region of the ramus and the mandibular condyle.

programmed directly into the bone, then control would be exercised at the level of the sutures and the periosteum. This seems unlikely, as a suture is designed to respond to traction rather than to produce an increase in size by pushing bones apart.

If control was exercised at the level of cartilage, then the final size and shape of a bone would be determined by the amount of activity in the cartilages associated with the bone. The nasal septum may well play a part in controlling the translation of the maxilla, pushing it downwards and forwards away from the cranial base. The synchondroses in the cranial base resemble the epiphyses that play an important part in the formation of the long bones. Though their inaccessibility makes them difficult to study, they probably determine the amount of anteroposterior growth in the cranial base. The cartilage in the mandibular condyle appears to be a secondary growth site, allowing growth of the condyle, rather than initiating such growth.

A third possibility is that the final size and shape of a bone is determined by the 'functional matrix' of its soft tissue environment. It is easy to accept that the size and shape of the cranium could be determined by the size and shape of the brain, or that the developing eyeball and its associated muscles determine the growth of the orbit. In the context of the face, it would be growth of the soft tissues of the face and the muscles of mastication that bring about the translation of the maxilla and the mandible, the cartilage of the nasal septum and the suture systems between the facial bones and the cranial base would simply provide a mechanism whereby this could be achieved.

This third possibility seems to be the main way in which growth of the facial skeleton and growth of the cranium is regulated. The cartilage in the cranial base is important in determining its final size and shape and the cartilage in the nasal septum may play some part in initiating the downward and forward translation of the maxilla; however, the growth of the brain, the soft tissues of the face, and the muscles of mastication seems to be the main factor regulating the growth of the craniofacial skeleton.

1.2.5 Normal variation

There is always variation between individuals. Variation in the pattern of facial growth is only to be expected and there are a number of compensatory mechanisms that operate to minimize the impact of such variation. Variation in the position or size of one structure is often compensated by corresponding change in another. The process of growth is constantly creating imbalances as related structures grow and develop at different rates, but the overall direction of growth is towards some position of overall balance or harmony.

Anteroposterior discrepancies can arise during facial growth because of the position of a bone, or as the result of an imbalance in the sizes of bones, or from a mixture of both. A class II skeletal pattern can be caused by insufficient growth in a backwards direction of the ramus of the mandible; alternatively, a class II skeletal pattern can be the result of a backwards tilt of the middle cranial fossa, as illustrated in Fig. 1.5. This change in angulation results in the maxilla having a more anterior position, relative to the glenoid fossa than would otherwise have been the case. The normal-sized mandible, occluding in the glenoid fossa, now has a class II relationship to the normal-sized maxilla. In a similar way, a converse alteration in the pattern of growth—excessive backwards growth of the ramus of the mandible, a more vertical tilt of the middle cranial fossa—can produce a class III skeletal relationship, with the accompanying dental malocclusion.

Vertical growth in the nasomaxillary region has to be combined with vertical growth of the mandibular ramus. Imbalances here will have the effect of producing a mandibular rotation. If there is an excess of vertical maxillary growth, which is not matched by vertical growth of the ramus, then the effect will be to produce

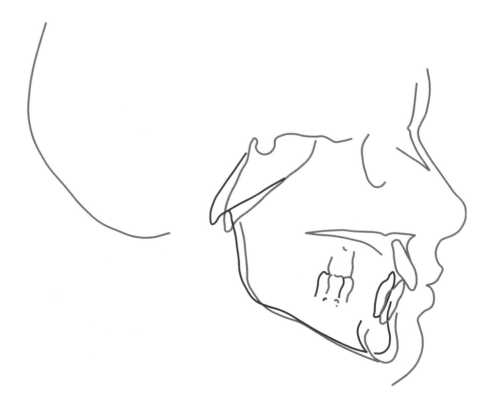

Fig. 1.5 A small change in the angle between the anterior cranial fossa and the middle cranial fossa can produce a class II skeletal relationship, with the resulting class II malocclusion of the teeth.

a downwards and backwards rotation of the mandible. This downwards and backwards rotation will, in turn, produce an anteroposterior discrepancy, with a tendency towards a class II relationship.

Horizontal and vertical discrepancies tend to be accompanied by dentoalveolar compensations. In the case of a class III skeletal pattern, the upper incisor teeth are frequently proclined and the lower incisor teeth retroclined, as illustrated in Fig. 1.6. These compensations are almost certainly brought about by muscular activity in the soft tissue integument affecting the position of the teeth, and they minimize what may otherwise have been a large reversed incisor overjet. In the case of class II skeletal patterns, the dentoalveolar compensation can take two forms. If the lips function in front of the upper incisor teeth, then these are generally retroclined, with the effect that the incisor overjet is virtually normal. If, however, the lower lip functions behind the upper incisors, then these teeth are usually proclined, and the lower incisors retroclined, to make way for the lip. This results in an increased incisor overjet.

Downward and backward mandibular rotations tend to be accompanied by a vertical drifting of the premolar, canine, and incisor teeth, to compensate for an arrangement that would otherwise have produced an anterior open bite. This vertical drifting should be distinguished from overeruption, which would produce a lengthening of the clinical crowns of the teeth.

1.2.6 Modification of the pattern of facial growth

Attempts to modify the pattern of facial growth have met with a certain amount of success. Orthodontic appliances have been designed that hold the mandible postured downwards and forwards. This moves the condyle out of the glenoid fossa and encourages upwards and backwards growth of the mandibular ramus. At the same time, the stretched muscles of mastication exert an upwards and backwards force (through the appliance) to the maxilla, which tends to inhibit its downwards and

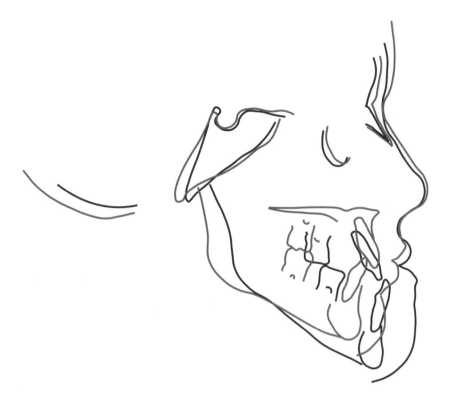

Fig. 1.6 Dentoalveolar compensation of a class III skeletal relationship, with proclination of the upper incisor teeth and retroclination of the lower.

forwards growth. The effect on the growing face is to help correct a developing class II skeletal pattern. If this developing class II skeletal pattern is being caused not so much by underdevelopment of the mandible (which seems to be the more common cause) but by excessive forwards growth of the maxilla, then an appliance may be used simply to exert an upwards and backwards force on the maxilla without involving the mandible, thus helping to influence the course of facial growth.

These appliances apply forces to the developing maxilla and mandible via the teeth—the appliances are attached to the teeth—and work partly by inducing a dentoalveolar compensation for the underlying skeletal discrepancy. This process is sometimes referred to as 'orthodontic camouflage'. There is likely to be some restraint of the downwards and forwards growth of the maxilla, but the appliances seem to have only a minimal effect on the eventual size of the mandible. The so-called 'myofunctional appliances', that derive their impetus from the muscles of mastication, are used most often to help correct class II malocclusions. The appliances work by maintaining a forwards and downwards posturing of the mandible; however, while it is possible to use myofunctional–functional appliances to correct a developing class III malocclusion, they are less often used in this context as it is difficult to obtain the necessary backwards posturing of the mandible. In addition, the dentoalveolar compensations that these appliances tend to produce are often already present in untreated class III occlusions.

1.3 TOOTH DEVELOPMENT

Teeth start to form during the fifth week of embryonic life and the process of tooth formation continues until the roots of the third permanent molars are completed at about the age of 20 years. The stages of tooth formation are the same whether the tooth is of the primary or the permanent dentition, although, obviously, the teeth develop at different times. The tooth-germs develop from the dental lamina, a sheet of

Table 1.1 The chronology of the development of the primary dentition

Stage of development	Central incisor		Lateral incisor		Canine		First molar		Second molar		Time
	Max	Mand	Max	Mand	Max	Mand	Max	Mand	Max	Mand	
Hard tissue formation begins	13–16	13–16	14.7–16.5	14.7–16.5	15–18	16–18	14.5–17	14.5–17	16–23.5	17–19.5	Weeks after ovulation
Crown formation complete	1.5	2.5	2.5	3	9	8–9	6	5–6	11	8–11	Months after birth
Beginning of eruption	8–12	6–10	9–13	10–16	16–22	17–23	13–19	14–18	25–33	23–31	Months after birth
Completion of root formation	33	33	33	30	43	43	37	34	47	42	Months after birth

(Adapted from Schroeder, 1991.)

Table 1.2 The chronology of the development of the permanent dentition

Stage of development	Central incisor		Lateral incisor		Canine		First premolar		Second premolar		Time
	Max	Mand	Max	Mand	Max	Mand	Max	Mand	Max	Mand	
Hard tissue formation begins (histology)	3–4		10–12	3–4	4–5		18–24		24–30		Months after birth
Hard tissue formation begins (radiology)	—		—		6		19		36		Months after birth
Crown formation complete	3.3–4.1	3.4–5.4	4.4–4.9	3.1–5.9	4.5–5.8	4.0–4.7	6.3–7.0	5–6	6.6–7.2	6.1–7.1	Years of age (decimal)
Beginning of eruption	6.7–8.1	6.0–6.9	7.0–8.8	6.8–8.1	10.0–12.2	9.2–11.4	9.6–10.9	9.6–11.5	10.2–11.4	10.1–12.1	Years of age (decimal)
Completion of root formation	8.6–9.8	7.7–8.6	9.6–10.8	8.5–9.6	11.2–13.3	10.8–13.0	11.2–13.6	11.0–13.4	11.6–14.0	11.7–14.3	Years of age (decimal)

Stage of development	First molar		Second molar		Third molar		Time
	Max	Mand	Max	Mand	Max	Mand	
Hard tissue formation begins (histology)	7–8 ao		30–36 mo		7–9yr	8–10yr	Months after ovulation (ao) or months (mo) and years (yr) after birth
Hard tissue formation begins (radiology)	2 mo		36–48 mo		9–10 yr		Months (mo) or years (yr) after birth
Crown formation complete	2.1–3.5	2.1–3.6	6.9–7.4	6.2–7.4	12.8–13.2	12.0–13.7	Years of age with decimal fractions
Beginning of eruption	6.1–6.7	5.9–6.9	11.9–12.8	11.2–12.2	17.0–19.0	17.0–19.0	Years of age with decimal fractions
Completion of root formation	9.3–10.8	7.8–9.8	12.9–16.2	11.0–15.7	19.5–19.6	20.0–20.8	Years of age with decimal fractions

Max = Maxilla
Mand = Mandible
(Adapted from Schroeder, 1991.)

epithelial cells which develops, itself, from the primary epithelial band. This is a layer of thickened epithelium which forms around the mouth in the area soon to be occupied by the upper and lower jaws. The primary epithelial band quickly organizes into two discrete epithelial ingrowths—the vestibular lamina and the dental lamina.

The vestibular lamina grows down into the underlying ectomesenchyme, the epithelial cells enlarge and then break down, thereby forming the cleft which becomes the sulcus between the cheeks and the alveolar processes.

The dental lamina forms a series of epithelial buds that grow outwards into the surrounding connective tissue. These buds represent the first stage in the development of the tooth-germs of the primary dentition. The epithelial bud continues to grow and becomes associated with a condensation of mesenchymal cells to form a tooth-germ at the cap stage of development. The epithelial bud develops into the enamel organ, the condensation of mesenchymal cells constitutes the dental papilla and comes to extend around the enamel organ to form the dental follicle. The cells at the margin of the epithelial bud continue to proliferate and grow to enfold the mesenchymal cells of the dental follicle, producing a tooth-germ at the bell stage of development. Around this time—the transition from cap stage to bell stage— a process of histodifferentiation produces the recognizable structures of the enamel organ, with its external and internal enamel epithelia, stratum intermedium, and stellate reticulum.

Further proliferation of the cells of the dental lamina, at a point adjacent to each primary tooth-germ, but on its lingual aspect, produces the tooth-germ of the permanent successor. The tooth-germs of the permanent molar teeth, which have no primary precursors are formed by distal extension of the dental lamina, which tunnels backwards as the jaws lengthen posteriorly.

The cells of the inner enamel epithelium lengthen to a columnar shape, with the cell nuclei occupying the portion of the cell beside the stratum intermedium, away from the dental papilla. The cells of the dental papilla adjacent to the internal enamel epithelium, also elongate to a columnar form, with their nuclei aligned away from the enamel organ and towards the centre of the dental papilla. These columnar cells of the dental papilla differentiate into odontoblasts, the cells which form dentine. Dentine formation, which is induced by the cells of the internal enamel epithelium, always precedes enamel formation. Although dentine is formed by the odontoblasts of the dental papilla, the process is initiated by the epithelial cells of the enamel organ. Once dentine formation begins, the cells of the internal enamel epithelium differentiate into ameloblasts and commence the formation of enamel. Dentine and enamel formation occurs initially in the region of the cusp tips and incisal edges of the teeth, then continues towards the cervical margin of their crowns.

Differentiation of odontoblasts and the formation of dentine is induced by the cells of the internal enamel epithelium. A similar process is involved in the production of dentine to form the roots of teeth. The epithelial cells at the cervical loop of the enamel organ proliferate and migrate in an apical direction to form a tubular epithelial sheath around the dental papilla. These epithelial cells—the root sheath of Hertwig—induce the formation of odontoblasts from the cells of the dental papilla and the production of dentine to form the roots of the teeth, a process which is not complete until 3–5 years after the eruption of the crown of the tooth.

The stages of tooth development are the same for both primary and permanent teeth, although progression through the stages occurs at different times and at varying rates for the different teeth. Tables 1.1 and 1.2 summarize the chronology of tooth development for the two dentitions.

1.4 TOOTH ERUPTION

There are several possible explanations to account for the phenomenon of tooth eruption. Some possibilities are more likely than others to play a part in the process, and some earlier theories have been largely discounted. Extrusion of pulp tissue through the apical foramen, arising from the growth of dentine and proliferation of cells in the pulp, has been suggested as a mechanism for providing a force that could be responsible for bringing about the eruption of teeth. The effect of blood pressure within the pulp or simple root lengthening have also been put forward as possible causative agents. However, observational and experimental studies of rootless teeth have shown that they erupt into a functional occlusion, so it is unlikely that these mechanisms have an important part to play in the process of eruption.

Remodelling of dentoalveolar bone has been proposed as a mechanism for tooth eruption, but the part it plays is difficult to assess. Bone remodelling has to occur as teeth erupt and it is hard to know whether the remodelling is a cause of tooth eruption or whether it is simply in response to the eruption of the teeth. Tooth eruption may occur in response to activity within the periodontal ligament, where contraction of fibroblasts could be capable of elevating the tooth root, but it is most likely that agents responsible for tooth eruption lie within the dental follicle itself, rather than the tooth. The connective tissue of the dental follicle is a rich source of factors that are responsible for the local mediation of bone deposition and resorption, and it seems probable that the dental follicle has a major part to play in the process of tooth eruption.

1.5 OCCLUSAL DEVELOPMENT

1.5.1 The primary dentition

The first tooth to erupt is usually the lower central incisor. Occasionally, this tooth is present at birth, but the average age for its eruption is about 7 or 8 months, although there is, inevitably, some individual variation. The other incisor teeth follow soon after, with the upper central incisors erupting at about 10 months followed by the upper lateral incisors at about 11 months and the lower lateral incisors at about 13 months. At about the age of 16 months the first primary molars put in an appearance, followed by the primary canine teeth at about 19 months. The second primary molars erupt at about 27–29 months, with the lower teeth usually erupting before the upper. While the eruption sequence—the order in which the teeth erupt— is usually as described above, there is considerable variation in the actual age at which the teeth erupt. In any event, there is almost a continuous process of tooth eruption between the ages of 7 and 29 months.

There are some occlusal features that occur relatively frequently in the established primary dentition.

1. The incisor teeth tend to be spaced. If the primary teeth are not spaced, then the permanent teeth will be crowded, because the larger permanent incisor teeth have to fit into the same space as their smaller primary predecessors. Crowding of the permanent incisor teeth is a relatively common occurrence, but the crowding is seldom so severe that there is no spacing of the primary incisors.

2. The so-called 'anthropoid' spaces between the upper lateral incisor and the canine and between the lower canine and the first primary molar are particularly common.

3. In the case of a class I occlusion, the mesiobuccal cusp of the primary upper second molar occludes in the mesiobuccal groove of the lower second molar, a situation analogous to the class I occlusion of first permanent molars. However, the lower, second primary molar is much longer, mesiodistally, than the upper second molar. Therefore the class I occlusion of the mesiobuccal cusp of the upper molar means that the distal surfaces of the teeth are in the same vertical plane.

The incisor relationship tends more towards edge-to-edge than is the case with permanent teeth (although with increasing wear of the primary teeth there may be a postural element in this) and the upper incisors tend to be more upright. There is sometimes an anterior open bite, associated with a sucking habit, and there may be cross-bites of the buccal segment teeth, but, in general, the teeth in the primary dentition tend to be well aligned. While there may be some anteroposterior, lateral, or vertical discrepancy, these deviations are seldom so marked that they give rise to comment.

1.5.2 The mixed dentition

The primary dentition erupts more or less continuously over a 2-year period. The permanent dentition, however, erupts in two stages as first the incisor teeth and the first permanent molars erupt, then the other teeth in the buccal segments. The lower central incisor and the first permanent molars erupt at about the age of 6 years. The upper central incisor and the lower lateral incisor erupt at about the age of 7 and the upper lateral incisor at about the age of 8 years. As with the primary teeth, while some variation in the timing of tooth eruption is only to be expected, this eruption sequence should not vary. In particular, the upper central incisor should erupt before the upper lateral incisor. If the upper lateral incisor erupts before the central then, almost certainly, there is something impeding the eruption of the central incisor, for example a supernumerary tooth, or dilaceration of the root of the central incisor.

The lower canine and the first premolar teeth are the next to erupt, at about 10 years of age, followed by the upper canine and the second premolar teeth at about the age of 11 and the second molar teeth at about the age of 12. Third molar teeth start to erupt from about the age of 16 onwards, but the eruption of third molars is very variable; not uncommonly, these teeth are impacted against their neighbours and fail to erupt at all.

The upper central incisors are more proclined than their primary counterparts. This allows some forward repositioning of the mandible when the first permanent molars erupt in a cusp-to-cusp relationship with their opponents. The distal surfaces of the second primary molars tend to be in the same vertical plane, so the first permanent molars, erupting behind them, tend to adopt a class II occlusal relationship. The forward repositioning of the mandible allows the establishment of a class I intercuspal position. The primary teeth in the buccal segments have a larger combined mesiodistal width than do the permanent teeth which replace them. This means that, provided the primary teeth are shed in the ordinary way, there should be no problem with a lack of space for the permanent teeth in the buccal segments of the dental arch. The 'leeway space', as it is sometimes called—the amount by which the combined size of the primary canine and molar teeth exceeds the combined mesiodistal widths of the permanent canine and pre-molar teeth—amounts to 1.5 mm in the upper arch and 2.5 mm in the lower, with its large second primary molar.

The size and shape of the anterior segments of the dentoalveolar arches do not change much following the eruption of the permanent incisor teeth; there is not much growth by deposition of bone on the labial aspect of the maxilla or mandible—these bones grow by forward and downward translation, with deposition of new bone on their posterior surfaces. If there is insufficient space to accommodate the teeth in the dental arches when the teeth erupt, then it is unlikely that the situation will improve as growth proceeds. There is a small expansion in the width of the dental arch, with deposition of bone on the lateral aspect of the maxilla and the mandible, and, while most of the 'leeway space' is taken up by mesial movement of the posterior teeth, this may allow for some improvement in the alignment of crowded incisors.

1.5.3 The permanent dentition

As with the primary dentition, it is possible to identify occlusal features of the established permanent dentition that occur consistently in ideal dental arches.

1. The mesiobuccal cusp of the upper first permanent molar occludes in the mesiobuccal groove of the lower first permanent molar, with the distal aspect of the upper first molar contacting the mesial aspect of the lower second molar.
2. The teeth should have a normal labiolingual inclination. In the case of the anterior teeth, the crown inclination must be sufficient to prevent overeruption of the teeth and an increased incisor overbite. In the case of the posterior teeth, the upper teeth should have a lingual inclination, which remains constant in the premolar and molar regions, while the lower teeth have a lingual inclination which becomes more pronounced towards the back of the arch.
3. The teeth should have a normal mesiodistal angulation, with the crowns of the teeth more mesially positioned than their roots.
4. There should be no rotated teeth.
5. There should be no spacing or crowding of the teeth.
6. The occlusal plane should be flat or with only a mild curve of Spee.

Not all these features are necessary for dental health, but taken together they provide a definition of the ideal class I occlusion.

1.6 SUMMARY

This chapter has set out to outline the pattern of normal craniofacial growth.

1. While normal variation of this pattern will produce the differences that occur between individuals, the underlying patterns of growth should not be radically different from those described here; that is, if development is to proceed in a normal fashion.
2. The growth of the brain and of the cranium is almost complete by the age of 5 years.
3. The facial skeleton grows downwards and forwards, relative to the cranial base—starting to grow rapidly at about the time of the pubertal growth spurt, and with facial growth virtually complete at about the age of 15.5 years in girls, slightly later in boys.
4. With regard to occlusal development, while the exact age at which structures form will vary from person to person, the overall pattern of tooth development and the process by which the dental occlusion becomes established should probably be much as described in this chapter.
5. The eruption sequence—the order in which the teeth erupt—is more important than the age at which they erupt. So that if there is a local problem with regard to the establishment of a normal occlusion, it is likely to become apparent, in the first instance, as a disturbance of the eruption sequence.

1.7 FURTHER READING

Enlow, D. H. (1990). *Facial growth* (3rd edn). W. B. Saunders, Philadelphia. (*This is a widely recommended textbook, which deals with the subject of facial growth, very much from a clinical point of view.*)

Schroeder, H. E. (1991). *Oral structural biology*. Georg Thieme Verlag, Stuttgart. (*A pocketsized book which presents a concise review of the subject, this text is best used as a reference rather than as an introduction to the subject. The points raised in the text are well documented by references to the academic literature.*)

Ten Cate, A. R. (2003). *Oral histology—development, structure and function* (6th edn). Mosby, St Louis. (*A popular, complete, and well-illustrated text, now in its 4th edition, which presents the subject clearly and in a modular, well-organized format.*)

2

Introduction to the dental surgery

2 Introduction to the dental surgery

A. S. Blinkhorn

2.1 INTRODUCTION

It is a common belief among many individuals that being 'good with people' is an inborn art and owes little to science or training. It is true that some individuals have a more open disposition and can relate well to others (Fig. 2.1). However, there is no logical reason why all of us shouldn't be able to put young patients at their ease and show that we are interested in their problems.

It is particularly important for dentists to learn how to help people relax, as failure to empathize and communicate will result in disappointed patients and an unsuccessful practising career. Communicating effectively with children is of great value, as 'being good with younger patients' is a practice-builder and can reduce the stress involved when offering clinical care.

All undergraduate and postgraduate dental training should include a thorough understanding of how children relate to an adult world, how the dental visit should be structured, and what strategies are available to help children cope with their apprehension about dental procedures. This chapter will consider these items, beginning with a discussion on the theories of psychological development, and following this up with sections on: parents and their influence on dental treatment; dentist–patient relationships; anxious and uncooperative children, and helping anxious patients to cope with dental care.

> Effective communication, good for patients and dentists.

2.2 PSYCHOLOGY OF CHILD DEVELOPMENT

At one time the psychological development of children was split into a series of well-defined phases, but more recently this division has been criticized and development

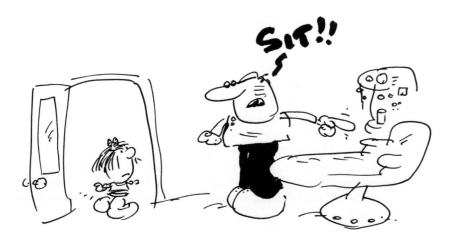

Fig. 2.1 Being good with patients is not necessarily an inborn art! (With thanks to David Myers and kind permission of Eden Bianchi Press.)

should now be seen as a continuum. The phases of development may well differ from child to child, so a rigidly applied definition will be artificial. Nevertheless, for the sake of clarity when describing a child's psychological development from infancy into adulthood, certain developmental milestones should be considered.

The academic considerations about psychological development have been dominated by a number of internationally known authorities who have, for the most part, concentrated on different aspects of the systematic progression from child to adult. However, the most important theoretical perspective now influencing thinking about child development is that of attachment theory—a theory developed by the psychoanalyst John Bowlby. In a series of writings over three decades, Bowlby developed his theory that child development could best be understood within the framework of patterns of interaction between the infant and the primary caregiver. If there were problems in this interaction, then the child was likely to develop insecure and/or anxious patterns that would affect the ability to form stable relationships with others, to develop a sense of self-worth, and to move towards independence. The other important concept to note is that development is a lifelong process, we do not switch off at 18, nor is development an even process. Development is uneven, influenced by periods of rapid bodily change.

The psychological literature contains many accounts of the changes accompanying development; therefore, this section will present a general outline of the major 'psychological signposts' of which the dental team should be aware. As the newborn child is not a 'common' visitor to the dental surgery no specific description of newborn behaviour will be offered, instead general accounts of motor, cognitive, perceptual, and social development from birth to adolescence will be included. It is important to understand that the thinking about child development has become less certain and simplistic in its approach; hence, dentists who make hard and fast rules about the way they offer care to children will cause stress to both their patients and themselves.

Quality of the interaction with primary care givers.

Psychological sign posts.

2.2.1 Motor development

A newborn child does not have an extensive range of movements, but these develop rapidly and by the age of 2 years the majority of children are capable of walking on their own. The 'motor milestones' occur in a predictable order and many of the tests used by paediatricians assess normal development in infancy in terms of motor skills. The predictability of early motor development suggests that it must be genetically programmed. Although this is true to some extent, there is evidence that the environment can influence motor development. This has led to a greater interest in the early diagnosis of motor problems so that remedial intervention can be offered. A good example of intervention is the help offered to Down syndrome babies, who have slow motor development. Specific programmes, which focus on practising sensory–motor tasks, can greatly accelerate motor development to almost normal levels.

Motor development is really completed in infancy, the changes which follow the walking milestone are refinements rather than the development of new skills. Eye–hand co-ordination gradually becomes more precise and elaborate with increasing experience. The dominance of one hand emerges at an early age and is usually linked to hemisphere dominance for language processing. The left hemisphere controls the right hand and the right hemisphere controls the left. The majority of right-handed people appear to be strongly left-hemisphere dominant for language processing, as are nearly all left-handers. Some children with motor retardation may fail to show specific right or left manual dominance and will lack good co-ordination between the hands.

Motor development—environment important.

Motor development completed early in life.

Children of 6–7 years of age usually have sufficient co-ordination to brush their teeth reasonably well. Below that age many areas of the mouth will be missed and there is a tendency to swallow relatively large amounts of toothpaste, hence parental supervision of brushing is important.

2.2.2 Cognitive development

The cognitive capability of children changes radically from birth through to adulthood, and the process is divided into a number of stages for ease of description. A Swiss psychologist called Piaget formulated the 'stages view' of cognitive development on the basis of detailed observations of his own children, and suggested that children pass through four broad stages of cognitive development, namely:

Piaget and his 'stages'.

1. *Sensorimotor*: this stage lasts until about 2 years of age. The prime achievement is 'object permanence'. The infant can think of things as permanent—which continue to exist when out of sight—and can think of objects without having to see them directly.

2. *Preoperational thought*: this runs from 2 to 7 years of age. The sensorimotor stage is further developed, allowing the child to predict outcomes of behaviour. Language development facilitates these changes. The thought patterns are not well developed, being egocentric, unable to encompass another person's point of view, single-tracked, and inflexible (sums up most politicians, some dental professors, and hospital administrators). Typically, children in this age band are unable to understand that areas and volumes remain the same despite changes in position or shape.

3. *Concrete operations*: this is the stage of thinking that occurs from about 7 to 11 years of age. Children are able to apply logical reasoning, consider another person's point of view, and assess more than one aspect of a particular situation (Fig. 2.2). Thinking is rooted in concrete objects, abstract thought is not well developed.

4. *Formal operations*: this is the last stage in the transition to adult thinking ability. It begins at about 11 years of age and results in the development of logical abstract thinking so that different possibilities for action can be considered.

Dogma bites the dust.

These stages have been highlighted because of the importance of Piaget's early work on cognitive development. However, an over-reliance on 'dogma' may well limit the development of a subject, and this was the case with cognitive development.

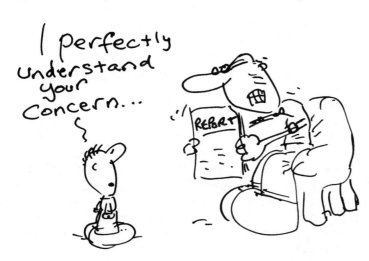

Fig. 2.2 Children aged 7–11 years are able to consider another person's point of view. (With thanks to David Myers and kind permission of Eden Bianchi Press.)

Few scientists challenged Piaget's findings so that the field of infant perception became a rather sterile area for a number of years, but this changed with the work of Bowlby. Enormous developments in research have since led to many doubts being raised about Piaget's original interpretation of his data. He underestimated the thinking abilities of younger children, and there is evidence to show that not all preschool thinking is totally egocentric. Of just as much interest is the modern view that not all adult thinking is logical, many of us are biased and illogical. A self-evident truth when one considers the arguments raised against water fluoridation!

There is, however, a serious point to this observation on adult illogicality. We must be prepared for parents who don't agree with our perceived wisdom (Fig. 2.3) or do not understand the basic tenets of specific programmes. Dentists will lead less stressful practising lives if they remember that not all their patients will always agree with or follow oral health advice.

So Piaget should be seen as a pioneer who really set in motion work on cognitive development, but it is now recognized that the developmental stages are not so clear-cut and many kids are smarter than we think!

2.2.3 Perceptual development

Clearly, it is very difficult to discover what babies and infants are experiencing perceptually, so much research has concentrated on eye movements. These types of studies have shown that with increasing age, scanning becomes broader and larger amounts of information are sought. Compared with adults, 6-year-old children cover less of the object, fixate on details, and gain less information. However, children do develop their selective attention, and by the age of 7 years can determine which messages merit attention and which can be ignored. Concentration skills also improve. Some dental advice can be offered to children of this age, but given the importance of the home environment parents should be the main focus of any information given on oral health care.

With increasing age children become more efficient at discriminating between different visual patterns and reach adult proficiency by about 9 years of age.

The majority of perceptual development is a function of the growth of knowledge about the environment in which a child lives, hence the necessity to spend time explaining aspects of dental care to new child patients (Fig. 2.4).

Are adults sensible?

Kids can pull the wool over our eyes!

Children are not vertically challenged adults!

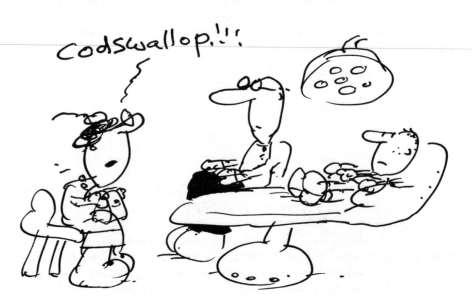

Fig. 2.3 Be prepared for parents who don't agree. (With thanks to David Myers and kind permission of Eden Bianchi Press.)

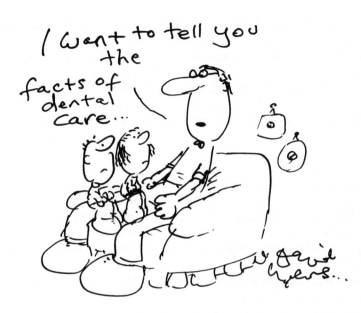

Fig. 2.4 Spend time explaining the facts about dental care. (With thanks to David Myers and kind permission of Eden Bianchi Press.)

2.2.4 Language development

A lack of the appropriate stimulation will retard a child's learning, particularly language. A child of 5 who can only speak in monosyllables and has no sensible sentence structure will not only be unable to communicate with others but will be unable to think about the things he/she sees and hears. Stimulation is important as language development is such a rapid process in childhood that any delay can seriously handicap a child. Newborn children show a remarkable ability to distinguish speech sounds and by the age of 5 years most children can use 2000 or more words. Language and thought are tied together and are important in cognitive development, but the complexities of the relationship between the two are not well understood.

Dentistry has a highly specialized vocabulary and it is unlikely that many children, even adolescents, will understand our meaning if we rely on jargon. The key to successful communication is to pitch your advice and instructions at just the right level for different age groups of children. There is a risk of being patronizing if every child patient is told that 'little pixies are eating away tiny bits of your tooth and I am going to run my little engine to frighten them away to fairyland'. A streetwise 10 year old who is a computer games officionado would probably call the police if you used such language! There is no universal approach to patients, so careful treatment planning and assessment are required before children or their parents are given specific written or verbal advice.

Keep jargon to a minimum.

Assess patients before offering advice.

2.2.5 Social development

Until fairly recently it was believed that newborn infants were individuals who spent most of their time sleeping. However, recent research reveals that babies interact quite markedly with their environment, often initiating interactions with other humans by movement of their eyes or limbs.

Babies tend to form specific attachments to people and are prone to separation anxiety. At about 8 months infants show a definite fear of strangers. This potential for anxiety separation remains high until about 5 years of age when separation anxiety declines quite markedly. This is consistent with studies of children in hospital, which show that after the age of 5 there is less distress on entering hospital. Separation anxiety should also be considered by dentists who insist that all young children must enter the dental surgery alone. Clearly, this will cause severe anxiety to patients under 5.

Separation anxiety.

It has been reported that a loving, early parental attachment is associated with a better social adjustment in later childhood and is a good basis for engendering trust and friendship with peers. This is important as a successful transition from home to school depends on the ability to interact with other individuals apart from parents. The home environment will play a major part in social development, but the effects of community expectations should not be underestimated. We are all products of our broad social environment, mediated to some extent by parental influences.

Love your parents—they made you!

2.2.6 Adolescence

The waning of parental influence can be seen in the final stage of child development, adolescence. This is the end of childhood and the beginning of adulthood. It is conceptualized as a period of emotional turmoil and a time of identity formation. This view is a 'Western' creation and is culturally biased. In many societies 'terrible teenagers' do not exist; childhood ends and adult responsibilities are offered at a relatively early age.

Teenagers are not always nasty.

It is interesting to note that even in Western industrialized societies there is little real evidence to support the idea that the majority of adolescents are rebellious and non-conformist. The main change is the evolution of a different sort of parental relationship. There is increasing independence and self-sufficiency. The research does show that young people tend to be moody, are oversensitive to criticism, and feel miserable for no apparent reason but do not on the whole rebel against their parental role models.

There are some clear messages to dentists who wish to retain their adolescent patients; don't criticize them excessively as this may compromise their future oral health. These patients are looking for support and reassurance. Many health professionals need to rethink their assumptions about young people, as personal behaviour patterns are not really related to health issues at all. Until there are acute problems 'health *per se*' is of little relevance to adolescents being a rather abstract concept. Future orientation is low and the major issues of concern are finding employment, exploring their sexuality, and having the friendship and support of their peers.

Health an abstract concept.

2.3 PARENTS AND THEIR INFLUENCE ON DENTAL TREATMENT

Children learn the basic aspects of everyday life from their parents, this process is termed socialization and is an ongoing and gradual process. By the age of 4 years children know many of the conventions current in their culture, such as male and female roles. The process of transmitting cultural information early in life is called primary socialization. In industrialized countries, obtaining information on many aspects of life is gained formally in schools and colleges rather than from the family. This is termed secondary socialization.

Socialization.

Interestingly, primary socialization can have a profound and lasting effect. For example, fear of dental treatment and when we first begin to clean our teeth can often be traced back to family influence. So parents can shape a child's expectations and attitudes about oral health; thus, every attempt should be made to involve them when attempting to offer dental care or change a child's health habits.

Involving parents means that the dentist must look to positive reinforcement rather than 'victim blaming'. Parents who are accused of oral neglect may well feel aggrieved or threatened. All too often children's oral health is compromised by a lack of parental knowledge so programmes have to be carefully designed to reduce any chances of making people feel guilty. Guilt often results in parents spending more time in seeking excuses for problems than trying to implement solutions.

Avoid victim blaming.

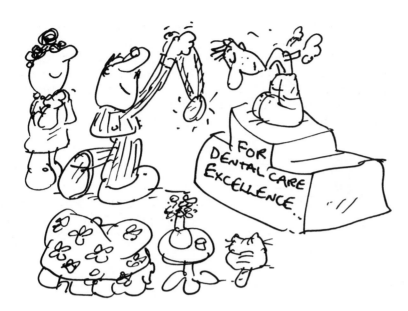

Fig. 2.5 Positive reinforcement is important. (With thanks to David Myers and kind permission of Eden Bianchi Press.)

Parents who are convinced that their child has an oral health problem which can be solved tend to react in a positive way, both to their dental advisor and the preventive programme itself. It is especially helpful if the preventive strategy can include a system of positive reinforcement for the child (Fig. 2.5). Features such as brushing charts, diet sheets, gold stars for brushing well, extra pocket money for curtailing thumb-sucking are all useful tips to help parents maintain a child's enthusiasm for a particular dental project.

It must be emphasized that preventive programmes must be carefully planned to include only one major goal at a time. Parents will be unable to cope if too much is expected of them at any one time. Programmes that involve families have much higher success rates than those which concentrate solely on the patient. Interestingly, families also have a profound influence on levels of dental anxiety among their children. Dentally anxious mothers have children who exhibit negative behaviour at the dentist. Hence, the need for dentists to look 'beyond' the child when assessing the reasons for dental anxiety.

One of the great debates in paediatric dentistry centres on whether parents should be allowed in the dental surgery while their child is receiving treatment. A child's family, it could be argued, can offer emotional support during treatment. There is no doubt that within the medical field there is great support for the concept of a parent actually 'living in' while a child is hospitalized. However, the issue is not so clear-cut in dentistry (Fig. 2.6).

The first issue that must be raised is whether dentists have the ethical/moral right to bar parents from sitting in with their children when dental care is being undertaken. Clearly, parents have views and anxiety levels may be raised if parents feel their familial rights are being threatened and a child may be stressed by tension between parents and the operator.

Wright *et al.* (1987) in their comprehensive book on child management summarize the advantages of keeping parents out of the surgery as:

(1) the parent often repeats orders, creating an annoyance for both dentist and child patient (Fig. 2.7);

(2) the parents intercept orders, becoming a barrier to the development of rapport between the dentist and the child;

(3) the dentist is unable to use voice intonation in the presence of the parent because he or she is offended;

Positive reinforcement is important.

Should parents join children in the surgery?

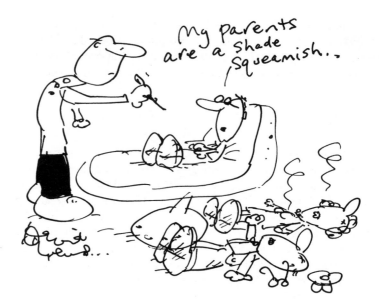

Fig. 2.6 Should we allow parents into the surgery? (With thanks to David Myers and kind permission of Eden Bianchi Press.)

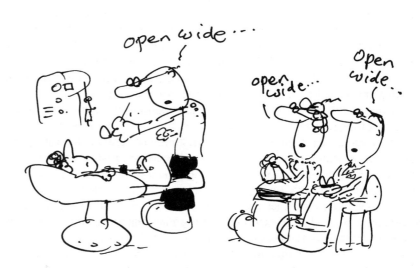

Fig. 2.7 Some parents can be very irritating by repeating all your requests. (With thanks to David Myers and kind permission of Eden Bianchi Press.)

(4) the child divides attention between the parent and the dentist;

(5) the dentist divides attention between the parent and the child;

(6) dentists are probably more relaxed and comfortable when the parent remains in the reception area.

These suggestions have merit but they do have a rather authoritarian feel to them, stressing the ordering and voice intonation rather than sympathetic communication. Practical research to support parents 'in or out' of the surgery is not available to suggest whether there is a right or wrong way to handle this particular question. In the end it is a personal decision taken by the dentist in the light of parental concerns and clinical experience. As in any branch of medicine there can be no 'hard and fast' rules for dealing with the general public, an adherence to any type of dogma 'come what may' is a recipe for confrontation and stress. Therefore, parents sitting in with children should be a decision taken for each individual rather than implementing a 'keep parents out' policy.

Patients with special needs require a high degree of parental involvement in oral health care, particularly for those children with educational, behavioural, and physical difficulties. For example, toothbrushing is a complex cognitive and motor

Each patient is a unique individual.

task which will tax the skills of many handicapped children. A parent will have to be taught how to monitor the efficiency of the plaque removal and intervene when necessary, to ensure the mouth is cleaned adequately. Diet is also important, so clear advice must be offered and reinforcement planned at regular intervals.

2.4 DENTIST–PATIENT RELATIONSHIP

The way a dentist interacts with patients will have a major influence on the success of any clinical or preventive care. Clearly, only broad guidelines can be presented on how to maintain an effective relationship with a patient, as all of us are unique individuals with different needs and aspirations. This is especially so in paediatric dentistry where a clinician may have to treat a frightened 3-year-old child at one appointment and an hour and a half later be faced with the problem of offering preventive advice on oral health to a recalcitrant 15 year old. There are, however, common research findings which highlight the key issues that will cause a dentist/patient consultation to founder or progress satisfactorily.

People like friendly dentists.

The first question that must be considered is 'Why me—what factors did the parents take into account before making an appointment at my practice?'

The obvious answers are that your practice is closest to the bus stop, has good parking, and you are the only one open after 6.00 p.m. Surprisingly, the choice is not so simple. Most people try to find out details about different dental practices from friends and colleagues. While the technical skill of the dentist is of some concern, the most important features people look for are, a gentle friendly manner, explains treatment procedures, and tries to keep any pain to a minimum.

As with any health issue the social class background of the respondents influences attitudes and beliefs. For example, parents of high socioeconomic status are more interested in professional competence and gaining information, whereas parents from poorer areas want a dentist to reassure and be friendly to their child.

So which dentist parents choose to offer care to their child will depend to some extent on reports about technical skill from family and friends, but the major driving force is well-developed interpersonal skills. A major point to emphasize is that technical skill is usually judged in terms of caring and sympathy, a finding which adds further weight to the importance of dentists developing a good 'chair-side manner'.

Explanation, 'taking the time to talk us through what our child's treatment will entail', is another factor which rates highly, and may actually influence the rate of attendance for follow-up appointments.

2.4.1 Structure of the dental consultation

To help students and new graduates improve their dentist/patient interaction skills it is possible to give an outline structure to a successful dental consultation. The proposed model consists of six stages, and is based on the work of Wanless and Holloway (1994).

1. *Greeting*. The dentist greets the child by name. Avoid using generalized terms such as 'Hi sonny, hello sunshine', which are general rather than specific to the patient (Fig. 2.8). If parents are present then include them in the conversation, but do not forget that the child should be central to the developing relationship. A greeting can be spoilt by proceeding too quickly to an instruction rather than an invitation. For example, 'Hello Sarah, jump in the chair' is rather abrupt and may prejudice an interactive relationship. The greeting should be used to put the child and parents at ease before proceeding to the next stage.

   Remember I have a name.

2. *Preliminary chat*. This phase has three objectives, to assess whether the patient or parents have any particular worries or concerns, to settle the patient into

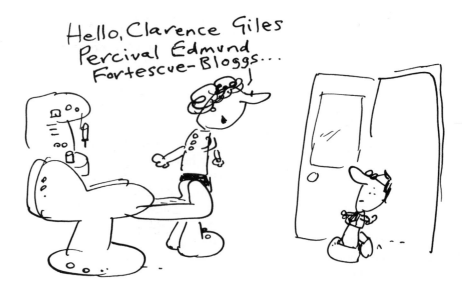

Fig. 2.8 Always greet your patient by name. (With thanks to David Myers and kind permission of Eden Bianchi Press.)

Talk and listen. Don't drill.

the clinical environment, and to assess the patient's emotional state. The following sequence represents one way of maximizing the effect of the 'preliminary chat':

(a) Begin with non-dental topics. For children who have been before it is helpful to record useful information such as the names of brothers/sisters, school, pets, and hobbies.

(b) Ask an open question such as, 'How are you/are you having any problems with your teeth?' Listen to the answer and probe further if necessary. All too often dentists ask questions and then ignore the answer!

By talking generally and taking note of what the child is saying you are offering a degree of control and reducing anxiety.

3. *Preliminary explanation.* In this stage the aim is to explain what the clinical or preventive objectives are in terms that parents and children will understand. This is a vital part of any visit as it establishes the credibility of the dentist as someone who knows what the ultimate goal for the treatment is, and is prepared to take the time and trouble to discuss it in non-technical language.

Full history vital.

While not wishing to labour the point, it must be stressed that sensible information cannot be offered to the patient or parents until the clinician has a full history and a treatment plan based on adequate information. This requires a broad view of the patient and should not be totally tooth-centred. It is all too easy to lose the confidence of parents and children if you find yourself making excuses for clinical decisions taken in a hurried and unscientific manner.

Thus the preliminary chat sets the scene prior to actual clinical activity.

4. *Business.* The patient is now in danger of becoming a passive object who is worked on rather than being involved in the treatment. Many jokes are made about dentists who ask questions of patients who are unable to reply because of a mouthful of instruments! (Fig. 2.9). This does not mean that the visit should enter a silent phase. It is important to remain in verbal contact. Check the patient is not in pain, discuss what you are doing, use the patient's name to show a 'personal' interest, and clarify any misunderstandings.

Is your patient still alive?

At the end of the business stage it is helpful to summarize what has been done and offer aftercare advice. If the parent is not present in the surgery, the treatment summary is particularly important, as it is a useful way of maintaining contact with the parents.

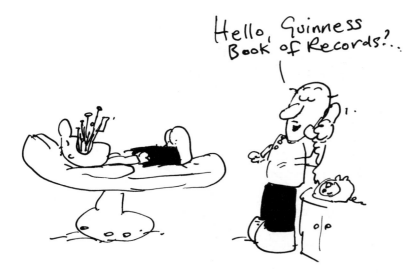

Fig. 2.9 Is your patient just a mouthful of instruments? (With thanks to David Myers and kind permission of Eden Bianchi Press.)

5. *Health education.* Oral health is, to a large extent, dependent upon personal behaviour and as such it would be unethical for dentists not to include advice on maintaining a healthy mouth. Although offering advice to parents and patients is useful, in many instances the profession treat health education in a 'throwaway' manner. This results in both patients and dentists being disappointed.

The key ways to improve the value of advice sessions are as follows:

(a) Make the advice specific, give a child a personal problem to solve.

(b) Give simple and precise information.

(c) Do not suggest goals of behaviour change which are beyond a patient's capacity to achieve.

(d) Check the message has been understood and not misinterpreted.

(e) Offer advice in such a way that the child and parents are not threatened or blamed.

(f) If you are trying to improve oral hygiene avoid theoretical discussions, offer a practical demonstration.

(g) At follow-up visits reinforce the advice and offer positive reinforcement.

Give advice as though you mean it.

The final part of the health education activity is goal setting. The dentist sets out in simple terms what the patient should try and achieve by the next visit. It implies a form of contract and as such helps both children and parents to gain a clearer insight into how they all can help to improve the child's oral health. Goal setting must be used sensibly. If goals are manifestly impossible then parents and child patients become disillusioned. Parents feel that the dentist does not understand their problems and complain that they are being blamed for any dental shortcomings. So always ensure that you plan goal setting carefully in a positive and friendly manner.

Set some realistic objectives.

6. *Dismissal.* This is the final part of the visit and should be clearly signposted so that everyone knows that the appointment is over. The patient should be addressed by name and a definite farewell offered (Fig. 2.10). The objective should be to ensure that wherever possible the patient and parents leave with a sense of goodwill.

Clearly, not all appointment sessions can be dissected into these six stages. However, the basic element of according the patient the maximum attention and personalizing your comments should never be forgotten.

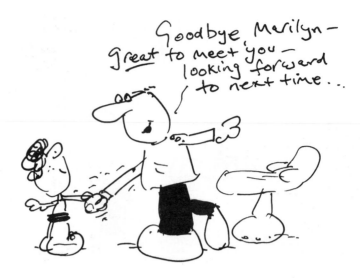

Fig. 2.10 Make sure you offer your patient a definite farewell. (With thanks to David Myers and kind permission of Eden Bianchi Press.)

2.5 ANXIOUS AND UNCOOPERATIVE CHILDREN

Dental anxiety should concern us as a profession because it not only prevents many potential patients from seeking care but it also causes stress to the dentists undertaking dental treatment. Indeed one of the major sources of stress for general dental practitioners is 'coping with difficult patients' (Fig. 2.11). Dentists do not want to be considered as people who inflict unnecessary anxiety on the general public. However, anxiety and dental care seem to be locked in the general folklore of many countries. In order to understand why, it is helpful to consider 'what is the nature of anxiety'.

Anxiety

Many definitions of anxiety have been suggested and it is a somewhat daunting task to reconcile them. However, it would seem sensible to consider the comments of Kent (see Kent and Blinkhorn 1991) who reported that anxiety is 'a vague unpleasant feeling accompanied by a premonition that something undesirable is going to happen'. In other words it relates to how people feel—a subjective definition. Another point of view is that anxiety manifests itself in behaviour. If, for example, a person is anxious, then she/he will act in a particular manner. A person will avoid visiting the dentist. Thus, anxiety should be seen as a multi-factorial problem made up of a number of different components, all of which can exert an effect.

Multifactorial.

Anxiety must also be seen as a continuum with fear—it is almost impossible to separate the two in much of the research undertaken in the field of dentistry, where the two words are used interchangeably. One could consider that anxiety is more a general feeling of discomfort, while fear is a strong reaction to a specific event. Nevertheless it is counterproductive to search for elusive definitions as both fear and anxiety are associated with dental visiting and treatment.

From a common-sense point of view it is clear that some situations will arouse more anxiety than others. For example, a fear of heights is relatively common, but it is galling to note that in the United States a study by Agras *et al.* (1969) found that visiting the dentist ranked fourth behind snakes, heights, and storms. Clearly then, anxiety about dental care is a problem that we as a profession must take seriously, especially as children remember pain and stress suffered at the dentist and carry the emotional scars into adult life. Some people may develop such a fear of dentistry that they are termed phobics. A phobia is an intense fear which is out of all proportion to the actual threat.

I'm not afraid just anxious!

Dental fear—a serious issue.

Research in this area suggests that the extent of anxiety a person experiences does not relate directly to dental knowledge, but is an amalgamation of personal experiences, family concerns, disease levels, and general personality traits. Such a complex

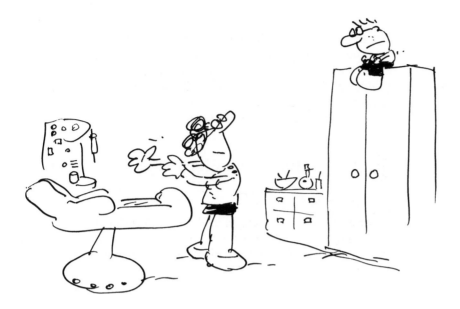

Fig. 2.11 Difficult patients can be a source of stress! (With thanks to David Myers and kind permission of Eden Bianchi Press.)

situation means that it is no easy task to measure dental anxiety and pinpoint aetiological agents.

Measuring dental anxiety is problematic because it relies on subjective measures, plus the influence of the parents, the dentist's behaviour, and the reason for a visit may all exert some effect on a child's anxiety levels.

Questionnaires and rating scales are the most commonly used means by which anxiety has been quantified, although there has been some interest in physiological data such as heart rate. Some questionnaires that have been used to measure anxiety can be applied to a whole variety of situations, such as recording 'exam nerves' or fear of spiders, while others are specific to the dental situation. The most widely used dental anxiety measure is Corah's Dental Anxiety Scale (see Kent and Blinkhorn 1991), which takes the form of a questionnaire. Patients are asked to choose an answer which best sums up their feelings. The answers are scored from 1 to 5 so that a total score can be computed. A high score should alert the dental team that a particular patient is very anxious.

However, patient-administered questionnaires have a limited value in evaluating a young child's anxiety because of their poorly developed vocabulary and understanding. Therefore there has been great interest in measuring anxiety by observing behaviour. One such scale was developed by Frankl to assess the effect of a parent remaining with a child in the surgery (see Kent and Blinkhorn 1991). It consists of four ratings from definitely negative to definitely positive. It is still commonly used in paediatric dental research. Another scale which is popular with researchers is one used by Houpt, which monitors behaviour by allocating a numerical score to items such as body movement and crying (see Kent and Blinkhorn 1991).

Recent studies have used the Frankl scale to select subjects for studies, and then more detailed behaviour evaluation systems are utilized to monitor the compliance with treatment (see Kent and Blinkhorn 1991). Behavioural observation research can be problematical as the presence of an observer in the surgery may upset the patient. In addition, it is difficult to be totally objective when different coping strategies are being used and some bias will occur. The development of cheap lightweight digital or video cameras has greatly helped observational research, as the patient's behaviour can be scored by a number of raters away from the surgery. Rescoring the videos is also possible to check the reliability of the index used.

Physiological measurements such as a higher pulse rate, perspiration, and peripheral blood flow have been used to quantify children's dental anxiety. However, few

Measuring dental fear difficult.

physiological signs are specific to one particular emotion and the measuring techniques often provoke anxiety in the child patient, so they are rarely used.

As yet, there is no standard measure of dental anxiety for children as the reproducibility and reliability of most questionnaires have not been demonstrated, plus observational and physiological indices are not well developed. This is a serious problem as the assessment of strategies to reduce anxiety is somewhat compromised by a lack of universally accepted measuring techniques.

> No standard measure of anxiety.

2.6 HELPING ANXIOUS PATIENTS TO COPE WITH DENTAL CARE

A number of theories have been suggested in an effort to explain the development of anxiety. Uncertainty about what is to happen is certainly a factor, a poor past experience with a dentist could upset a patient, while others may learn anxiety responses from parents, relations, or friends.

A dentist who can alleviate anxiety or prevent it happening in the first place will always be popular with patients. Clearly, the easiest way to control anxiety is to establish an effective preventive programme so that children do not require any treatment. In addition to an effective preventive regimen it is important to establish a trusting relationship, listening to a child's specific worries and concerns. Every effort must be taken to ensure that any treatment is pain-free. All too often we forget that local analgesia requires time and patience. With the use of a topical anaesthetic paste and slow release of the anaesthetic solution most 'injections' should be painless. There is no excuse for the 'stab and squirt method' (Fig. 2.12).

> Injections should be painless.

Children are not 'little adults', they are vulnerable and afraid of new surroundings so effective time management is important. Try to see young patients on time and do not stress yourself or the child by expecting to complete a clinical task in a short time on an apprehensive patient.

> Children have short attention span.

Despite the dental team's best efforts anxiety may persist and routine dental care is compromised. Other options will then have to be considered to help the child. An increasingly popular choice is the use of pharmacological agents; these will be discussed in Chapter 4. The alternatives to the pharmacological approach are:

> Pharmacological alternatives.

(1) reducing uncertainty;

(2) modelling;

(3) cognitive approaches;

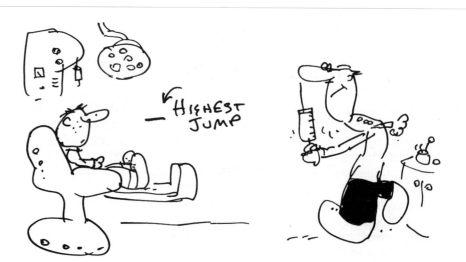

Fig. 2.12 Stab and squirt has no place in our anaesthetic technique. (With thanks to David Myers and kind permission of Eden Bianchi Press.)

(4) relaxation; and

(5) systematic desensitization.

(6) hand over mouth exercise (HOME).

These are discussed in more detail below.

2.6.1 Reducing uncertainty

The majority of young children have very little idea of what dental treatment involves and this will raise anxiety levels. Most children will cope if given friendly reassurance from the dentist, but some patients will need a more structured programme.

One such structured method is the tell–show–do technique. As its name implies it centres on three phases:

1. *Tell*: explanation of procedures at the right age/educational level.
2. *Show*: demonstrate the procedure.
3. *Do*: following on to undertake the task. Praise being an essential part of the exercise (Fig. 2.13).

While it is a popular technique there is little experimental work to support its use.

Another technique to reduce anxiety among very worried children is to send a letter home explaining all the details of the proposed first visit so that uncertainty will be reduced. The evidence for this approach is not clear-cut as parental anxiety is changed by preinformation rather than the child's.

Acclimatization programmes gradually introducing the child to dental care over a number of visits have been shown to be of value. This approach is rather time consuming and does little for the really nervous child.

2.6.2 Modelling

This makes use of the fact that individuals learn much about their environment from observing the consequences of other people's behaviour. You or I might repeat an action if we see others being rewarded, or if someone is punished we might well decide not to follow that behaviour. Modelling could be used to alleviate anxiety. If a child could be shown that it is possible to visit the dentist, have treatment, and then leave in a happy frame of mind (Fig. 2.14), this could reduce anxiety due to 'fear of the unknown'. A child would see behind that forbidding surgery door!

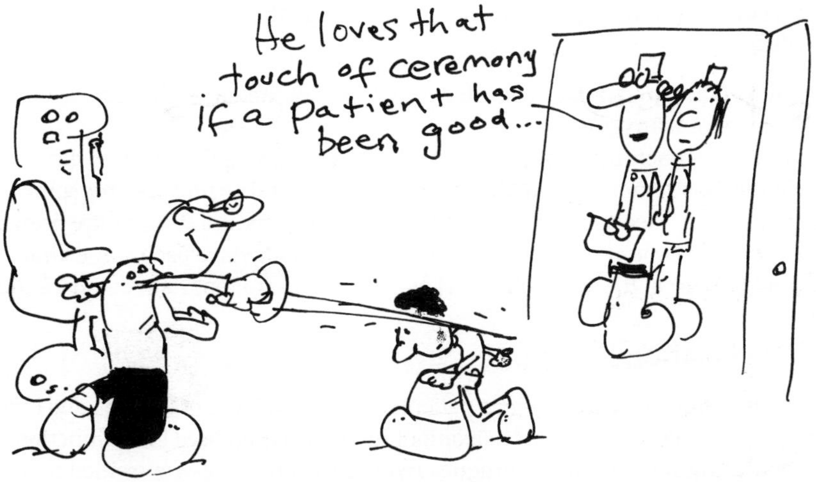

Tell–show–do.

More information for parents.

Modelling reduces fear of unknown.

Fig. 2.13 Praise costs little, but does show you to be a caring person. (With thanks to David Myers and kind permission of Eden Bianchi Press.)

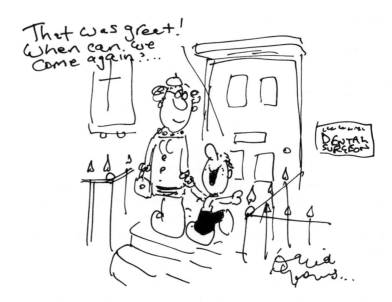

Fig. 2.14 We want our patients to leave us in a happy frame of mind. (With thanks to David Myers and kind permission of Eden Bianchi Press.)

It is not necessary to use a live model, videos of co-operative patients are of value. However, the following points should be taken into consideration when setting up a programme.

1. Ensure that the model is close in age to the nervous child or children involved.
2. The model should be shown entering and leaving the surgery to prove treatment has no lasting effect.
3. The dentist should be shown to be a caring person who praises the patient.

2.6.3 Cognitive approaches

Modelling helps people learn about dental treatment from watching others, but it does not take account of an individual's 'cognitions' or thoughts. People may heighten their anxiety by worrying more and more about a dental problem so creating a vicious reinforcing circle. Thus there has been great interest in trying to get individuals to identify and then alter their dysfunctional beliefs. A number of cognitive modification techniques have been suggested, the most common ones including:

(1) asking patients to identify and make a record of their negative thoughts;
(2) helping patients to recognize their negative thoughts and suggesting more positive alternatives—'reality based';
(3) working with a therapist to identify and change the more deep-seated negative beliefs.

Cognitive therapy is useful for focused types of anxiety—hence its value in combating dental anxiety.

Another approach that could be considered a cognitive approach is distraction. This technique attempts to shift attention from the dental setting towards some other kind of situation. Distracters such as videotaped cartoons and stories have been used to help children cope with dental treatment. The results have been somewhat equivocal and the threat to switch off the video was needed to maintain co-operation.

2.6.4 Relaxation

Relaxation training is of value where patients report high levels of tension, and consists of bringing about deep muscular relaxation. It has also been used in conjunction with biofeedback training. As the techniques require the presence of a trained therapist, the potential value in general paediatric dentistry has still to be assessed.

Worrying increases anxiety.

Distraction helps to reduce anxiety.

2.6.5 Systematic desensitization

The basic principle of this treatment consists of allowing the patient gradually to come to terms with a particular fear or set of fears by working through various levels of the feared situation, from the 'mildest' to the 'most anxiety' programme.

This technique relies on the use of a trained therapist and in most instances a simple dentally based acclimatization programme should be tried first.

Work through fears.

2.6.6 Hand over mouth exercise (HOME)

The physical restraint of children in order to undertake clinical dental care has prompted much debate. Hosey (2002) and Manley (2004) note that in the United Kingdom the use of physical restraint is presently unacceptable. However, some authors are suggesting (Connick *et al.*, 2000; Kupietsky, 2004) that restraint in combination with inhalation sedation may be a helpful procedure if general anaesthesia is not readily available.

In this section other options to restraint have been suggested and, although time consuming, are likely to provoke less of a nervous reaction and avoid associating dental care with an unpleasant experience. For those readers who wish to study the topic in more detail, comprehensive clinical guidelines collated by The American Academy of Paediatric Dentistry have been published in the *Journal of Paediatric Dentistry* (2002).

2.7 SYNOPSIS OF THE GUIDELINES BY THE AMERICAN ACADEMY OF PAEDIATRIC DENTISTRY ON BEHAVIOUR MANAGEMENT

To help those readers who wish to have an overview of the key elements in the guidelines, a brief summary of the objectives and indications/contraindications for a number of behaviour management techniques, available to dental practitioners, are listed.

2.7.1 Communication management

1. Voice control is a controlled alteration of voice volume, tone, or pace to influence and direct the patient's behaviour.

Objectives:

  (i) To gain the patient's attention and compliance.

  (ii) To avert negative or avoidance behaviour.

  (iii) To establish appropriate adult–child roles.

Indications: May be used with any patient.
Contraindications: None.

2. Non-verbal communication is the reinforcement and guidance of behaviour through appropriate contact, posture, and facial expression.

Objectives:

  (i) To enhance the effectiveness of other communicative management techniques.

  (ii) To gain or maintain the patient's attention and compliance.

Indications: May be used with any patient.
Contraindications: None.

3. Tell–show–do is a technique of behaviour shaping used with both verbal and non-verbal communication.

Objectives:

  (i) To teach the patient important aspects of the dental visit and familiarize the patient with the dental setting.

(ii) To shape the patient's response to procedures through desensitization and well-described expectations.

Indications: May be used with any patient.
Contraindications: None.

4. Positive reinforcement is the process of establishing desirable patient behaviour through appropriate feedback.

Objectives:

(i) To reinforce desired behaviour.

Indications: May be useful for any patient.
Contraindications: None.

5. Parental presence/absence involves either allowing or removing the parent(s) from the dental surgery in order to gain cooperation.

Objectives:

(i) To gain the patient's attention and compliance.

(ii) To avert negative or avoidance behaviours.

(iii) To establish appropriate adult–child roles.

(iv) To enhance the communication environment.

Indications: May be used with any patient.
Contraindications: None.

6. Hand over mouth exercise is a technique for managing unsuitable behaviour that cannot be modified by the more straightforward techniques. It is often used with inhalation sedation (conscious sedation).

Objectives:

(i) To redirect the child's attention, enable communication with the dentist so that appropriate behavioural expectations can be explained.

(ii) To extinguish excessive avoidance behaviour and help the child regain self-control.

(iii) To ensure the child's safety in the delivery of quality dental treatment.

(iv) To reduce the need for sedation or general anaesthesia.

Indications:

(i) A healthy child who is able to understand and co-operate, but who exhibits obstreperous or hysterical avoidance behaviours.

Contraindications:

(i) In children who, due to age, disability, medication, or emotional immaturity are unable to verbally communicate, understand, and co-operate.

(ii) Any child with an airway obstruction.

Other techniques such as sedation in all its forms and general anaesthesia are described elsewhere.

2.8 SUMMARY

1. To prevent the development of anxiety it is more important to maintain trust than concentrate on finishing a clinical task.

2. The reduction in dental caries means that children with special psychological, medical, and physical needs can be offered the oral health care they require. We are not being swamped by overwhelming clinical demand.

3. The care of children who are very anxious can be improved by using the techniques described in this chapter.

4. Preventing dental disease should always be given the same status as clinical intervention. However, it is important to ensure that preventive care is appropriate and relevant. The key messages are outlined in *The scientific basis of oral health education* (Levine and Stillman-Lowe, 2004).

2.9 FURTHER READING

Blinkhorn, A. S. and Mackie, I. C. (1992). *Treatment planning for the paedodontic patient.* Quintessence, London. (*There is a comprehensive question and answer section in this book which will help you check up on your treatment planning knowledge.*)

Freeman, R. (1999). The determinants of dental health attitudes and behaviours. *British Dental Journal*, **187**, 15–18. (*This paper examines the role of psychosocial factors on health behaviour, and case-based examples highlight the psychology of patient care in a practical way.*)

Humphris, G. M., Milsom, K., Tickle, M., Holbrook, H., and Blinkhorn, A. S. (2002). A new dental anxiety scale for 5 year old children (DA5): description and concurrent validity. *Health Education Journal*, **61**, 5–19. (*This paper describes the development of a new dental anxiety scale for children and highlights the key elements associated with measuring anxiety.*)

Rutter, M. and Rutter, M. (1993). *Developing minds.* Penguin Books, London. (*A fascinating insight into how we develop throughout life.*)

Weinman, J. (1987). *An outline of psychology as applied to medicine* (2nd edn), pp. 132–4. Butterworth–Heineman, London. (*This book is for those students who want to take a broader view on the subject of psychology and medicine.*)

2.10 REFERENCES

Agras, S., Sylvester, D., and Oliveau, D. (1969). The epidemiology of common fears and phobias. *Comprehensive Psychiatry*, **10**, 151–56. (*This paper will show you that fear of dentistry is a problem the dental profession must take seriously.*)

Clinical guideline on behaviour management (2002). *Journal of Paediatric Dentistry*, **24**, 68–73. (*An American perspective on behaviour management in paediatric dentistry.*)

Connick, C., Palat, M., and Puliese, S. (2000). The appropriate use of physical restraints: considerations. *Journal of Dentistry for Children*, **67**, 256–62. (*A useful discussion on the role of restraint in clinical paediatric dental practice.*)

Hosey, M. T. (2002). Managing anxious children: the use of conscious sedation in paediatric dentistry. *International Journal of Paediatric Dentistry*, **12**, 359–72. (*A useful guide to managing anxious children.*)

Kent, G. G. and Blinkhorn, A. S. (1991). *The psychology of dental care* (2nd edn). Wright, Bristol. (*This short book highlights the important psychological aspects of providing clinical care, as well as giving details of the Houpt, Frankl, and Corah dental anxiety scales.*)

Kupietzky, A. (2004). Strap him down or knock him out: is conscious sedation with restraint an alternative to general anaesthesia? *British Dental Journal*, **196**, 133–8. (*A discussion on the role of conscious sedation allied to the use of restraint in paediatric dentistry.*)

Levine, R. S. and Stillman-Lowe, C. (2004). *The scientific basis of oral health education.* BDJ Books, London (*A comprehensive guide to dental health education and promotion, including the key preventive messages.*)

Manley, M. C. G. (2004). A UK perspective. *British Dental Journal*, **196**, 138–9. (*A view on the use of HOME in the United Kingdom.*)

Wanless, M. B. and Holloway, P. J. (1994). An analysis of audio-recordings of general dental practitioners' consultations with adolescent patients. *British Dental Journal*, **177**, 94–8. (*This article gives advice on how to improve communication skills in the surgery and reminds clinicians that our livelihood depends on effective communication.*)

Wright, G., Starkey, P. E., Gardener, D. E., and Curzon, M. E. J. (1987). *Child management in dentistry.* Wright, Bristol. (*A detailed account of child management, including advice on how to introduce different clinical techniques.*)

3

History, examination, risk assessment, and treatment planning

3 History, examination, risk assessment, and treatment planning

M. L. Hunter and H. D. Rodd

3.1 INTRODUCTION

The provision of dental care for children presents some of the greatest challenges (and rewards) in clinical dental practice. High on the list of challenges is the need to devise a comprehensive yet realistic treatment plan for these young patients. Successful outcomes are very unlikely in the absence of thorough short- and long-term treatment planning. Furthermore, decision-making for children has to take into account many more factors than is the case for adults. This chapter aims to highlight how history-taking, examination, and risk assessment are all critical stages in the treatment planning process. Principles of good treatment planning will also be outlined.

3.2 CONSENT

Consent to examination, investigation, or treatment is fundamental to the provision of dental care. The most important element of the consent procedure is ensuring that the patient/parent understands the nature and purpose of the proposed treatment, together with any alternatives available, and the potential benefits and risks. In this context, where clinician and patient/parent do not share a common language, the assistance of an interpreter is essential.

> **Key Point**
> A signature on a consent form is not consent if the patient/parent has not been given and understood the relevant information.

In the United Kingdom, for the purposes of medical and dental treatment, a child is defined as being less than 16 years of age. If a child is subjected to examination, investigation, or treatment without the consent of an individual who has parental responsibility, this can constitute an assault, actionable in civil or criminal law as a breach of the human right. While most children will attend the dental surgery accompanied by an adult, it is important to bear in mind that this individual will not always have parental responsibility (the Children Act 1989 sets out the persons who may have parental responsibility for a child).

> **Key Point**
> It is essential to establish what relationship exists between the child and the accompanying adult at the outset. Foster parents do not automatically have parental responsibility. In circumstances where a child is a ward of Court, the prior consent of the Court is required for significant interventions.

In an emergency, it is justifiable to treat a child without the consent of the person with parental responsibility if the treatment is vital to the health of the child. For example, while it may be acceptable to replant an avulsed permanent incisor, the parent should be contacted before proceeding to other forms of treatment.

Using the principle of Gillick competence, a child under the age of 16 years can give valid consent provided that the clinician considers him or her to be mature enough to fully understand the proposed intervention. However, as the understanding required for different interventions will vary, a child aged less than 16 years may have the capacity to consent to some interventions but not to others.

> **Key Point**
>
> If a child is considered to be Gillick competent, his or her consent will be valid. Additional consent by a person with parental responsibility will not be required.

Young people aged 16 or 17 years are entitled to consent to their own dental treatment and anaesthetic where the treatment offers direct benefit to the individual. However, the refusal of a competent individual of this age to undergo treatment may in certain circumstances be over-ridden by either a person who has parental responsibility or by a Court.

3.3 HISTORY

Taking a comprehensive case history is an essential prelude to clinical examination, diagnosis, and treatment planning. It is also an excellent opportunity for the dentist to establish a relationship with the child and his or her parent. Generally speaking, information is best gathered by way of a relaxed conversation with the child and his or her parent in which the dentist assumes the role of an interested listener rather than that of an inquisitor. While some clinicians may prefer to employ a proforma to ensure the completeness of the process, this is less important than the adherence to a set routine.

A complete case history should consist of:

- personal details;
- presenting complaint(s);
- social history;
- medical history;
- dental history.

Table 3.1 summarizes the key information that should be included under each heading.

3.3.1 Personal details

A note should be made of the patient's name (including any abbreviated name or nickname), age, address, and telephone number. Where these details have been entered in the case notes prior to the appointment they should be verified. Details of the patient's medical practitioner should also be noted.

3.3.2 Presenting complaint(s)

It is important to ascertain from the child and his or her parent why the visit has been made or what they are seeking from treatment. It is good practice to ask this question to the child before involving the parent as this establishes the child's importance

Table 3.1 History-taking for the paediatric dental patient

1 Personal details	Name	Abbreviated name/nickname
	Contact details	Address, telephone number
	Date of birth	Age
	GMP details	Name and address
2 Presenting complaint	Planned/emergency appointment	
	Pain or swelling	Duration, nature,
		Exacerbating and relieving factors
	Trauma	Detailed history of event
	Particular concerns	Colour, shape, position of teeth
3 Social history	With whom does the child live?	Parental responsibility (consent)
	Parental occupation	Ease of dental attendance
	Siblings	Number and ages
	School	
	Interests	
4 Medical history		
Pregnancy/birth/neonatal	Maternal health	
	Birth details	Delivery, complications, weight
	Neonatal period	Icterus, feeding or respiratory problems, neonatal teeth
	Development	Somatic, psychomotor
	Trauma injuries and childhood illnesses	Age, severity
Systems	Respiratory	Asthma, hayfever
	Cardiovascular	SBE risk factors
	Haematological	Anaemia, bleeding, bruising
	Immunological	Predisposition to infections
	Endocrine	Diabetes
	Gastrointestinal	Abnormal bowel habits
	Neuromuscular	
	Skeletal	
Hospitalization	Age and cause of admission	
	Operations	
	Experience of GA	
Medication	Regular prescriptions	Format—tablets, liquid, inhalers
	Recent/current medication allergies	
Additional information	Learning difficulties	
	Behavioural problems	ADHD, autistic spectrum disorders
Relevant family medical history	Problems with GA, allergies, bleeding disorders, any siblings with significant medical problems	
5 Dental history		
Professional care	Attendance pattern	Regular or irregular attender
	Previous treatment	Prevention, restorations, extractions
	LA/GA/sedation	Any problems encountered
	Previous co-operation	
Home care	Diet	Bottle/breast feeding, snacks, drinks
	Oral hygiene	Frequency, type of brush and paste, assistance
	Fluoride	Fluoridated water, drops, tablets, mouthrinses
Habits	Sucking/biting	Dummy, digit sucking, nail biting
	Parafunction	Bruxism

LA—local anaesthesia; GA—general anaesthesia.

in the process, though the dentist should be prepared to receive different answers from these two sources.

Where a child presents in pain or has a particular concern, this should be recorded in the child's own words and, if relevant, the history of the present complaint (e.g. duration, mode of onset, progression) should be documented. It should be recognized that, even where other (perhaps more important) treatment is required, failure to take into consideration the patient's/parent's needs or wishes at this stage may be detrimental to both the development of the dentist/patient/parent relationship and the outcome of care.

3.3.3 Social (family) history

A child is a product of his or her environment. Factors such as whether both parents are alive and well, the number and age of siblings, the parents' occupations, ease of travel, as well as attendance at school or day-care facilities are all important if a realistic treatment plan is to be arrived at. However, since some parents will consider this kind of information confidential, the dentist may need to exercise considerable tact in order to obtain it.

This stage of history-taking also presents an opportunity to engage the child in conversation. In this way, the dentist gains an insight into the child's interests (e.g. pets, favourite subjects at school, favourite pastimes) and is able to record potential topics of conversation that can act as 'ice-breakers' in future appointments.

3.3.4 Medical history

Various diseases or functional disturbances may directly or indirectly cause or predispose to oral problems. Likewise, they may affect the delivery of oral and dental care. Conditions that will be of significance include allergies, severe asthma, diabetes, cerebral palsy, cardiac conditions, haematological disorders, and oncology.

Wherever possible, a comprehensive medical history should commence with information relating to pregnancy and birth, the neonatal period, and early childhood. Indeed, asking a mother about her child's health since birth will not infrequently stimulate the production of a complete medical history! Previous and current problems associated with each of the major systems should be elicited through careful questioning, and here a proforma may well be helpful. Details about previous hospitalizations, operations (or planned operations), illnesses, allergies (particularly adverse reactions to drugs), and traumatic injuries should be recorded, as well as those relating to previous and current medical treatment.

Key Point

If any relevant conditions become apparent, these may need to be investigated in greater detail, contacting the child's general medical practitioner or hospital consultant where necessary.

It is useful to end by asking the parent whether there is anything else that they think the dentist should know about their child. (Sometimes, important details are not volunteered until this point!) This is a particularly useful approach in relation to children who suffer from behavioural or learning problems, such as attention deficit and hyperactivity disorder (ADHD) or autism.

Key Point

Sensitive questioning is required if the child appears to have a behavioural problem that has not been mentioned by the parent during the formal medical history.

It is important to bear in mind that many children with significant medical problems will have been subjected to multiple hospital admissions/attendances. These experiences may have a negative effect on the attitude of both the child and his or her parents towards dental treatment; in addition, dental care may not be seen as a priority in the context of total care.

Finally, a brief enquiry should also be made regarding the health of siblings and close family. Significant family medical problems, for instance problems in relation to general anaesthesia, may not only alert the practitioner to potential risks for the child, but may also be factors to consider when treatment planning. Likewise, if the patient has a sick sibling, it may not be possible for the parents to commit to a prolonged course of dental treatment.

3.3.5 Dental history

A child's previous dental experiences may affect the way in which he or she reacts to further treatment. Evaluation of a child's previous behaviour requires the dentist to obtain information about the kind of dental treatment a child has received (including the method of pain and anxiety control which has been offered) and the way in which he or she has reacted to this. In so doing, specific procedures may emerge as having proved particularly problematic; such prior knowledge will enable the dentist to modify the treatment plan appropriately.

The dental history should also identify factors that have been responsible for existing oral and dental problems as well as those which might have an impact on future health. These include dietary, oral hygiene, dummy/digit sucking, and parafunctional habits. Specific questions should be asked about drinks (particularly the use of a bottle at bedtime in the younger age group,), between-meal snacks, frequency of brushing, and type of toothpaste used.

Finally, a thorough dental history is an opportunity to evaluate the attitude of the parent to his or her child's dental treatment. For example, the regularity of previous dental care may be an indicator of the value that the parent places on his or her child's dental health.

> **Key Point**
> Embarking on a treatment plan that is at significant variance with parental attitudes and expectations without clear explanation and justification invites non-completion.

3.4 EXAMINATION

3.4.1 First impressions

An initial impression of the child's overall health and development can be gained as soon as he or she is greeted in the waiting room or enters the surgery. In particular, it is useful to note:

- general health—does the child look well?
- overall physical and mental development—does it seem appropriate for the child's chronological age?
- weight—is the child grossly under- or overweight?
- co-ordination—does the child have an abnormal gait or obvious motor impairment?

While the history is being taken, the clinician should also be making an 'unofficial' assessment of the child's likely level of co-operation in order that the most appropriate

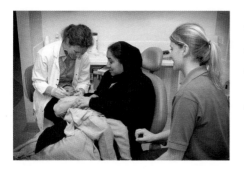

Fig. 3.1 Controlled examination of a young boy laid across his mother's knee.

approach for the examination can be adopted right from the start (hopefully saving both time and tears). Broadly speaking, prospective young patients may fall into one of the following categories:

- happy and confident—this child is likely to hop into the chair for a check-up without further coaxing;
- a little anxious or shy but displaying some rapport with the dental team—this child will probably allow an examination after some simple acclimatization and reassurance (if the child is very young, the option of sitting on the mother's knee could be given);
- very frightened, crying, clutching their parent, avoiding eye contact, or not responding to direct questions—this child is unlikely to accept a conventional examination at this visit (though the child may allow a brief examination while sitting on a non-dental chair, perhaps even in the waiting room); further acclimatization will be required before a thorough examination can be undertaken;
- severe behavioural problem or learning disability—in a few cases, this may preclude the child from ever voluntarily accepting an examination; restraint (with or without pharmacological management) may be indicated to facilitate an intraoral examination.

3.4.2 Restraint

> **Key Point**
>
> It is not good practice to formulate a definitive treatment plan, especially one involving a general anaesthetic, without first performing a thorough examination.

In an ideal world, unco-operative children would be given the time and opportunity to voluntarily accept a dental examination over a series of desensitizing visits. In reality, if a child presents with a reported problem but remains unco-operative after gentle coaxing and normal behaviour management strategies, restraint may be necessary.

Physical restraint should only be considered for infants/very young children, or children with severe learning difficulties (providing they are not too big or strong to make any restraint potentially dangerous or uncontrolled). The issue of informed consent is important here, as it is imperative that the need for the examination and the manner in which it is going to be conducted is clearly understood by all concerned. It is best to:

- explain in advance how the child is to be positioned,
- ask parents for their active help,
- give reassurance that the child is not going to be hurt in any way.

In the most controlled approach, the child is laid across the parent's knees with his or her head on those of the operator (Fig. 3.1). The parent is able to hold the child's arms though a dental nurse may need to restrain the child's legs. It may be easier to examine bigger children who have special needs while they are restrained in their own wheelchair, the dental nurse supporting the child's head during the examination. (See also Chapter 17 page 419.)

3.4.3 Extraoral examination

General examination

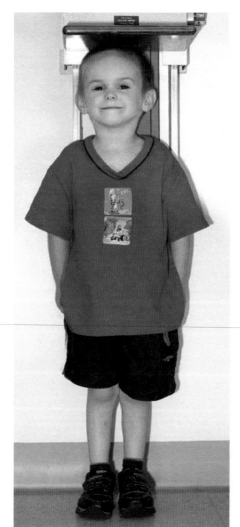

Fig. 3.2 Use of a wall-mounted stediometer to take an accurate height measurement (the patient's shoes should be removed!).

Before carrying out a detailed examination of the craniofacial structures, a more general physical assessment should be undertaken. Valuable information about a

47

child's overall health, development, or even habits can often be determined by noting:

- height—is the child very tall or very small for their age? In a few cases, it may be appropriate to take an accurate height measurement (Fig. 3.2) and plot data on a standard growth chart (Fig. 3.3). Children whose height lies below the third

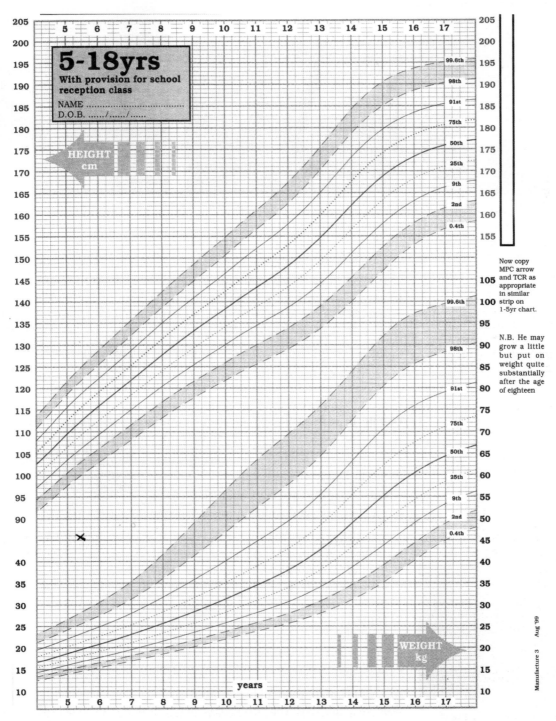

Fig. 3.3 Standard growth chart showing plot of height against age for boy in Fig. 3.2 who has a severe growth deficiency.

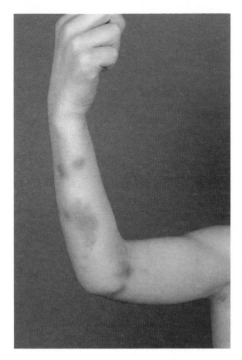

Fig. 3.4 Multiple bruises on arm of child with a platelet disorder.

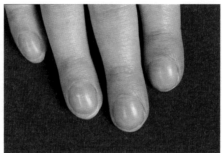

Fig. 3.5 Finger clubbing in child with a congenital heart disorder.

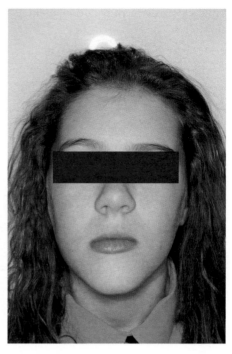

Fig. 3.6 Facial asymmetry in a teenage girl.

centile, above the ninety-seventh centile, or who exhibit less than 3–5 cm growth per year should be referred to a paediatrician for further investigation;

• weight—could there be an underlying eating disorder? Is general anaesthesia contraindicated due to the child's obesity? Is there an underlying endocrine problem?

• skin—look for any notable bruising or injury on exposed arms or legs (Fig. 3.4);

• hands—assess for evidence of digit sucking or nail biting, warts, finger clubbing, abnormal nail, or finger morphology (Fig. 3.5).

The head and neck

During the examination of the head and neck, the following structures should be briefly assessed:

• head—note size, shape (abnormalities may be seen in certain syndromes), and any facial asymmetry (Fig. 3.6);

• hair—note if sparse (look out for head lice!);

• eyes—is there any visual impairment or abnormality of the sclera?

• ears—record any abnormal morphology or presence of hearing aids;

• skin—document any scars, bruising, lacerations, pallor, birthmarks (Fig. 3.7) and be aware of contagious infections, such as impetigo;

• temporomandibular joint—is there any pain, crepitus, deviation, or restricted opening?

• lymph nodes—palpate for enlarged submandibular or cervical lymph nodes (bear in mind that lymphadenopathy is not uncommon in children, due to frequent viral infections) (Fig. 3.8);

• lips—note the presence of cold sores, swelling, or abnormal colouring (Fig. 3.9).

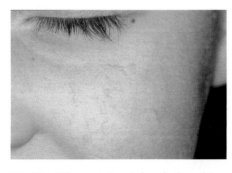

Fig. 3.7 Telangiectasia noted on the face of a young boy.

Any positive findings should be recorded carefully. Clinical photographs or annotated sketches (Fig. 3.10) may be very helpful for future reference, particularly with respect to medico-legal purposes, or in cases of suspected child physical abuse (see

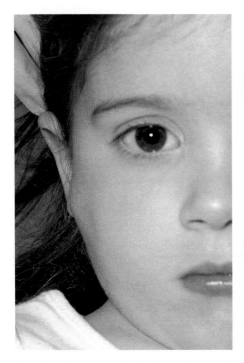
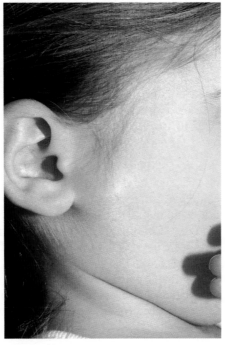

Fig. 3.8 Three-year-old girl with swelling possibly in pre-auricular lymph node or parotid gland.

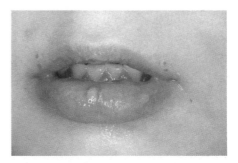

Fig. 3.9 Multiple vesicles on lip of young patient with acute herpetic gingivostomatitis.

Chapter 12). Obviously, when the child presents with a specific problem, such as a facial swelling, a more thorough examination of the presenting condition is needed (see Chapter 15).

3.4.4 Intraoral examination

A systematic approach should be adopted for the intraoral examination. The following is a suggested order:

- soft tissues
- gingival and periodontal tissues
- teeth
- occlusion.

Soft tissues

An abnormal appearance of the oral soft tissues may be indicative of an underlying systemic disease or nutritional deficiency. In addition, a variety of oral pathologies may be seen in children (see Chapter 15). It is therefore important to carefully examine the tongue, palate, throat, and cheeks, noting any colour changes, ulceration, swelling, or other pathology (Fig. 3.11).

It is also sensible to check for abnormal frenal attachment or tongue-tie, which may have functional implications. If a tongue-tie or abnormal tongue function is observed, some consideration should be given to the child's speech. During examination of the soft tissues, an overall impression of salivary flow rate and consistency should also be gained.

Gingival and periodontal tissues

A visual examination of the gingival tissues is usually all that is indicated for young children, as periodontal disease is very uncommon in this age group. The presence

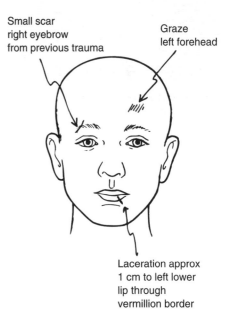

Small scar
right eyebrow
from previous trauma

Graze
left forehead

Laceration approx
1 cm to left lower
lip through
vermillion border

Fig. 3.10 Example of annotated sketch used to record trauma.

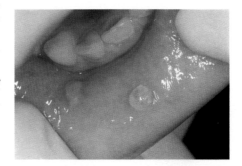

Fig. 3.11 Mucocoele of labial mucosa: an incidental finding.

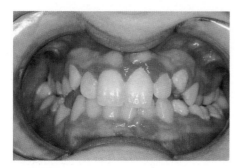

Fig. 3.12 Plaque-induced gingival inflammation.

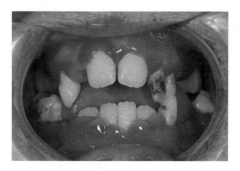

Fig. 3.13 Severe gingival inflammation in patient with cyclical neutropenia.

of colour change (redness), swelling, ulceration, spontaneous bleeding, or recession (Figs 3.12 and 3.13.) should be carefully noted, and the aetiology sought.

> **Key Point**
>
> The presence of profound gingival inflammation in the absence of gross plaque deposits, lateral periodontal abscesses, prematurely exfoliating teeth, or mobile permanent teeth may indicate a more serious underlying problem, warranting further investigation.

During inspection of the gingival tissues, an assessment of oral cleanliness should also be made, and the presence of any plaque or calculus deposits noted. A number of simple oral hygiene indices have been developed to provide an objective record of oral cleanliness. One such index, the oral debris index (Green and Vermillion, 1964), requires disclosing prior to an evaluation of the amount of plaque on selected teeth (first permanent molars, and upper right and lower left central incisors) as shown in Fig. 3.14.

Systematic periodontal probing is not routinely practised in young children, unless there is a specific problem (see Chapter 11). However, it is prudent to carry out some selective probing for teenagers in order to detect any early tissue attachment loss, which may indicate the onset of adult periodontitis.

Teeth

Following assessment of the oral soft tissues, a full dental charting should be performed. A thorough knowledge of eruption dates for the primary and permanent dentition is essential as any delayed or premature eruption may alert the clinician to a potential problem. However, simply recording the presence or absence of a tooth is not adequate: closer scrutiny of each tooth's condition, structure, and shape is also required. Suggested features to note are briefly listed below:

- caries—is it active/arrested, restorable/unrestorable? Check for the presence of a chronic sinus associated with grossly carious teeth;

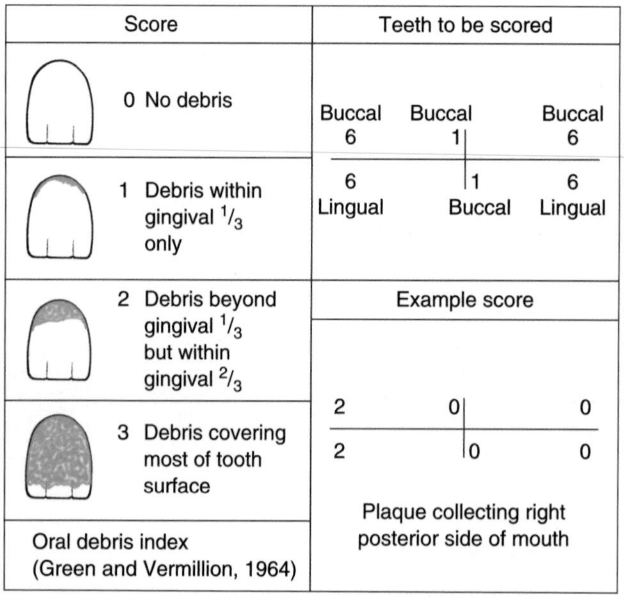

Score	Teeth to be scored
0 No debris	Buccal Buccal Buccal 6 1 6
1 Debris within gingival ⅓ only	6 1 6 Lingual Buccal Lingual
2 Debris beyond gingival ⅓ but within gingival ⅔	Example score
3 Debris covering most of tooth surface	2 0 0 2 0 0
Oral debris index (Green and Vermillion, 1964)	Plaque collecting right posterior side of mouth

Fig. 3.14 Oral debris index by Green and Vermillion (1964).

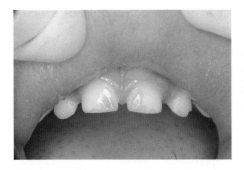

Fig. 3.15 Unusual pattern of erosion affecting labial surface of maxillary primary incisors attributed to use of lemon tea in feeder cup.

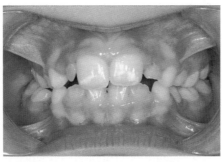

Fig. 3.16 Localized white enamel opacities affecting permanent maxillary central incisors.

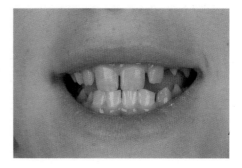

Fig 3.17 Generalized inherited enamel defect (amelogenesis imperfecta).

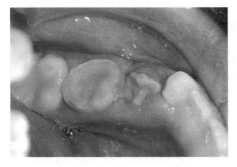

Fig. 3.18 Partially erupted mandibular first premolar showing severe enamel hypoplasia.

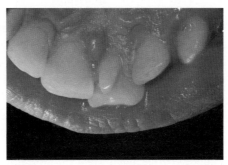

Fig. 3.19 Maxillary central incisor with talon cusp.

- restorations—are they intact/deficient?
- fissure sealants—are they intact/deficient?
- tooth surface loss—note any erosion/attrition, site, extent (Fig. 3.15);
- trauma—note extent, site, or signs of loss of vitality;
- tooth structure—record any enamel opacities/hypoplasia (are defects localised/ generalised?) (Figs. 3.16–3.18);
- tooth shape/size—note presence of double teeth, conical teeth, macrodontia/ microdontia, talon cusps, deep cingulum pits (Fig. 3.19);
- tooth number—any missing/extra teeth?
- tooth mobility—is it physiological or pathological?
- tooth eruption—are there any impactions, infraoccluded primary molars, or ectopically erupting first permanent molars?

Occlusion

Clearly, a full orthodontic assessment is not indicated every time a child is examined. However, tooth alignment and occlusion should be briefly considered, as these may provide an early prompt as to the need for interceptive orthodontic treatment. It is certainly worth noting:

- severe skeletal abnormalities;
- overjet and overbite;
- first molar relationships;
- presence of crowding/spacing;
- deviations/displacements.

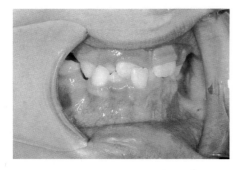

Fig. 3.20   Cross-bite in early mixed dentition.

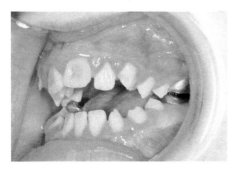

Fig. 3.21   Severe anterior open bite (in association with amelogenesis imperfecta).

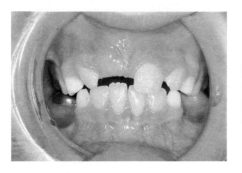

Fig. 3.22   Failure of eruption of maxillary left central incisor: time to be concerned!

There are also two key stages of dental development, when the clinician should be particularly vigilant in checking tooth eruption and position:

1. Age 8–9 years—eruption of upper permanent incisors
    - increased overjet—may predispose to trauma
    - cross-bite—need for early intervention? (Fig. 3.20)
    - traumatic bite—associated with localized gingival recession of lower incisor?
    - anterior open bite—skeletal problem, digit-sucking habit, or tongue thrust? (Fig. 3.21)
    - failure of eruption—presence of a supernumary, crown/root dilaceration, retained primary incisor, congenitally missing lateral incisors? (Fig. 3.22).

2. Age 10+ years—eruption of upper permanent canines
    - are the permanent canines palpable buccally—if not, they may be heading in a palatal direction
    - are the primary canines becoming mobile—if not, the permanent canines may be ectopic.

3.5 FURTHER INVESTIGATIONS

Having carried out a thorough extra- and intraoral examination as described above, the clinician may feel that further investigations are indicated for diagnostic purposes. Table 3.2 highlights the range of dental (and more general) investigations that may be employed to aid diagnosis of the presenting complaint. The use of radiographs is more fully described in the following section.

3.5.1 Radiographs

> **Key Point**
>
> Since patients should not be over-exposed to ionizing radiation, every radiographic investigation should be clinically justified and have a clear diagnostic purpose.

Comprehensive clinical guidelines for radiographic assessment of children have been proposed by the European Academy of Paediatric Dentistry (2003). 'Routine' radiographic screening is certainly not indicated for children. However, radiographs may be indicated in order to facilitate:

- caries diagnosis;
- trauma diagnosis;
- orthodontic treatment planning;
- identification of any abnormalities in dental development;
- detection of any bony or dental pathology.

Caries diagnosis

Bitewing radiographs are invaluable for the detection of early interproximal carious lesions (Fig. 3.23), or occult occlusal lesions. Indeed, bitewing radiography will increase the identification of interproximal lesions by a factor of between 2 and 8, compared to visual assessment alone. Bitewing radiographs are usually recommended for all new patients, especially high caries risk individuals, to provide a baseline caries assessment. However, they may not be necessary for very young patients with open primary molar contacts.

The bitewing radiograph is the view of choice for interproximal caries detection, but it does require a reasonable degree of patient co-operation. For patients unable to tolerate intraoral films, the lateral oblique radiograph provides a useful alternative

Table 3.2 Special investigations for the paediatric dental patient

Investigation	Comment
Intraoral	
Sensibility testing	Use of ethyl chloride or electric pulp tester maybe useful for determining pulpal status following trauma. Caution should be exercised in interpretation of results
Transillumination	Useful for interproximal caries detection, or trauma-related sequelae, such as pulpal haemorrhage or enamel infractions
Mobility	Gentle finger pressure will reveal any pathological or physiological mobility
Percussion	A 'cracked tea-cup' sound on gentle tapping of tooth indicates likely ankylosis
Periodontal probing	Indicated in specific periodontal conditions or to detect presence of foreign body
Saliva tests	May be appropriate to test salivary flow rate and buffering capacity in cases of suspected xerostomia
Oral microbial tests	*Streptococcus mutans* or *Lactobacillus* counts may be indicated in children presenting with rampant caries
	Culture and sensitivity of micro-organisms from intra-oral pus sample may aid antibiotic selection
	Cytology of intraoral swab may confirm suspected candidal infection
Tooth measurement	Space analysis and measurement of tooth size may be necessary for treatment planning
Oral histology/pathology	Specialist examination of soft or hard tissue specimens may be essential to obtain diagnosis of presenting complaint
Study models	May be useful for treatment planning ($\pm$ Kesling set-up) or providing record of presenting problems, such as erosion, infraocclusion, orthodontic status
Photographs	Provide record of presenting problem and pre- and post-treatment status
General	
Specialist imaging	Computerized axial tomography (CAT), ultrasound, magnetic resonance imaging (MRI), or sialography may be indicated in special cases
Haematology	Full blood picture, electrophoresis (for sickle-cell status), clinical chemistry, or immunological tests may be requested in certain cases
Height and weight	Assessment of height may be indicated where there is an obvious deviation from normal or where detection of pubertal growth spurt is indicated for orthodontic purposes (use of functional appliances). Weight assessment may be necessary to determine suitability of patient for out-patient general anaesthesia
Dietary assessment	A 3-day dietary record may be analysed to identify potential cariogenic and/or erosive components and provide basis for dietary advice
Temperature	Assessment of any pyrexia is indicated when a child presents with an acute orofacial infection

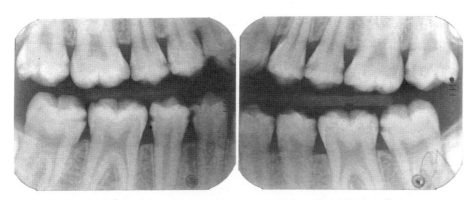

Fig. 3.23 Left and right bitewing radiographs showing multiple approximal carious lesions not evident clinically.

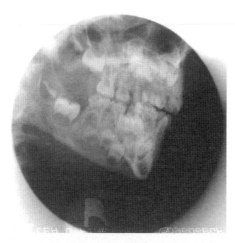

Fig. 3.24 Right lateral oblique radiograph showing caries in lower primary molars.

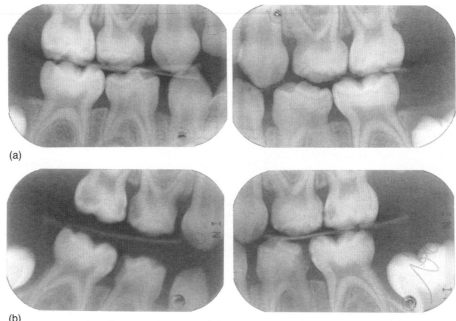

(a)

(b)

Fig. 3.25 Left and right bitewing radiographs of young boy from high carious-risk family at (a) 3 years 10 months and (b) 4 years 10 months demonstrating rapid carious development.

(Fig. 3.24). This view has the added advantage of including the developing permanent dentition.

Following the initial radiographic investigation of caries, a decision should be made regarding the frequency of any future assessment. The interval will depend on the patient's individual caries risk (see Section 3.6) as follows:

*   high caries risk—repeat bitewings in 12 months (Fig. 3.25)
*   low caries risk—repeat bitewings in 24–36 months

Trauma assessment

Radiographs may be indicated for patients who have sustained facial or dental trauma. This topic will be discussed in more detail in Chapter 12.

Orthodontic treatment planning

A discussion of radiographic views for orthodontic treatment planning is not within the remit of this chapter. However, a panoral radiograph is usually mandatory prior to any orthodontic treatment. The need for other views, such as an upper standard occlusal or lateral cephalometric radiograph, is dependent on the individual clinical situation (Chapter 14).

Dental development

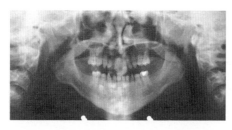

Fig. 3.26 Panoral radiograph of 10-year-old boy with severe hypodontia (only two permanent units are present). Note taurodont mandibular second primary molars.

The need for radiographic assessment of the developing dentition may be prompted by any of the following clinical features:

(1) delayed/premature dental development;
(2) suspected missing/extra teeth (Fig. 3.26);
(3) potential ectopic tooth position (especially upper maxillary canines);
(4) first permanent molars of poor prognosis—in cases where first permanent molars are to be extracted it is mandatory to check for the radiographic presence of all other permanent teeth, including third molars, and to assess the stage of dental development of the lower second permanent molars in order to determine the optimum time for any first permanent molar extractions (see Chapter 14).

The panoral radiograph provides the optimum view for an overall assessment of normal or abnormal dental development. Furthermore, accurate determination of chronological age can be achieved by calculating dental age, using a panoral radiograph and a technique for dental aging, such as that described by Demirjian (1973).

A panoral radiograph may be supplemented with an intraoral radiograph, such as an upper standard occlusal, when an 'abnormality' presents in the anterior maxilla. The combination of these two views provides the opportunity to confirm the exact position of any unerupted maxillary canines or supernumary teeth, using the vertical parallax technique (Fig. 3.27).

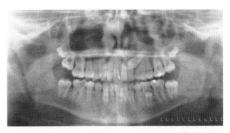

(a)

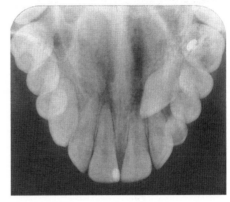

(b)

Fig. 3.27 (a) Panoral radiograph and (b) upper standard occlusal radiograph used to confirm the palatal position of the unerupted maxillary left canine by the vertical parallax technique.

> **Key Point**
>
> The 'SLOB' rule: if the tooth in question moves in the **s**ame direction as the xray tube, then the tooth is **l**ingually or palatally positioned (in relation to the reference point). However, if the tooth moves in the **o**pposite direction to the X-ray tube, it is **b**uccally placed.

Detection of pathology

Selected radiographs may be required in cases of suspected pathology. The actual view is obviously dictated by the presenting complaint, but a periapical radiograph is frequently indicated for localized pathologies, such as:

- periapical or interadicular infection (primary molars) associated with non-vital teeth;
- periodontal conditions;
- trauma-related sequelae, such as root resorption.

A panoral view is particularly valuable where the pathology involves more than one quadrant or has extensive bony involvement. A sectional panoral radiograph may be prescribed in some situations since this approach helps to reduce ionizing exposure.

3.6 RISK ASSESSMENT

Having gathered relevant information by taking a history, conducting an examination, and carrying out any special investigations, there is one final consideration to make prior to treatment planning: that is, risk assessment.

> **Key Point**
>
> Risk assessment is simply an assessment of the likelihood of a disease or condition developing in an individual patient.

Risk assessment is certainly not a new concept, but it has now become a more recognized step in the decision-making process. When conducting a risk assessment, the clinician needs to consider all factors that may have a negative or positive effect on oral health. Generally, risk assessments are undertaken with respect to caries, but there are other recognized 'risks' to consider for the young dental patient including:

- periodontal disease;
- erosion;
- orofacial trauma.

The rationale for risk assessment is to target resources to those who most need them! Ideally, any preventive or operative treatment programme should be directed by an appreciation of the patient's risk status, thus ensuring that service delivery is both effective and cost-efficient. Risk assessment is also relevant when determining an optimum recall interval, as not all patients need to be seen with the same frequency. Furthermore, a child's risk status is not static; it may change due to any number of changes in personal circumstances. It is therefore important to continually re-assess risk status at future visits.

3.6.1 Caries

The aim of caries risk assessment is to predict whether the disease is likely to develop in an as yet caries-free individual, or to determine the rate of disease progression in a patient who already has some caries experience. It has been proposed that a reasonable model for caries risk assessment should have a combined sensitivity and specificity of 160% where:

- sensitivity = proportion of people actually with a disease who have a positive test result;
- specificity = proportion of people without a disease who have a negative test result.

In general, caries prediction models have higher specificity than sensitivity. However, the 'science' of caries risk assessment is still in its developmental stages and, to date, no single model provides a 100% accurate prediction of caries risk. Indeed, due to the complex nature of caries, it may not be possible to devise the perfect risk assessment model for clinical use.

Interestingly, research has shown that the experienced clinician can actually achieve a high level of prediction simply on the basis of a socio-demographic history and clinical examination. Thus the need for specific testing, such as microbiological investigation, may not confer significant additional benefit. In particular, past caries experience has proved to be the most useful clinical predictor of caries risk. Additionally, poor oral hygiene (visible plaque on maxillary incisors) in very young children has also been found to be a reliable indicator of high caries risk. Table 3.3 highlights the key risk factors that should be taken into consideration when conducting a risk assessment.

Very simply, children may be categorized as low, moderate, or high caries risk according to the following criteria:

- low risk—intact dentition, good oral hygiene, well-educated affluent family background, good dietary control, and use of fluoride regimens;
- moderate risk—1–2 new lesions per year, poor oral hygiene, and non-optimum fluoride use;
- high risk—three or more new lesions per year, poor oral hygiene and dietary control, significant medical history, immigrant status, poverty, low education, and poor uptake of fluoride regimens.

It is also important to bear in mind that the risk of caries development also varies significantly for:

- different age groups: children aged 1–2 years and 5–7 years are considered high risk age groups;
- individual teeth: first primary molars and first permanent molars are high risk;
- different tooth surfaces: interproximal primary molar surfaces and occlusal surfaces of first permanent molars are high risk.

Table 3.3 Factors relevant to caries risk assessment.

Socio-demographic	Dental	Other
Low risk status Affluent Well-educated mother	No previous caries experience Good oral hygiene Low family caries experience Regular brushing with fluoride toothpaste from early age	Fluoride exposure (water, milk, toothpaste) No significant medical history Good dietary control
High risk status Poverty Poorly educated mother Immigrant status	Past caries experience (especially in first permanent molars) Current caries experience (especially if involving smooth surfaces, lower incisors) Plaque accumulation (especially primary maxillary incisors) Matrilinear transmission of *Streptococcus* mutans in early childhood Low salivary flow Family history of high caries experience Caries-prone sites: deep pits and fissures Hypomineralised/ hypoplastic enamel	Limited/no exposure to fluoride Use of sweetened drinks in bottles in young children Significant medical history (especially if associated with xerostomia) Frequent intake of fermentable carbohydrates

3.6.2 Periodontal disease

While periodontal disease is not common in children, a few recognized risk factors are associated with increased likelihood of its development. These include:

- smoking;
- diabetes;
- plaque accumulation—although this is not such a reliable indicator at an individual level;
- family history (genetic factors).

Hormonal changes around puberty, low vitamin C or calcium intake, socio-economic status, psychosocial factors, tooth position, and occlusal relationships may also influence periodontal health, but are not considered reliable risk indicators.

3.6.3 Erosion

There is no established model for risk prediction in relation to erosion. However it has been suggested that:

- intake of more than 6 carbonated drinks weekly is associated with moderate erosion risk;
- intake of more than 14 carbonated drinks weekly is associated with high erosion risk.

In addition, the following risk factors have been reported to have some association with erosion:

- intake of more than two citrus fruits daily;
- frequent sports participation;
- eating disorders;
- gastric reflux, rumination.

3.6.4 Orofacial trauma

The majority of orofacial trauma cannot be prevented, as it usually results from an unavoidable accident! However, there are some recognized trauma risk factors that warrant consideration and appropriate prevention where possible:

- increased overjet: children with an overjet of >9 mm are twice as likely to sustain dental trauma;
- contact sports: active participation in sports, such as rugby, hockey, and martial arts, carries an increased risk of sustaining orofacial trauma;
- previous dental trauma: there is a significant risk of sustaining further trauma!
- motor disabilities: children with poor co-ordination are more at risk of sustaining trauma;
- neurological disabilities: uncontrolled epileptics are high trauma risk candidates;
- age: peak ages for sustaining orofacial trauma are around 1-2 years and 8–10 years;
- gender: boys are more at risk than girls.

3.7 PRINCIPLES OF TREATMENT PLANNING

In planning dental care for child patients, the dentist must satisfy two, sometimes apparently conflicting, objectives. First, it is clearly necessary to ensure that the child reaches adulthood with the optimum achievable dental health. Second, it is essential that the child both learns to trust the dental team and develops a positive attitude towards dental treatment. At any point in time, therefore, the desirability of the 'ideal' care (whatever this might be) must be carefully balanced against

- the child's potential to cope with the proposed treatment;
- the ability and willingness of the child and parent to attend for care;
- parental preference.

Thus, the dentist may be required to exercise a degree of compromise which those more used to treating adults may find unfamiliar and even a little uncomfortable. However, it is important to accept that there will be no winners if, at the outset, a treatment plan is unrealistic or insufficiently flexible to allow modification, should this become necessary, as treatment progresses.

From the foregoing comments, it should be evident that it is not possible to take a 'one size fits all' approach to treatment planning: very different treatment plans may be drawn up for children who present with very similar problems. However, basic principles pervade all treatment plans and these are set out in Fig. 3.28. (The reader should note the emphasis that has been placed on repeated assessment and discussion.) Several aspects of this approach are worthy of special comment.

3.7.1 Management of acute dental problems

The management of acute problems present at the time of the child's first visit is undoubtedly a priority. However it is important that any treatment that is provided sits well in the context of a holistic treatment plan and does not jeopardize its completion. In most cases, therefore, pain relief should be provided without recourse to extraction.

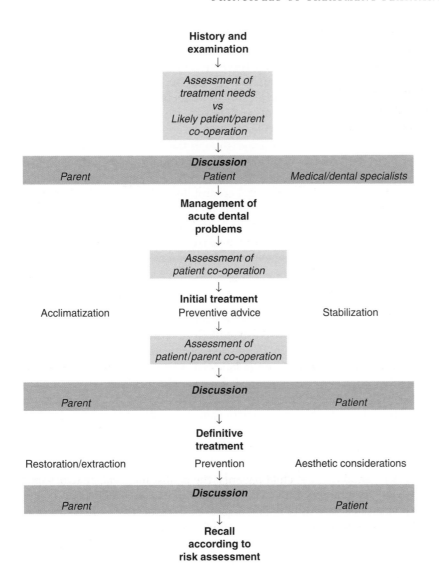

History and examination
↓
Assessment of treatment needs vs Likely patient/parent co-operation
↓
Discussion
Parent   *Patient*   *Medical/dental specialists*
↓
Management of acute dental problems
↓
Assessment of patient co-operation
↓
Initial treatment
Acclimatization   Preventive advice   Stabilization
↓
Assessment of patient/parent co-operation
↓
Discussion
Parent   *Patient*
↓
Definitive treatment
Restoration/extraction   Prevention   Aesthetic considerations
↓
Discussion
Parent   *Patient*
↓
Recall according to risk assessment

Fig. 3.28 Principles of treatment planning for a paediatric dental patient.

3.7.2 Prevention

Any treatment plan relies for its support on a 'spine' of prevention (Chapter 6). Restorations placed in a mouth in which the caries process is still active are prone to failure: repeated restorations may be detrimental to the child's ability to co-operate and the dentist–parent relationship (as well as frustrating to the dental team). Likewise, managing a child's grossly carious teeth by multiple extractions without ensuring that he or she receives appropriate preventive input does nothing to assist that child in maintaining dental health in the future.

An added advantage of a 'prevention first approach' is its importance in behaviour management, acclimatizing the child to future treatment. Procedures such as fluoride varnish applications or disclosing are good confidence-building steps.

Key Point

Preventive advice, whether this is in relation to diet, oral hygiene, fluoride supplementation, or even the prevention of dental trauma, should be realistic and specifically tailored to the individual child and parent.

Any preventive strategy should be dictated by an individual's risk assessment: for instance low caries risk children do not routinely require fissure sealants.

The delivery of preventive advice and interventions should not be restricted to the commencement of treatment. Rather, prevention should be reinforced as treatment progresses, modifications being incorporated should these become necessary.

Clearly, prevention is not simply a job for the members of the dental team. It demands the creation of a partnership in which both the child and the parent are key players, though the relative role and prominence of each will differ with the age of the child. In the case of young children, parents are (or, at least, should be) responsible for food choices and oral hygiene, though the latter responsibility is not infrequently abdicated before the child has sufficient manual dexterity to brush adequately alone. As the child approaches the teenage years (and particularly when he or she enters secondary schooling), parental control inevitably decreases. Any discussion of the proposed treatment plan should, therefore, include an agreement as to what is required of the child and/or parent as well as what will be offered by various members of the dental team (including professionals complementary to dentistry). It may be helpful to document this agreement in the form of a written 'contract'.

3.7.3 Stabilization

Where a child has open cavities, a phase of stabilization should precede the provision of definitive treatment, whether this is to be entirely restorative in nature or a combination of restorations and extractions. In this process, no attempt is made to render the cavities caries free; rather, minimal tissue is removed without local anaesthesia, allowing placement of an appropriate temporary dressing. The inclusion of such a phase in a holistic treatment plan reduces the overall bacterial load and slows caries progression, renders the child less likely to present with pain and sepsis, and buys time for the implementation of preventive measures and for the child to be acclimatised to treatment.

However, one word of caution is offered: it is essential that the parent understands the purpose of stabilization and that what have been provided are not permanent restorations. Otherwise, it is possible that they will perceive that treatment is failing to progress.

Following stabilization, the child's response to acclimatization and compliance with the suggested preventive regime should be assessed. This is particularly important before proceeding with definitive treatment. For example, in a scenario in which a child has not responded to acclimatization and has either refused stabilization or accepted this only with extreme difficulty, the dentist may be entirely justified in considering extractions. This will allow the child and his or her family to enjoy a period where no active treatment is required and in which prevention can be established (always provided, of course, they return for continuing care).

3.7.4 Scheduling operative treatment

In any treatment plan, it is necessary to give careful consideration to the order in which items of operative care are provided. The following are general rules of thumb:

- small, simple restorations should be completed first;
- maxillary teeth should be treated before mandibular ones (since it is usually easier to administer local anaesthesia in the upper jaw);
- posterior teeth should be treated before anteriors (this usually ensures that the patient returns for treatment);
- quadrant dentistry should be practised wherever possible (this reduces the number of visits to a minimum) but only if the time in chair is not excessive for a very young patient;
- endodontic treatment should follow completion of simple restorative treatment;
- extractions should be the last items of operative care (at this stage, patient co-operation can more reliably be assured) unless the patient presents with an acute problem mid-treatment.

3.7.5 Recall

Treatment planning (in its broadest sense) clearly does not end with the completion of one treatment journey. The determination of a recall schedule tailored to the needs of the individual child is an essential part of the treatment-planning process.

It is generally accepted that children should receive a dental assessment more frequently than adults since

- there is evidence that the rate of progression of dental caries can be more rapid in children than in adults;
- the rate of progression of caries and erosive tooth wear is faster in primary than in permanent teeth;
- periodic assessment of orofacial growth and the developing occlusion is required.

In the latter context, there is considerable merit in ensuring that recall examinations coincide with particular milestones in dental development, for example, around 6, 9, and 12 years. Generally speaking, recall intervals of no more than 12 months offer the dentist the opportunity to deliver and reinforce preventive advice during the crucial period when a child is establishing the basis for their future dental health. However, the exact recall interval (3, 6, 9, or 12 months) should be tailored to meet, and vary with the child's needs. This requires an assessment of disease levels as well as risk of/from dental disease.

3.7.6 Treatment planning for general anaesthesia

Treatment planning for general anaesthesia is an extremely complex area that merits special mention. However, a full discussion lies outside the scope of the current chapter. It is sufficient to emphasize here that, in this context, a comprehensive approach must be taken. Providing treatment under general anaesthesia for a child who has been shown to be unable to cope with operative dental care under local anaesthesia (with or without the support of conscious sedation) will do absolutely nothing to improve his or her future co-operation. Such treatment should, therefore, include the restoration or extraction (as appropriate) of ALL carious teeth.

> **Key Point**
>
> The practice of extracting only the most grossly carious or symptomatic teeth (and assuming that other carious teeth can be restored under local anaesthetic at a later stage) predisposes to a high rate of repeat general anaesthesia and should be discouraged.

The orthodontic implications of any proposed treatment should always be considered. This is particularly so when the loss of one or more permanent units is to be included in the treatment plan. In such cases, the latter should ideally be drawn up in consultation with a specialist in orthodontics.

Treatment under general anaesthesia, irrespective of whether this includes restorative treatment or is limited to extractions, should be followed with an appropriate preventive programme. Failure to provide this almost inevitably leads to the child undergoing further treatment (usually extractions) under general anaesthesia.

3.7.7 Treatment planning for complex cases

The clinician should always have a clear long-term 'vision' for the management of the individual patient. In creating this, appropriate specialist input to treatment planning should be sought where indicated. At the simplest level, an orthodontic opinion should be obtained before committing a child to multiple visits to restore first permanent molars of poor prognosis. However, it is in the treatment planning of complex cases (such as those presenting with generalized defects of enamel or dentine formation, hypodontia, or clefts of lip and palate) that interdisciplinary specialist input is essential. For example, such input may result in

- the retention of anterior roots to maintain alveolar bone in preparation for future implants;
- the use of preformed metal crowns to maintain clinical crown height in preparation for definitive crowns;
- the use of direct/laboratory-formed composite veneers in preparation for porcelain veneers when growth (and any orthodontic treatment) is complete.

> **Key Point**
> The one over-riding consideration is this: management in early adulthood should never be compromised by inappropriate treatment at a young age.

3.8 SUMMARY

Treatment planning for young patients should not only address current needs but should plan ahead for those of the future, thus ensuring that every child reaches adulthood with a healthy, functional, and aesthetic dentition as well as positive attitudes towards dentistry. Meticulous history-taking, clinical examination, and risk assessment contribute to the decision-making process, but one should never lose sight of what is realistic and practical for the child in the context of his or her environment. To do otherwise not only courts non-compliance but also fails to recognize the most important aspect of all—a child's individuality.

3.9 FURTHER READING

Demirjian, A., Goldstein, H., and Tanner, J. M. (1973). A new system of dental age assessment. *Human Biology*, **45**, 211–27. (*This paper describes how to undertake an accurate dental age assessment for patients using a panoral radiograph.*)

Espelid, I., Mejàre, I., and Weerheijm, K. (2003). EAPD guidelines for the use of radiographs in children. *European Journal of Paediatric Dentistry*, **4**, 40–8. (*This excellent and comprehensive paper describes the appropriate use of dental radiographs for young patients.*)

Mascarenhas, A. K. (1998). Oral hygiene as a risk indicator of enamel and dentine caries. *Community Dentistry and Oral Epidemiology*, **26**, 331–9. (*This study reviews the clinical indicators employed in caries risk assessment and highlights the relationship between poor oral hygiene and caries.*)

Powell, L. V. (1988). Caries risk assessment: relevance to the practitioner. *Journal of the American Dental Association*, **129**, 349–53. (*This comprehensive paper reviews the practical aspects of caries risk assessment.*)

Rodd, H. D., and Wray, A. (2004). *Treatment planning for the developing dentition.* Quintessence Publishing, London. (*This practical and easily read book covers all aspects of treatment planning for children.*)

3.10 REFERENCE

The Children Act (1989). Department of Health. HMSO London.

Pharmacological management of pain and anxiety

4 Pharmacological management of pain and anxiety

G. J. Roberts and M. T. Hosey

4.1 INTRODUCTION

Effective pain management of a child, especially an anxious one, is a challenge to every dentist. The need for good management of anxiety and pain in paediatric dentistry is paramount. A common cause of complaint from parents and their children is that a dentist 'hurt' unnecessarily. Such a complaint can jeopardize access to life-long dental care.

Children are anatomically and physiologically different from adults. The anatomy of the airway means that breathing is through a narrower, more fixed 'wind pipe'. Physiologically, a child is less capable of taking in a bigger volume of air even when urgently required. Coupled with this, both the demand for oxygen (consumption) and the incidence of periodic breathing and apnoeas are higher compared to adults. These differences mean that a child can become hypoxic more easily.

4.2 CHILDREN'S PERCEPTION OF PAIN

A child's perception of pain is purely subjective and varies widely, particularly with age. Infants up to about 2 years of age are unable to distinguish between pressure and pain. After the age of approximately 2 and up to the age of 10, children begin to have some understanding of 'hurt' and begin to distinguish it from pressure or 'a heavy push'. The problem is that it is not always possible to identify which children are amenable to explanation and who will respond by being co-operative when challenged with local anaesthesia and dental treatment in the form of drilling or extractions. Children over the age of 10 are much more likely to be able to think abstractly and participate more actively in the decision to use local anaesthesia, sedation, or general anaesthesia. Indeed, as children enter their teenage years they are rapidly becoming more and more like adults and are able to determine more directly, sometimes aggressively, whether or not a particular method of pain control will be used. The response is further determined by the child's coping ability influenced by family values, level of general anxiety (trait), and intelligence.

Key Points
- Children are anatomically and physiologically different from adults this results in them becoming hypoxic more easily.
- Children's response to pain is influenced by age, memory of previous negative dental experience, and coping ability.

4.3 CONSENT

Before you can do anything to a patient, even a simple examination, consent must be obtained. Consent may be implied, verbal, or written. The main purpose of written consent is to demonstrate *post hoc*, in the event of a dispute, that informed consent was obtained. It has the considerable advantage of making clinicians and patients pause to consider the implications of what is planned and to weigh the advantages and disadvantages so that a reasoned and informed choice can be made. The responsibility for informed consent is often shared between the referring primary care dentist and the secondary care service provider, especially where sedation and general anaesthesia are involved. Many health trusts and other employing authorities are increasingly demanding that written consent is obtained for all procedures. This is especially difficult now as the lower age of consent is no longer specifically limited. The sole criterion is whether or not the patient is 'able to understand' the procedures and their implications. If so, the patient is considered 'competent' and the child may give (or refuse) consent. It is usual to arrive at a consensus view among parents, child, and dental surgeon. A sufficiently informative entry should be placed in the patient's case records. As a pragmatic rule the age of 16 years still acts as a guide. But if a procedure is proposed and a child under 16 years says 'no' then consent has been refused. Fortunately, in paediatric dentistry the prospect of a life-saving operation is rare so a refusal of consent can be managed by a change in the procedure or by establishing a temporal respite. The current advice from the protection societies is that written consent must be obtained for a course of treatment. The plan of treatment proposed must indicate the nature and extent of the treatment and the approximate number of times that local anaesthesia and/or sedation is to be used. There is no need to obtain written consent for each separate time that sedation is used. If the plan of treatment changes and along with it the frequency or nature of sedation, then it is prudent to obtain written consent for the change. The greater risks associated with general anaesthesia require specific written consent for each and every occasion that treatment is carried out under general anaesthesia. Examples of suitably worded forms are available from the Medical Defence Societies.

Key Points

- A conference that involves both the parent and child helps to gain informed consent:
  –discuss the dental problems;
  –discuss the treatment options/alternatives;
  –agree the treatment plan.
- Write-up in the case record.
- Obtain written (signed) consent

4.4 SYSTEMIC PAIN CONTROL

Children may need pain control for 'toothache' for a day or two before the removal of carious teeth. Often, the teeth are also abscessed so that it is necessary to combine antibiotic therapy with analgesia to obtain optimum pain relief. Additionally, analgesia is required postoperatively usually after dento-alveolar surgery.

The most common method of administration is by mouth. Small children, and some recalcitrant adolescents, refuse to take tablets so liquid preparations are needed. If other methods of administration, such as intramuscular or intravenous, are required then these injections should be administered by clinical staff experienced with these special techniques. Rectal administration is increasingly common as absorption from the rectal mucosa is rapid. If such a route of administration is to be used, specific consent must be obtained. It should be remembered that the dose for children of different ages needs to be carefully estimated to avoid the risk of an overdose (dangerous) or of an underdose (ineffective). The parents must be advised that all drugs must be stored in a safe place, in a child-proof container. Bathroom cabinets or kitchen cabinets are the safest places as they are out of reach and out of sight of small children. Specific advice on prescribing for children can be obtained from a local pharmacist or the British National Formulary (BNF).

The dosages for children can be calculated on the basis of a percentage chart (Table 4.1). Often 'average' doses are used but the prescriber has the absolute responsibility to confirm that the dosages recommended are correct.

The common drugs used for pain control in children are paracetamol BNF and ibuprofen BNF. The potential side-effects and the dosages should be checked with the formulary before prescribing. Aspirin should not be used on children because of the risk of Reye's syndrome. The increase in asthma among children requires that this be considered before ibuprofen is prescribed. Narcotic analgesics such as codeine or morphine can be used on children but only after less powerful analgesics have been shown to be ineffective. As above, the dosage should be checked with the BNF.

4.5 METHODS OF PAIN CONTROL

The different methods of pain control vary from simple behaviour management to full intubational general anaesthesia in a hospital operating theatre (Fig. 4.1). There is a strong relationship between the perception of pain experienced and the degree of anxiety perceived by the patient. Painful procedures cause fear and anxiety; fear and anxiety intensify pain. This circle of cause and effect is central to the management of all patients. Good behaviour management reduces anxiety, which in turn reduces the perceived intensity of pain, which further reduces the experience of anxiety.

Behaviour management have been covered in detail in Chapter 2 and local anaesthetic techniques in Chapter 5. The majority of dental procedures on children can be carried out using a combination of these two techniques. This chapter will

Table 4.1 Percentage method for calculating doses

Age (years)	Mean weight (kg)	Approximate percentage of adult dose
1	10	25
3	15	33
5	18	40
7	23	50
12	39	75
Adult	68	100

Abstracted from The British National Formulary, p. 11 No. 47, March 2004.

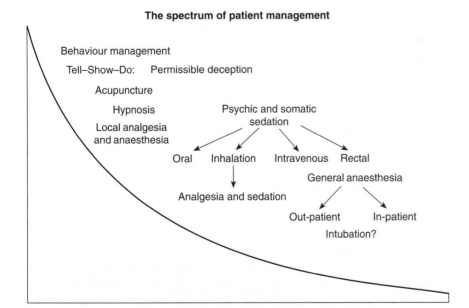

The spectrum of patient management

Behaviour management

Tell–Show–Do: Permissible deception

Acupuncture

Hypnosis

Local analgesia and anaesthesia

Psychic and somatic sedation

Oral   Inhalation   Intravenous   Rectal

General anaesthesia

Analgesia and sedation

Out-patient   In-patient

Intubation?

Fig. 4.1 The figure shows, on the left-hand scale, the approximate frequency with which a particular pain control technique is used, and on the bottom scale the increasing degree of physiological intrusion from local analgesia, through sedation to general anaesthesia.

deal with the methods of sedation and general anaesthesia that are applicable to dental treatment in children.

4.6 MEDICAL STATUS

The wide variety of medical problems makes it difficult to be precise about the management strategy appropriate for each patient. Detailed descriptions of management of a variety of medical problems appear in a comprehensive book by Scully and Cawson (1998). With regard to sedation, the American Society of Anesthesiologists' (ASA) classification provides an excellent guide to the type of sedation or anaesthesia appropriate to an individual patient's medical and behavioural problems (Table 4.2).

The decision as to whether a patient should be treated under general anaesthesia or local anaesthesia, or local anaesthesia with sedation depends on a combination of factors, the most important of which are:

(1) the age of the child;
(2) the degree of surgical trauma involved;
(3) the perceived anxiety and how the patient may (or has) responded to similar levels of surgical trauma;
(4) the complexity of the operative procedure;
(5) the medical status of the child.

There are no hard and fast rules, and every procedure in every child must be assessed individually and the different elements considered in collaboration with the parent and, where appropriate, with the child. For example, the younger the child the greater the likelihood of a need for general anaesthesia. At the other end of the age range it is unlikely that a 15-year old will need general anaesthesia for simple orthodontic extractions, although this might be required for moderately complex surgery, such as exposing and bonding an impacted canine. The degree of trauma involved is also another factor; a single extraction is most likely to be carried out under local anaesthesia, removal of the four first permanent molars is most likely to be carried out under general anaesthesia. Anxiety perceived as excessive, especially after an attempt at treatment under local anaesthesia and sedation, would lead to simple treatment such as conservative dentistry being carried out under a general anaesthetic usually involving endotracheal intubation. Serious medical problems,

Table 4.2   The American Society of Anesthesiologists' (ASA) physical status classification

Classification	Description
Class I	A healthy patient
Class II	A patient with mild systemic disease, for example, diet controlled diabetes,asthma well controlled with drugs
Class III	A patient with severe systemic disease that is not incapacitating, for example, insulin-dependent diabetes, congenital heart disease
Class IV	A patient with incapacitating systemic disease that is a constant threat to life, for example, cystic fibrosis, congenital heart disease with cyanosis
Class V	A moribund patient not expected to survive for 24 h with or without operation

American Society of Anesthesiologists (1963). New classification of physical status. *Anesthesiology*, 24, 111.

for example, cystic fibrosis with the associated respiratory problems would justify using sedation instead of general anaesthesia even for more traumatic surgery, such as removal of impacted canines, but it would be appropriate to carry out this sedation in a hospital environment. The degree of intellectual and/or physical impairment in handicapped children would also be a factor to be considered.

General anaesthesia carries with it a finite risk of serious morbidity such as psychological trauma and even death (3 to 4 per million). No child should be submitted to a general anaesthetic without consideration of this potentially devastating outcome. Intermediate between the minimally intrusive techniques of local anaesthesia and the major intrusion of general anaesthesia are the techniques of conscious sedation (Fig. 4.1).

Key Points

- Each child should be assessed on their merits and an appropriate method of pain control used.
- The vast majority of children are amenable to satisfactory treatment using behaviour management and local anaesthesia alone.
- No child should be submitted to a general anaesthetic without consideration of potential risk.

4.7 CONSCIOUS SEDATION TECHNIQUES

Conscious sedation is defined as:

A technique in which the use of a drug or drugs produces a state of depression of the central nervous system enabling treatment to be carried out, but during which verbal contact with the patient is maintained throughout the period of sedation. The drugs and techniques used to provide conscious sedation for dental treatment should carry a margin of safety wide enough to render unintended loss of consciousness unlikely. The level of sedation must be such that the patient remains conscious, retains protective reflexes, and is able to understand and respond to verbal commands.

The routes of administration of sedative drugs used in clinical paediatric dentistry are oral, inhalational, intravenous, and transmucosal (e.g. nasal, rectal, sublingual). However, the transmucosal routes are little used in the United Kingdom and currently, intravenous sedation is considered unsuitable for the operator/sedationist when working on children. Current developments in intravenous techniques, especially the use of target-controlled infusion pumps and patient-controlled sedation (PCS) may prove to be sufficiently effective and safe for use by the operator/sedationist, but further research is required.

Key Point

- The goal of conscious sedation is to use a pharmacological agent to augment behavioural management to decrease anxiety levels while maintaining a responsive patient.

4.7.1 General facilities

The use of sedative drugs carries the risk of inadvertent loss of consciousness. Although the techniques are designed to reduce this risk to a minimum it should always be borne in mind that every time a sedative is given to a patient there is a risk of an idiosyncratic reaction to the drug, which may result in hypoxia or unexpected loss of consciousness. The clinician must arrange the clinical session so that sedation, irrespective of complications, can proceed smoothly and safely. This includes the need for all patients who are having sedation to be accompanied. This can be any adult, who understands the implications and potential problems of caring for a child during the later stages of recovery. In addition, the clinical facilities need to include suitable resuscitation equipment coupled with the knowledge and skills to use them.

> **Key Points**
> - The main complications related to paediatric conscious sedation are:
>   - hypoxia,
>   - nausea,
>   - vomiting,
>   - inadvertent loss of consciousness (general anaesthesia/over sedation).
> - Morbidity and mortality increase with:
>   - young age,
>   - worsening ASA classification.

4.7.2 Emergency equipment

Suitable emergency equipment must be available easily to hand since time is of the utmost importance. For this reason emergency equipment and drugs should be within arms reach of the operator and ready for immediate use. Training of the dental team is a requirement, irrespective of whether conscious sedation is practised. Training should be updated at regular intervals of not more than 1 year. It is essential that each member of the dental team knows exactly what is required of them in an emergency. The dental surgeon has the responsibility of ensuring the easy availability of drugs, particularly oxygen, and to see that the drugs in the emergency kit are not past their 'use by' date.

4.7.3 Emergency equipment for the dental surgeon

The following are items of equipment that a dental surgeon should be prepared to use in an emergency.

1. High volume suction for clearing the airways of saliva, debris, and blood. This must be capable of reaching the floor as a patient may be removed from the dental chair to lie on the floor to enable resuscitation.
2. An emergency supply of oxygen. A regular working supply of oxygen from an inhalation sedation unit is an alternative.
3. Positive pressure ventilation apparatus with a self-inflating bag.
4. Face masks to fit children and adolescents.
5. Three sizes of oral airways.

Note: These items should form part of an armamentarium of any dentist when treating patients using local anaesthesia alone.

4.7.4 Emergency drugs

Suitable emergency drugs must be available and because of the need for speed, the drugs must be stored with the emergency equipment. Training of the dental surgeon and their staff in the use of drugs has the same requirements as for equipment.

The nature and content of 'emergency drugs' kits are usually determined by a local resuscitation adviser.

4.7.5 Emergency drugs for the dental surgeon

The following are drugs that the dentist should be prepared to use in an emergency:

1. Oxygen.
2. Adrenaline hydrochloride 1 mg/ml (1000 mg/ml), that is, 1 : 1000 on a 1 ml ampoule for subcutaneous or intramuscular injection. The IMS Min-I-Jet system is particularly quick and easy to use.
3. Hydrocortisone sodium phosphate 100 mg per vial. To be made up to 1 ml with physiological saline immediately before use. For intravenous injection.
4. In addition to the above drugs suitable needles and syringes should be available to enable drugs to be drawn up and administered parenterally.
5. Flumazenil (benzodiazepine anatagonist) for reversing unexpected over-sedation from orally, intravenously, or rectally administered benzodiazepine.

4.7.6 Emergency equipment for medically qualified and those staff trained in advanced life support

1. A laryngoscope, endotracheal tubes, and forceps to manipulate the endotracheal tubes during intubation.
2. A cricothyrotomy kit.
3. An electrocardiograph.
4. A defibrillator.

4.7.7 Emergency drugs for medically qualified and/or specially trained staff

1. Adrenaline 1 : 10, 000 (10 ml vials).
2. Atropine 1 mg/10 ml (10 ml vials).
3. Calcium chloride 10% (10 ml vials).
4. Lignocaine 100 mg/10 ml (1%) (10 ml vials).
5. Isoprenaline 0.2 mg/ml (10 ml vials).
6. Frusemide 80 mg/8 ml (8 ml vials).
7. Sodium bicarbonate 8.4% (50 ml vials).
8. Glucose 50% (50 ml vials).
9. Naloxone 4 mg/ml (1 ml vials).
10. Aminophylline 250 mg/10 ml (10 ml vials).
11. Diazemuls 10 mg/2 ml (2 ml vials).
12. Flumazenil 500 μg/5 ml (5 ml vials).

Many of these drugs are available in prefilled syringes. It is the responsibility of the dentist to ensure the availability of the drugs required by the medical staff who may be called to deal with an emergency. Equally, it is the responsibility of the same medical staff to advise the dental surgeon of his or her precise requirements with regard to emergency drugs. This advice must be in writing. These can be reviewed by reading the following: European Resuscitation Council (1992). Guidelines for basic and advanced life support. *Resuscitation*, **24**, 103–10.

Key Points

- Dental surgeons and their staff should at least be capable of providing basic life support:
  –**A**irways;
  –**B**reathing;
  –**C**irculation;
  –**ABC**.
- The dental team should have at least yearly basic life support training.
- The dental surgeon is responsible for ensuring the readiness of emergency equipment and drugs.

4.8 PREPARATION FOR CONSCIOUS SEDATION

4.8.1 Environment

There should be a suitable area where the child can sit quietly before the operation so that the sedative can be administered and the child monitored while it is taking effect. As a general rule it is not wise to let children have medication at home as quiet supervision of the child within the surgery premises is prudent. A journey to the surgery under the increasing influence of a mood-altering drug is not the most propitious way of preparing distressed children for treatment. These strictures do not apply to inhalation sedation or intravenous sedation. However, the facilities suitable for providing care apply equally to oral, inhalational, and intravenous sedation. During treatment there must be effective suction equipment and in the event of a power failure, a mechanically operated backup. Sedated patients often hallucinate or misinterpret words and actions and so, a chaperone to safeguard the operator–sedationist is also essential. Once treatment is complete the child should be able to sit (or lie) quietly until sufficiently recovered to be accompanied home.

A further important strategy is to have a checklist so that the dental surgeon can be sure that all important elements of sedation have been properly considered.

4.8.2 Preoperative instructions

These should be provided in writing and cover such points as ensuring that a suitable companion brings the child to and from the surgery, that only a light meal is eaten 2 h or more before an appointment for sedation. In this context, a light meal is a cup of tea and a slice of toast. Postoperatively, suitable arrangements need to be in place for travel and to ensure that the child plays quietly at home. In addition to these specific points 'local' rules are likely to apply.

Key Points

To carry out conscious sedation:
- informed consent is mandatory;
- preoperative and postoperative instructions should be given prior to the sedation visit;
- patient assessment includes medical, dental, and anxiety history;
- appropriate facilities, child-friendly environment and sedation trained staff are essential;
- the operator–sedationist, irrespective of gender, must be chaperoned at all times;
- the child must be accompanied by an adult escort;
- a checklist is important to ensure all preparations are in place.

4.9 MONITORING THE SEDATED CHILD

4.9.1 Clinical status

Sedative drugs are also central nervous system and respiratory depressants and as such, cause a variety of effects from mild sedation, deep sedation, and general anaesthesia and, in excessive concentrations, even death. For this reason, the facilities outlined above are necessary in the unlikely event of unexpected loss of consciousness. It is important that dental surgeons working with children have a very clear idea of the clinical status of sedated patients. These are:

(1) the patient's eyes are open;
(2) the patient is able to respond verbally to questions;
(3) the patient is able to independently maintain an open mouth (this may preclude the use of a mouth-prop);
(4) the patient is able to independently maintain a patent airway;
(5) the ability to swallow;
(6) the child is a normal pink colour.

All these criteria are evidence of conscious sedation. For this reason it is important not to let a child go to sleep in the dental chair while receiving treatment with sedation as closed eyes may be a sign of sleep, over-sedation, loss of consciousness, or cardiovascular collapse.

4.9.2 Pulse oximetry

Pulse oximetry is a non-invasive method of measuring arterial oxygen saturation using a sensor probe placed on the patient's finger or ear lobe, which has a red light source to detect the relative difference in the absorption of light between saturated and desaturated haemoglobin during arterial pulsation. The probe is sensitive to patient movement, relative hypothermia, ambient light, and abnormal haemoglobinaemias, so false readings can occur. In room air, a child's normal oxygen saturation (SaO_2) is 97% to 100%. Adequate oxygenation of the tissues occurs above 95% while oxygen saturations lower than this are considered hypoxaemic.

> **Key Points**
> Monitoring a sedated child involves:
> - alert clinical monitoring—skin colour, response to stimulus, ability to keep mouth open, ability to both swallow and to maintain an independent airway, normal radial pulse;
> - the use of a pulse oximeter (except for nitrous oxide inhalation sedation).

4.10 ORAL SEDATION

The onset of the effect of oral sedatives is variable and is largely dependent on the individual's rate of absorption from the gastro-intestinal tract, which can be affected by the rate of gastric clearance, the amount of food in the stomach, and even the time of the day. In addition, the dosage is determined by the body weight. Therefore, a set of properly calibrated bathroom scales is needed to enable the correct dose of sedative to be estimated for each patient. Despite this, some children may spit out the drug, leaving the clinician uncertain about the exact dosage that was administered. To combat this, some sedationists administer the liquid sedative using a syringe placed in the buccal mucosa or mix the drug with a flavoured elixir. The patient may require up to an hour of supervised postoperative recovery.

4.10.1 Oral sedatives

Diazepam

The most familiar of the benzodiazepines is diazepam, usually administered at a dosage of 250 μg/kg. For a 6-year-old child this is approximately 5 mg but could be as low as 3.9 mg or as high as 6.6 mg. For a much older patient, for example, a 15-year old, the average dose would be 13.6 mg and may vary from 9.7 mg to 18.9 mg.

Midazolam

Midazolam is another benzodiazepine that is more commonly used as an intra-venous agent. However, its use as an oral sedative is growing though, currently it does not have a product licence for this application. The intravenous liquid is bitter to taste and so the preparation is often mixed with a fruit flavoured drink. The oral dose is higher (0.3–0.7 mg/kg) than the intravenous dose because the oral midazolam reaches the systemic circulation via the portal circulation which decreases the drug's bioavailability, necessitating a higher oral dosage. Evidence is still relatively scant, especially in children under 8 years of age, and so the use of oral midazolam is still largely restricted to specialist hospital practice.

Chloral hydrate

Chloral hydrate is a chlorinated derivative of ethyl alcohol, the 'Micky Finn'. It is a weak analgesic and psychosedative with an elimination half-life of about 8 h. In small doses (40–60 mg/kg, but not exceeding 1 g), mild sedation occurs but it can be ineffective in the management of the more anxious child. Nausea and vomiting are common due to gastric irritation. The drug also depresses the blood pressure and the respiratory rate, myocardial depression and arrhythmia can also occur. Recently, there has been concern that there is a risk of carcinogenesis. Although it is still in widespread use around the world it is gradually becoming obsolete.

Other drugs

There are other oral sedative drugs that are commonly reported in the literature in relation to paediatric dental sedation. These include: hydroxyzine hydrochloride and promethazine hydrochloride (psychosedatives with an antihistaminic, antiemetic, and antispasmodic effect), and ketamine which is a powerful general anaesthetic agent which, in small dosages, can produce a state of dissociation while maintaining the protective reflexes. Common side-effects of hydroxyzine hydrochloride and promet-hazine hydrochloride are dry mouth, fever, and skin rash. Side-effects of ketamine include hypertension, vivid hallucinations, physical movement, increased salivation, and risk of laryngospasm, advanced airway proficiency training is, therefore, essential. Ketamine carries the additional risk of increase in blood pressure, heart rate, and a fall in oxygen saturation when used in combination with other sedatives.

Evidence to support the single use of either hydroxyzine hydrochloride, promethazine hydrochloride, or ketamine is poor.

Monitoring during oral sedation

This involves alert clinical monitoring and at least the use of a pulse oximeter.

4.10.2 Clinical technique

The following regimen, using the example of diazepam, was found to be effective in clinical practice:

(1) on arrival of the patient check whether, preoperative instructions have been followed;

(2) weigh the patient and estimate the dose of diazepam;

(3) have the dosage checked by a second person;

(4) administer diazepam ~1 h before the treatment;

(5) allow the patient to sit in a 'quiet' room;

(6) once ready, start and complete the treatment with (or without) local anaesthesia;

(7) once the treatment is complete, allow the patient to recover in the quiet room until ready to return home;

(8) reiterate the postoperative instructions to escort.

4.11 INHALATION SEDATION

This is synonymous with inhalation of an oxygen–nitrous oxide gas mixture in relatively low concentrations, usually 20–50% nitrous oxide. The technique is unique as the operator is able to titrate the gas against each individual patient. That is to say, the operator increases the concentration to the patient, observes the effect, and as appropriate, increases (or sometimes decreases) the concentration to obtain optimum sedation in each individual patient.

Inhalation sedation consists of three elements (Fig. 4.2):

1. The administration of low-to-moderate concentrations of nitrous oxide in oxygen to patients who remain conscious. The precise concentration of nitrous oxide is carefully titrated to the needs of each individual patient.

2. As the nitrous oxide begins to exert its pharmacological effects, the patient is subjected to a steady flow of reassuring and semi-hypnotic suggestion. This establishes and maintains rapport with the patient.

3. The use of equipment that exceeds the current BSI Standard for safety cut-out devices installed within inhalation sedation equipment. This means that it is not possible to administer 100% nitrous oxide either accidentally or deliberately (the cut-off point is usually 70%). This is an important and critical clinical safety feature that is essential for the operator/sedationist.

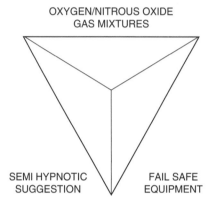

Fig. 4.2 The triad of elements of inhalation sedation.

4.11.1 Equipment for inhalation sedation with oxygen–nitrous oxide gas mixture

The most widely used equipment for inhalation sedation is the Quantiflex MDM (Fig. 4.3), which enables the operator to deliver carefully controlled volumes and concentrations of gases to the patient. In addition to the machine head that controls the delivery of gases, it is also necessary to have a suitable scavenging system, and an assembly for the gas cylinders, either a mobile stand (Fig. 4.4) or a pipeline system with cylinders stored remote from the machine head (Fig. 4.5).

4.11.2 Clinical technique

Of the inhalation sedation techniques available, the following is the easiest, the most flexible, and the least likely to cause surgery pollution. The control unit for the Quantiflex MDM (Fig. 4.3) has a single control for the total flow of gases (Fig. 4.3 '1'), and a central, vertically placed, dial is turned to regulate simultaneously the percentage flow of both gases (Fig. 4.3 '2'). Either of these controls can be changed without altering the other. The actual percentage of gases being delivered is monitored by observing the flow meters for oxygen and nitrous oxide, respectively (Fig. 4.3: '3' & '4'). There are 15 steps for the technique:

1. Check the machine.

2. Select the appropriate size of nasal mask and clean it with alcohol.

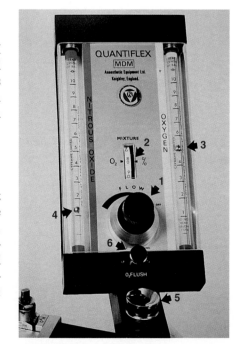

Fig. 4.3 The MDM inhalation sedation unit.

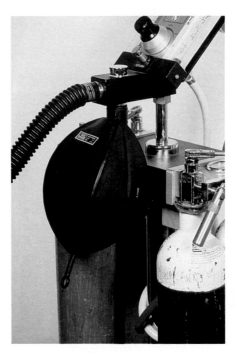

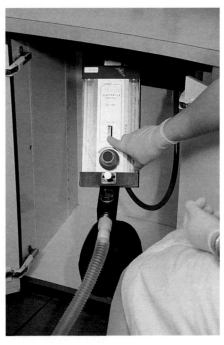

Fig. 4.4　The mobile cylinder stand showing the upper part of the oxygen and nitrous oxide cylinders and the reservoir bag.

Fig. 4.5　The MDM unit mounted unobtrusively under a worktop.

3.　Connect up the scavenging pipe.

4.　Set the mixture dial to 100% oxygen. (Fig. 4.3 '2')

5.　Settle the patient in the dental chair.

6.　Turn the flow control (Fig. 4.3 '1') to 3 l/min and allow the reservoir bag to fill with oxygen.

7.　With the patient's help, position the nasal mask gently and comfortably to preclude any leaks. If necessary explain the way the mask is used.

8.　Turn the flow control knob to the left until the flow rate of oxygen (l/min) matches the patient's tidal volume. This can be monitored by watching the reservoir bag, and should take 15–20 s. When the patient inspires, the reservoir bag gets smaller. When the patient breathes out the reservoir bag gets larger as it fills with the mixture of gases emanating from the machine.

9.　Simultaneously, reassure the patient about the sensations that will be felt. Encourage the patient to concentrate on breathing gently through the nose. If the reservoir bag appears to be getting too empty then the flow of oxygen should be increased until the flow rate in l/min matches the patient's minute volume.

10.　Turn the mixture dial vertically to 90% oxygen (10% nitrous oxide) (Fig. 4.3 '2'). Wait for 60 s.

11.　Turn the mixture dial to 80% oxygen (20% nitrous oxide) (Fig. 4.3 '2'). Wait 60 s, above this level the operator should exercise more caution and consider whether further increments should be only 5%. With experience, operators will be able to judge whether further increments are needed.

12.　At the appropriate level of sedation dental treatment can be started.

13.　To bring about recovery turn the mixture dial to 100% oxygen and oxygenate the patient for 2 min before removing the nasal mask.

14.　Turn the flow control to zero and switch off the machine.

15.　The patient should breathe ambient air for a further 5 min before leaving the dental chair. The patient should be allowed to recover for a total period of 15 min before leaving.

At all times the patient must remain conscious. This is judged by the five clinically discernible signs described previously.

The above method of administration is the basic technique that is required in the early stages of clinical experience for any operator. This method ensures that the changes experienced by the patient do not occur so quickly that the patient is unable to cope. Once the operator has sufficient skill and confidence the stages can be 'concertinaed', for example, by starting at 20% nitrous oxide and reducing the time intervals between increments.

The initial time intervals of 60 s are used because clinical experience shows that shorter intervals between increments can lead to too rapid an induction and over-dosage.

4.11.3 The correct level of clinical sedation with nitrous oxide

One of the problems for the inexperienced clinician is to determine whether or not the patient is adequately sedated for treatment to start. By careful attention to signs and symptoms experienced by the patient the dentist will soon be able to decide whether the patient is ready for treatment.

The very rapid uptake and elimination of nitrous oxide requires the operator to be acutely vigilant so that the patient does not become sedated too rapidly.

4.11.4 Objective signs

The objective signs showing the patient is ready for treatment are (Fig. 4.6):

 (1) the patient is awake;
 (2) the patient is relaxed and comfortable;
 (3) the patient responds coherently to verbal instructions;
 (4) pulse rate is normal;
 (5) blood pressure is normal;
 (6) respiration is normal;
 (7) skin colour is normal;
 (8) pupils are normal and contract normally if a light is shone into them;
 (9) the laryngeal reflex is normal;
(10) the gag reflex is reduced;
(11) reaction to painful stimuli is lessened;
(12) there is a general reduction in spontaneous movements;
(13) the mouth is maintained open on request (Fig. 4.7).

4.11.5 Subjective symptoms

Subjective symptoms experienced by the patient are (Fig. 4.8):

(1) mental and physical relaxation;
(2) a tingling sensation (paraesthesia) singly or in any combination of lips, fingers, toes, or over the whole body;
(3) mild intoxication and euphoria;
(4) lethargy;
(5) a sense of detachment, sometimes interpreted as a floating or drifting sensation;
(6) a feeling of warmth;
(7) indifference to surroundings and the passage of time;

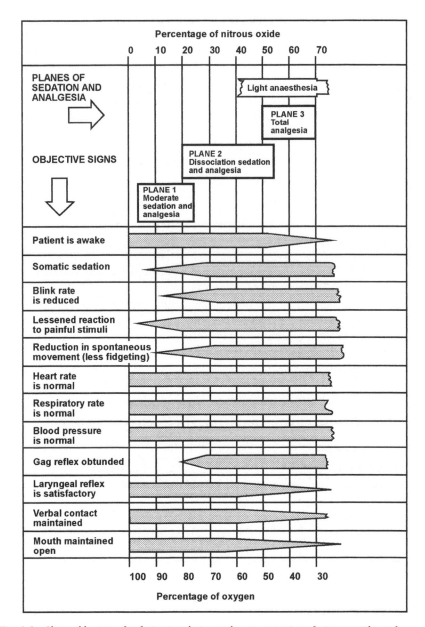

Fig. 4.6   Observable signs of sedation in relation to the concentration of nitrous oxide used.

(8)   dreaming;

(9)   lessened awareness of pain.

If the patient tends to communicate less and less, and is allowing the mouth to close, then these are signs that the patient is becoming too deeply sedated. The concentration of nitrous oxide should be reduced by 10 or 15% to prevent the patient moving into a state of total analgesia.

4.11.6 Monitoring during nitrous oxide sedation

During inhalation sedation it is essential that the clinician monitors both the patient and the machinery. For healthy patients with ASA I or II, use of a radial pulse is sufficient. For patients with ASA III or IV, treatment within a hospital environment and pulse oximetry, blood pressure cuff, and/or electrocardiograph monitoring

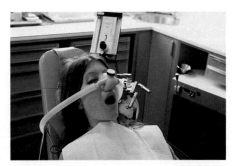

Fig. 4.7   The 'mouth open' sign.

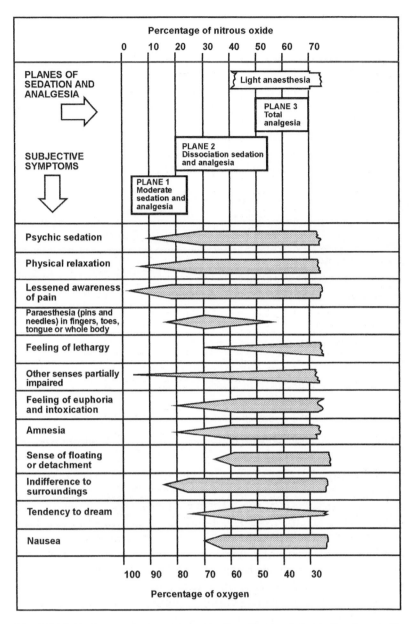

Fig. 4.8 Subjective symptoms experienced by the patient in relation to the nitrous oxide concentration.

would be prudent. This applies to only a very small proportion of patients such as those with cystic fibrosis with marked lung scarring or children with severe congenital cardiac disease where there is high blood pressure or cyanosis.

The patient

The clinician should pay careful attention to the patient's level of anxiety. This is achieved by assessing the patient's responses to an operative stimulus such as the dental drill. The level of sedation is assessed by the patient's demeanour compared with his or her presedation behaviour. It is important to note that different patients exhibit similar levels of impairment at different concentrations of nitrous oxide. If the patient appears to be too heavily sedated then the concentration of nitrous oxide should be reduced. There is no need to use pulse oximetry or capnography (to measure exhaled carbon dioxide levels) as is currently recommended for patients being sedated with intravenously administered drugs.

The machinery

At all stages of inhalation sedation, it is necessary to monitor intermittently the oxygen and nitrous oxide flow meters to verify that the machine is delivering the gases as required. In addition, it is essential to look at the reservoir bag to confirm that the patient is continuing to breathe through the nose the nitrous oxide gas mixture. Little or no movement of the reservoir bag suggests that the patient is mouth breathing, or that there is a gross leak, for example, a poorly fitting nasal mask.

> **Key Points**
> For nitrous oxide inhalation sedation:
> * set the flow;
> * slowly titrate the dose;
> * monitor the patient's response;
> * monitor the equipment.

4.11.7 The planes of inhalation sedation

The administration of oxygen–nitrous oxide gas mixture for sedating child patients induces three levels or planes of analgesia and sedation.

Plane 1: moderate sedation and analgesia

This plane is usually obtained with concentrations of 5–25% nitrous oxide (95–75% oxygen). As the patient is being encouraged to inhale the mixture of gases through the nose, it is necessary to reassure him or her that the sensations described by the clinician may not always be experienced. The patient may feel tingling in the fingers, toes, cheeks, tongue, back, head, or chest. There is a marked sense of relaxation, the pain threshold is raised, and there is a diminution of fear and anxiety. The patient will be obviously relaxed and will respond clearly and sensibly to questions and commands.

Other senses, such as hearing, vision, touch, and proprioception, are impaired in addition to the sensation of pain being reduced. The pupils are normal in appearance and contract when a light is shone into them. The peri-oral musculature, so often tensed involuntarily by the patient during treatment, is more easily retracted when the dental surgeon attempts to obtain good access for operative work. The absence of any side-effects makes this an extremely useful plane when working on moderately anxious patients.

Plane 2: dissociation sedation and analgesia

This plane is usually obtained with concentrations of 20–55% nitrous oxide (80–45% oxygen). As with plane 1, patients do not always experience all the symptoms. This should be remembered when reassuring and encouraging them.

As the patient enters this plane, psychological symptoms, described as dissociation or detachment from the environment, are experienced. Sometimes this dissociation is minimal, at other times it is profound. It may also take the form of a euphoria similar to alcoholic intoxication (witness the laughing gas parties of the mid-nineteenth century). The patient may feel suffused by a warm wave, and may experience a slight humming or buzzing in the ears, and a drowsiness or light-headedness sometimes described by the patient as a 'floaty' or 'woozy' feeling.

The overall demeanour of the patient will be relaxed and acquiescent. Apart from the overall appearance of relaxation, one of the few tangible physical signs is a reduction in the blink rate. At the deeper level of this plane of sedation the psychological effects become more pronounced. Occasionally, a patient will repeat words or phrases several times in succession. The words repeated may or may not make sense.

There is a noticeable tendency for the patient to dream, the dreams usually being of a pleasant nature. It is believed by many operators that the dreams experienced by the patient are to some extent conditioned by the ideas and thoughts introduced by the dental surgeon during the induction phase of sedation. The sedative effect is considerably pronounced, with both psychosedation and somatic sedation being present.

The psychosedation takes the form of a relaxed demeanour, and a willingness on the part of the previously unwilling patient to allow treatment regarded as frightening or especially traumatic. The somatic sedation takes the form of physical relaxation, unresisting peri-oral musculature, and occasionally an arm or leg sliding off the side of the dental chair indicating profound relaxation. The analgesic effect is probably accentuated by the sedation and sense of detachment. The patient is still able to respond to questions and commands, although there may be a considerable mental effort involved in thinking out the answer. The response is usually delayed and sluggish. Paraesthesia may be more pronounced and cover a greater area of the body than in plane 1. The patient is nevertheless obviously conscious and can demonstrate this by keeping the mouth wide open to assist the dental surgeon during operative treatment. On recovery, the patient may exhibit total amnesia. Nausea is a rare side-effect and very occasionally (in less than 0.003% of administrations) a patient may vomit.

Plane 3: total analgesia

This plane is usually obtained with concentrations of 50–70% nitrous oxide (50–30% oxygen). It has been claimed, that analgesia is so complete that extraction of teeth may be carried out in this plane. This has not been our experience. In this plane there is an increased tendency to dream. It is important to recognize that in a small number of patients as little as 50% nitrous oxide may bring about loss of consciousness. It is for this reason that dentists must exercise considerable caution if the concentration of gas coming from the machine rises above 40% nitrous oxide.

If the patient does become too deeply sedated and enters this third plane of total analgesia, he or she begins to lose the ability to independently maintain an open mouth and will be unable to co-operate or respond to the dentist's requests. If this 'open mouth' sign is lost, the operator can be sure that the patient is too deep in the plane of total analgesia and within a few minutes is likely to enter the plane of light anaesthesia. It is for this reason that a mouth prop must never be used, for if a prop is used the open mouth sign would not function.

If sedation is too deep and the patient shows signs of failing to co-operate, then the dentist should reduce the concentration of nitrous oxide by 10 or 15% for a couple of minutes. If it is considered necessary to lighten the sedation even more rapidly, the nasal hood should be removed and the patient allowed to breathe ambient air. The patient will return to a lighter plane within 15–20 s.

This plane of total analgesia is regarded as a buffer zone between the clinically useful planes of moderate and dissociation sedation and analgesia, and the potentially hazardous plane of light anaesthesia.

4.11.8 Clinical application

The technique of nitrous oxide sedation can be used for a wide range of procedures involving the cutting of hard or soft tissue where local anaesthesia will usually be needed to supplement the general analgesia from the nitrous oxide. The major disadvantage (or minor if handled properly) is the inconvenience of the nasal hood restricting access to the upper incisor area if an apicectomy is required. This problem can be overcome by careful retraction of the upper lip and counterpressure from the thumb held on the bridge of the nose.

4.11.9 Scavenging

Repeated exposure to environmental pollution with nitrous oxide can cause megaloblastic anaemia and problems with both conception and pregnancy. The Control of Substances Hazardous to Health (COSHH) advises that over a time-weighted average (TWA) of 8 h, the exposure should not exceed 100 p.p.m. This is five times lower than the safest dose found in animal studies.

Surgery contamination is affected by the *modus operandi* of the dental surgeon. Considerable care needs to be taken to discourage the patients from mouth breathing, to use rubber dam whenever possible, and ensure that full recovery is carried out with the nasal hood in place. Effective scavenging equipment is extremely simple in design (Fig. 4.9). This design of scavenger can be used on a normal relative analgesia machine without any specific modifications to the machine itself. All that is required is a change in the design of the nasal hood and the tubing leading from the machine to the hood. First, the expiratory and/or air entrainment valve on the nasal hood itself is removed and replaced with a simple blank because the use of this valve is obsolete. The efferent tube that leads away from the nasal mask is doubled in diameter to reduce resistance and connects to a specially devised exhaust pipe built into the wall or floor of the surgery. If considered essential, negative pressure can be applied at this connection to increase the efficiency of the scavenging (active scavenging).

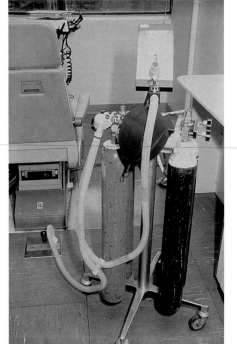

Fig. 4.9 Scavenging system applied to an inhalation sedation machine with outlet in the floor.

> **Key Points**
>
> To reduce nitrous oxide pollution
>
> - use a scavenging system;
> - use a scavenging nasal hood (block air entrainment valves in older nasal hoods);
> - discourage mouth breathing (do not let the child talk);
> - use rubber dam.

4.12 INTRAVENOUS SEDATION

The circumstances when intravenous sedation can be used in paediatric dentistry are limited, although there is a slow but steady trend to extending its use especially in adolescents.

4.12.1 Intravenous agents

There are many intravenous agents available in the BNF, but for dental purposes the practical choice is between midazolam, a benzodiazepine that is water soluble and well tolerated by tissues (important if some midazolam inadvertently becomes deposited outside rather than inside a vein) and propofol, which leads to rapid sedation and rapid recovery. Unfortunately, the risk of unintended loss of consciousness is high with propofol because of the narrow therapeutic range of the drug that leads quickly to anaesthesia. Therefore, propofol is used only when there is an anaesthetist present.

4.12.2 Equipment for intravenous sedation

The general surgery set up is the same as for inhalation sedation. A disposable tray should be prepared with the following:

(1) a 5 ml syringe;
(2) a venflon;
(3) adhesive tape;
(4) a green needle gauge 21;
(5) isopropyl alcohol swab;
(6) a single ampoule of the intravenous sedation drug;
(7) an ampoule of flumazenil (for urgent reversal of benzodiazepine sedation);
(8) a tourniquet.

The technique can be carried out as shown in the following sections.

4.12.3 Intravenous technique

The standard regimen is to use 0.07 mg/kg of midazolam infused slowly until the signs of satisfactory sedation are reached. This usually entails a loading dose of 2 mg followed by further increments as appropriate.

The technique requires the insertion of a venflon that is allowed to remain *in situ* until the treatment for that visit is complete. This applies to manual infusion by the dental surgeon, diffusion pump infusion supervised by the dental surgeon, and patient controlled anaesthesia (PCA). For anxious children this is an almost insuperable problem as 'the needle' is the cause of their fear. Nevertheless, there appears to be a group of older children, usually adolescents requiring dento-alveolar surgery, who are willing to allow the placement of a needle in the dorsum of the hand or the antecubital fossa for infusion of benzodiazepine drugs.

Intravenous access

The two most common sites of access are the antecubital fossa and the dorsum of the hand. In children especially, the antecubital fossa carries with it the danger of the needle causing damage to the vein and surrounding structures if the arm is bent during sedation. For this reason the dorsum of the hand is the preferred site.

Procedure

1. The patient's medical history is checked.
2. The arm is extended and a tourniquet applied.
3. The pulse oximeter is applied to the contralateral arm. *Note*: a very anxious patient might be distressed by these procedures so they can be left until the patient is sedated.
4. The venflon is inserted into the vein and taped into place.
5. The patient is asked to touch the tip of the nose to demonstrate good neuromotor control.
6. The first dose of drug is administered over 30 s (Fig. 4.10).
7. The patient's response is assessed after 2 min to determine whether further (smaller) increments of the sedative agent are required.
8. Dental treatment is carried out. If sedation becomes inadequate further increments of the sedative agent may be given.

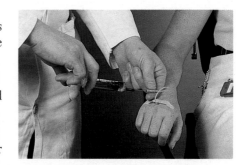

Fig. 4.10 Intravenous administration of midazolam through a vein in the dorsum of the hand.

9. Once dental treatment is complete, the patient is allowed to recover sufficiently to be helped to the recovery area.
10. Recovery must be under the supervisory eye of a specially trained personnel.
11. Once the patient is 'street fit', they are discharged into the care of an accompanying adult.
12. Postoperative instructions are reiterated.

Monitoring during intravenous sedation

This involves alert clinical monitoring and at least the use of a pulse oximeter.

4.12.4 Unexpected loss of consciousness

On the rare occasions when the patient becomes unconscious the dentist and their staff should follow the following routine.

1. Cease the operative procedure immediately.
2. Ensure that the mouth is cleared of all fluids by using high-volume suction.
3. Turn the patient on to his or her side in the 'recovery' position (Fig. 4.11).
4. Consider the administration of 100% oxygen.
5. If intravenous sedation is being used, leave the venflon in place so that emergency drugs can be administered through it if required.
6. Consider monitoring pulse, blood pressure, and respiration. Be ready to start resuscitation.
7. Dentist to stay with the patient until full signs of being awake are present (eyes open, independent maintenance of the airways, and verbal contact).
8. Follow-up of the patient by review within 3 days.
9. Full documentation of the incident.
10. Inform the patient's general medical practitioner of the incident.

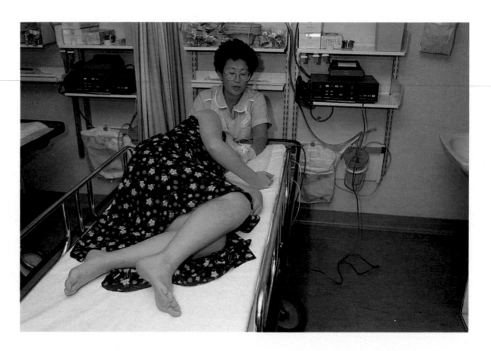

Fig. 4.11   Recovery position.

4.13 GENERAL ANAESTHESIA

The use of general anaesthesia in paediatric dentistry has a wide application, usually for the extraction of teeth. Fortunately, referrals have reduced, due to both the reduction in dental disease and to the use of sedation. Nevertheless, there will always be a need for general anaesthesia in dentistry, especially for pre-co-operative children.

Key Points

- In the United Kingdom, general anaesthesia can now only take place in a hospital setting, and be administered by a consultant anaesthetist.
- Risk of general anaesthesia:
  –mortality— $\sim$ 3 per million;
  –morbidity—symptoms associated with the procedure, distress at induction and during recovery, prolonged crying, nausea, sickness, and postoperative bleeding.
- Referring dentists are obliged to:
  –explain the risks of general anaesthesia;
  –discuss the alternative treatment modalities;
  –explain why the option of general anaesthesia has been selected;
  –keep a copy of their referral letter;
  –the referring dentist must be assured of the appropriateness of the care provided by sedation or general anaesthetic service.
- Indications for general anaesthesia
  –the child is pre cooperative (too young to cope)
  –uncontrolled fear
  –complexity of procedure.

4.13.1 Type of anaesthesia

In dentistry, anaesthesia falls into three main groups:

(1) out-patient short-case 'dental chair' anaesthesia traditionally with a nose mask but now more often with a laryngeal mask

(2) out-patient/day-stay 'intubation' anaesthesia;

(3) in-patient/hospital-stay 'intubation' anaesthesia.

Within these categories there are variations determined by anaesthetistic preference. Anaesthesia for dental treatment requires the help of a consultant anaesthetist. The organization of dental general anaesthesia lists, at least in the preliminary stages, is performed by a dental surgeon who therefore must understand the type of anaesthesia and the implications of any underlying medical condition.

4.13.2 Definition of anaesthesia

The state of anaesthesia is defined as: 'The absence of sensation artificially induced by the administration of gases or the injection of drugs or a combination of both'. The important feature of anaesthesia is that the patient is completely without the ability to independently maintain physiological function, such as breathing and protective reflexes, and is acutely vulnerable to the loss of any foreign bodies or fluids down the throat.

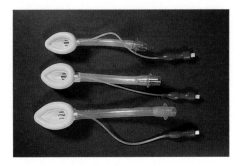

Fig. 4.12 Different sizes of laryngeal masks.

4.13.3 Out-patient 'short-case' general anaesthesia

This is used for ASA class I or class II patients requiring short, 2–10 min, procedures with rapid induction and early recovery, for example, dental extractions. Anaesthesia is induced either by inhalation of an anaesthetic vapour in an oxygen–nitrous oxide mixture using a face mask or by an intravenous injection for example, propofol. Occasionally, the child is premedicated with a benzodiazepine. The parent commonly accompanies the child to help them cope with the anaesthetic induction. Irrespective of the induction method, anaesthesia is maintained by the anaesthetic vapour, for example, sevofluorane, carried in a mixture of oxygen and nitrous oxide, and the face mask is exchanged for a nose mask or a laryngeal mask (Fig. 4.12 different sizes of laryngeal masks). Following this, the oropharynx is packed with gauze to protect the airway. This gauze is the reason why children sometimes later complain of a sore throat. Monitoring for this type of anaesthesia usually consists of an electrocardiograph, pulse oximeter, and a blood pressure cuff.

On completion of treatment, the gauze is removed and the patient turned into the recovery position and removed to a quiet recovery room so that he/she can be monitored during their final recovery. The child is discharged when he or she is able to drink a glass of water without being sick and able to stand without swaying or appearing dizzy. Although the child is deemed 'street fit', once he or she has arrived home the combined effects of anxiety, the general anaesthetic, and the dental surgery, make it necessary for the child to play 'quietly at home' for the rest of that day.

4.13.4 Out-patient 'day-stay' general anaesthesia

This is usually reserved for ASA class I or class II patients who require dental treatment that lasts more than 10 min, for example, removal of supernumeraries, complex and compound odontomes, exposing and bonding impacted teeth, or extensive conservative dentistry. Day surgery units commonly offer premedication and pre-anaesthetic visits to facilitate the child's ability to cope with the visit.

Anaesthetic induction is similar to that for 'short case' anaesthesia but an endotracheal tube is used, instead of a nose mask, either inserted through the nose (nasotracheal tube) or through the mouth (orotracheal tube). To insert it, a short-acting neuromuscular paralysing agent needs to be used, when this wears off the patient then breaths spontaneously. Occasionally, a longer-acting neuromuscular paralysing agent is selected to enable the anaesthetist to ventilate the patient artificially. These forms of anaesthesia have a greater intrusion upon the patient's physiological state. However, the use of a laryngeal mask instead of an endotracheal tube is gaining in popularity because it avoids the use of the paralysing agent reducing postoperative muscle pain. Nevertheless, the same principles of protecting the airways apply. In addition to the tube, the throat will be packed with gauze. If conservation is required it is prudent to use a rubber dam, as good isolation is essential for a high standard of operative dentistry (Fig. 4.13). For surgical procedures, local anaesthesia infiltration (2% lignocaine with 1 : 80,000 adrenaline) reduces bleeding and aids visibility during surgery while reducing the risk of cardiac dysrhythmias.

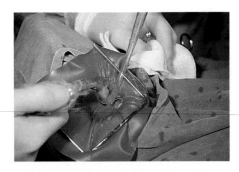

Fig. 4.13 Rubber dam applied during general anaesthesia.

Once the treatment is complete the patient is placed in the recovery position and wheeled to a recovery suite. The recovery from such extensive anaesthesia is such that the patient may not be able to return home for several hours. Usually it is necessary to have access to a car as the children are never quite as 'street fit' as those who have had a short anaesthetic, so public transport is best avoided.

4.13.5 In-patient/hospital-stay 'intubation' anaesthesia

Patients who are unfit for short or medium length general anaesthetics are usually in ASA class III. These patients have a medical problem that constitutes a significant increased risk, so anaesthetists advise that they are treated in a hospital operating theatre, which is always close to the facilities of an intensive care unit. The dental surgery is no more complex than that carried out for 'short-' and 'day-stay' anaesthesia, but the underlying medical condition requires the increased level of care that may be needed in the operating theatre environment and during post-operative recovery, and even later on the ward.

> **Key Points**
> - There are different types of dental anaesthesia, dependent on the complexity and length of time for the planned dental procedure.
> - Children with a medical condition may require hospital admission.

4.14 SUMMARY

1. Most patients can be treated using local anaesthesia and good behaviour management.
2. A significant minority of patients will require some form of sedation to enable them to undergo dental treatment.
3. A small minority of patients require general anaesthesia.
4. All techniques require careful and systematic assessment of the patient before being used.
5. Dentists and their staff require careful training and regular updates in the techniques of anaesthesia and sedation for children.

4.15 FURTHER READING

Chadwick, B. L. and Hosey, M. T. (2003). *Child taming: how to manage children in dental practice* (Quintessentials series number 9). Quintessence publishers, London. (*An easy read for the whole dental team that also provides insight on how to incorporate inhalation sedation into a treatment plan.*)

Cote, C. J., Notterman, D. A., Karl, H. W, Weinberg, J. A., and McCloskey, C. (2000). Adverse sedation events in pediatrics: a critical incident analysis of contributing factors. [see comments]. *Pediatrics*, **105**, 805–14. (*A rather scary paper that highlights the need for appropriate training, facilities and resuscitation skill.*)

Craig D. and Skelly M. (2004). *Practical conscious sedation* (Quintessentials Series number 15). Quintessence publishers, London. (*A user-friendly guide for the dental team that mainly focuses on intravenous sedation.*)

European Resuscitation Council (1992). Guidelines for basic and advanced life support. *Resuscitation*, **24**, 103–10. (*Guidelines that all practitioners should read and put into effect.*)

Health Services Advisory Committee. (1995). *Anaesthetic agents: controlling exposure under COSHH*. HMSO. (*The current UK safety standard of nitrous oxide environmental exposure.*)

Lindsay, S. J. E. and Yates, J. A. (1985). The effectiveness of oral diazepam in anxious child dental patients. *British Dental Journal*, **159**, 149–53. (*An objective study on the efficacy of oral premedication.*)

Report of the Working Party on Training in Dental Anaesthesia. (1993). Standing Dental Advisory Committee, Department of Health, United Kingdom. (*An excellent guide to sedation and anaesthesia in general dental practice and community dental practice.*)

Roberts, G. J. and Rosenbaum, N. L. (1990). *A colour atlas of dental analgesia and sedation*. Wolfe Publishing, London. (*All you need to know about local analgesia and sedation.*)

Standards in Conscious Sedation for Dentistry. (2000). Report of an Independent Expert Working Group. October. Available from SAAD 53 Wimpole Street London. W1G 8YH www.saaduk.org (*A matter-of fact document that outlines the facilities and training expected in the UK.*)

Wilson, K. E., Welbury, R. R., and Girdler, N. M. (2002). A randomised double blind crossover trial of oral midazolam for paediatric dental sedation. *Anaesthesia* **57**, 860–7. (*One of the few oral midazolam trials conducted in children.*)

Scully, C. and Cawson, R. A. (2004). *Medical problems in dentistry*. Churchill Livingstone, Edinburgh (5th edn). (*The most comprehensive account of how to cope with medical problems.*)

Local anaesthesia for children

5 Local anaesthesia for children

J. G. Meechan

5.1 INTRODUCTION

This chapter considers the use of local anaesthesia in children and describes methods of injection that should produce minimal discomfort. The complications and contraindications to the use of local anaesthesia in children are also discussed. The major use of local anaesthetics is in providing operative pain control. It should not be forgotten, however, that these drugs can be used as diagnostic tools and in the control of haemorrhage.

5.2 SURFACE ANAESTHESIA

Surface anaesthesia can be achieved by physical or pharmacological methods (topical anaesthetics). One physical method employed in dentistry involves the use of ethyl chloride. It relies on the latent heat of evaporation of this volatile liquid to reduce the temperature of the surface tissue to produce anaesthesia. This method is rarely used in children as it is difficult to direct the stream of liquid accurately without involving associated sensitive structures such as teeth. In addition, the general anaesthetic action of ethyl chloride should not be forgotten.

5.2.1 Intraoral topical agents

The success of topical anaesthesia is technique dependent. Topical anaesthetic agents will anaesthetize a 2–3 mm depth of surface tissue when used properly. The following points are worth noting when using intraoral topical anaesthetics:

1. The area of application should be dried.
2. The anaesthetic should be applied over a limited area.
3. The anaesthetic should be applied for sufficient time.

A number of different preparations varying in the active agent and in concentration are available for intraoral use. In the United Kingdom the agents most commonly employed are lidocaine (lignocaine) and benzocaine. Topical anaesthetics are provided as sprays, solutions, creams, or ointments. Sprays are the least convenient as they are difficult to direct. Some sprays taste unpleasant and can lead to excess salivation if they inadvertently reach the tongue. In addition, unless a metered dose is delivered, the quantity of anaesthetic used is poorly controlled. It is important to limit the amount of topical anaesthetic used. The active agent is present in greater concentration in topical preparations compared with local anaesthetic solutions and uptake from the mucosa is rapid. Systemic uptake is even quicker in damaged tissue. An effective method of application is to spread some cream on the end of a cotton bud (Fig. 5.1). All the conventional intraoral topical anaesthetics are equally effective when used on reflected mucosa. The length of time of administration is crucial

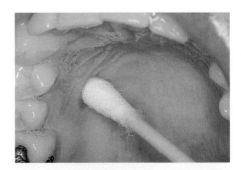

Fig. 5.1 Use of a cotton bud to apply a topical anaesthetic over a limited area.

for the success of topical anaesthetics. Applications of around 15 s or so are useless. An application time of around 5 min is recommended. It is important that topical anaesthetics are given sufficient time to work, because for many children this will be their initial experience of intraoral pain-control techniques. If the first method encountered is unsuccessful then confidence in the operator and his armamentarium will not be established. Although the main use of topical anaesthetics is as a preinjection treatment, these agents have been used in children as the sole means of anaesthesia for some intraoral procedures including the extraction of deciduous teeth.

5.2.2 Topical anaesthetics that will anaesthetize skin

EMLA cream (a 5% eutectic mixture of the anaesthetic agents prilocaine and lidocaine (lignocaine)) was the first topical anaesthetic to be shown to produce effective surface anaesthesia of intact skin. Therefore it is a useful adjunct to the provision of general anaesthesia in children as it allows pain-free venepuncture. When used on skin it has to be applied for 1 h and is thus only appropriate for elective general anaesthetics. Clinical trials of the use of EMLA intraorally have shown it to be more effective than conventional local anaesthetics when used on attached gingiva such as the hard palate and interdental papillae. It appears to be no more effective than conventional topical agents when applied to reflected mucosa. At present, the intraoral use of EMLA is not recommended by its manufacturers. An intraoral formulation of the combination of prilocaine and lidocaine (Oraqix®) has shown promise in clinical trials but at the time of writing was not available for use.

Tetracaine (amethocaine) 4% gel is another skin topical anaesthetic that may be useful prior to venepuncture. Unlike EMLA, which consists of amide local anaesthetics, tetracaine (amethocaine) is an ester-type anaesthetic agent.

5.2.3 Controlled-release devices

The use of topically active agents incorporated into materials that will adhere to mucosa and allow the slow release of the agent is a potential growth area in the field of local anaesthetic delivery. Such techniques might prove to be of value in paediatric dentistry. Clinical studies investigating the release of lidocaine (ligno-caine) from intraoral patches have shown some promise.

5.2.4 Jet injectors

Jet injectors belong to a category somewhere between topical and local anaesthesia but will be discussed here for completeness. These devices allow anaesthesia of the surface and to a depth of over 1 cm without the use of a needle. They deliver a jet of solution through the tissue under high pressure (Fig. 5.2). Conventional local anaesthetic solutions are used in specialized syringes and have been successful in children with bleeding diatheses where deep injection is contraindicated. Jet injection has been used both as the sole means of achieving local anaesthesia and prior to conventional techniques. This method of anaesthesia has been used alone and in combination with sedation to allow the pain-free extraction of primary teeth. The use of jet injection is not widespread for a number of reasons. Expensive equipment is required, soft tissue damage can be produced if a careless technique is employed, and the specialized syringes can be frightening to children both in appearance and in the sound produced during anaesthetic delivery. In addition, the unpleasant taste of the anaesthetic solution, which can accompany the use of this technique, can be off-putting. Although no needle is employed the technique is not painless.

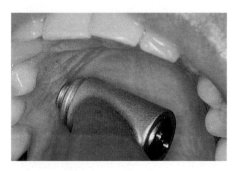

Fig. 5.2 The jet injector. (By kind permission of *Dental Update*.)

5.3 NON-PHARMACOLOGICAL PAIN CONTROL

A number of non-pharmacological methods for reducing the pain of operative dentistry are now available, including the use of electrical stimulation and radio waves. Hypnosis also belongs to this category.

Electroanalgesia or TENS (transcutaneous electrical nerve stimulation) has been shown to be very effective in providing anaesthesia for restorative procedures in children aged 3–12 years. The technique has also been used to provide pain control during the extraction of primary teeth. It can also be used as a 'deep topical' agent to reduce the pain of local anaesthetic injections. In younger children the level of stimulation is controlled by the operator. Children over 10 years can sufficiently understand the method to be able to control the level of stimulus themselves. The basis of TENS blocking transmission of the acute pain of dental operative procedures is due to the fact that large myelinated nerve fibres (such as those responding to touch) have a lower threshold for electrical stimulation than smaller unmyelinated pain fibres. Stimulation of these fibres by the current from the TENS machine closes the 'gate' to central transmission of the signal from the pain fibres. This is quite different from the use of TENS in the treatment of chronic pain where the release of endogenous painkillers such as β-endorphins is stimulated. In addition, if the patient operates the machine, the feeling of control can allay anxiety and aid in pain management.

Non-pharmacological methods of pain control offer two advantages. First, systemic toxicity will not occur, and, second, the soft tissue anaesthesia resolves at the end of the procedure. This reduces the chances of self-inflicted trauma. Hypnosis can be used as an adjunct to local anaesthesia in children by decreasing the pulse rate and the incidence of crying. It appears to be most effective in young children.

5.4 LOCAL ANAESTHETIC SOLUTIONS

A number of local anaesthetic solutions are now available that can provide anaesthesia lasting from 10 min to over 6 h. There are few, if any, indications for the use of the so-called 'long-acting' agents in children. The gold standard is lidocaine (lignocaine) with epinephrine (adrenaline). Unless there is a true allergy to lidocaine then 2% lidocaine with 1 : 80,000 epinephrine is the solution of choice in the United Kingdom. 'Short-acting' agents such as plain lidocaine are seldom employed as the sole agent because, although pulpal anaesthesia may be short-lived, soft tissue effects can still last over an hour or so. More importantly, the efficacy of plain solutions is much less than those containing a vasoconstrictor.

5.5 TECHNIQUES OF LOCAL ANAESTHESIA

There are no techniques of local anaesthetic administration that are unique to children; however, modifications to standard methods are sometimes required. As far as positioning the child is concerned the upper body should be around 30 degrees to the vertical. Sitting upright can increase the chances of a faint, while at the other extreme (fully supine) the child may feel ill at ease. When there is a choice of sites at which to administer the first local anaesthetic injection the primary maxillary molar area should be chosen. This is the region that is most easily anaesthetized with the least discomfort.

5.5.1 Infiltration anaesthesia

Infiltration anaesthesia is the method of choice in the maxilla. The infiltration of 0.5–1.0 ml of local anaesthetic is sufficient for pulpal anaesthesia of most teeth in children. The objective is to deposit local anaesthetic solution as close as possible to the apex of the tooth of interest—however, the presence of bone prevents direct apposition. As the apices of most teeth are closer to the buccal side, a buccal approach is employed and the needle is directed towards the apex after insertion through reflected mucosa. Direct deposition under periosteum can be painful, therefore a compromise is made and the solution is delivered supraperiosteally. The one area where pulpal anaesthesia can prove troublesome in the child's maxilla is the upper first permanent molar region where the proximity of the zygomatic buttress can inhibit the spread of solution to the apical area (see further). In the mandible, the use of buccal infiltration anaesthesia will often produce pulpal anaesthesia of the primary teeth; however, it is usually unreliable when operating on the permanent dentition with the exception of the lower incisor teeth. The most dependable form of anaesthesia in the posterior mandible is inferior alveolar nerve block anaesthesia.

5.5.2 Regional block anaesthesia

Inferior alveolar and lingual nerve blocks

The administration of the inferior alveolar and lingual nerve block is easier to perform successfully in children compared to adults. A common fault in adults is placing the needle too low on the ramus of the mandible with deposition of solution inferior to the mandibular foramen. In children, the mandibular foramen is low in relation to the occlusal plane (Fig. 5.3), and it is difficult to place the needle inferior to the mandibular foramen if it is introduced parallel to the occlusal plane. Thus in children it is easier to ensure that the solution is deposited around the nerve before it enters the mandibular canal. The technique of administration is identical to that used in adults and is best performed with the child's mouth fully open. The direct approach—introducing the needle from the primary molars of the opposite side—is recommended as less needle movement is required after tissue penetration with this method compared to the indirect technique. The operator's non-dominant hand supports the mandible with the thumb intraorally in the retromolar region of the mandible. The index or middle finger is placed extraorally at the posterior border of the ramus at the same height as the thumb. The needle is advanced from the primary molar region of the opposite side with the syringe held parallel to the mandibular occlusal plane. The needle is inserted through mucosa in the mandibular retromolar region lateral to the ptery-gomandibular raphe midway between the raphe and the anterior border of the ascending ramus of the mandible, aiming for a point halfway between the operator's thumb and index finger. The height of insertion is about 5 mm above the mandibular occlusal plane, although in young children entry at the height of the occlusal plane should also be successful. The needle should be advanced until the medial border of the mandible is reached. In young children bone will be reached after about 15 mm and thus a 25-mm needle can be used; however, in older children a long (35 mm) needle should be employed as penetration up to 25 mm may be required. Once bone has been touched the needle is withdrawn slightly until it is supraperiosteal, aspiration is performed, and 1.5 ml of solution deposited. The lingual nerve is blocked by withdrawing the needle halfway, aspirating again, and depositing most of the remaining solution at this point. The final contents of the cartridge are expelled as the needle is withdrawn through the tissues. A common fault is to contact bone only a few millimetres following insertion. In most children this will lead to unsuccessful anaesthesia. This usually occurs due to entry at too obtuse an angle. If this occurs the needle should not be completely withdrawn but pulled back a couple of millimetres, and then advanced parallel to the ramus for about 1 cm with the barrel of the syringe over the mandibular teeth of the same side. The body of the syringe is then repositioned across the primary molars or premolars of the opposite side and advanced towards the medial border of the ramus.

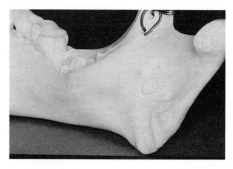

Fig. 5.3 The mandibular foramen is below the occlusal plane in children. (By kind permission of *Dental Update*.)

Long buccal, mental, and incisive nerve blocks

The long buccal injection usually equates to a buccal infiltration in children. The mental and incisive nerve block is readily administered in children as the orientation of the mental foramen is such that it faces forward rather than posteriorly as in adults (Fig. 5.4). Thus it is easier for solution to diffuse through the foramen when approached from an anterior direction. The needle is advanced in the buccal sulcus and directed towards the region between the first and second primary molar apices. Blockade of transmission in the mental nerve provides excellent soft tissue anaesthesia; however, anaesthesia of the incisive nerve (which supplies the dental pulps) by this approach is not as reliable as an inferior alveolar nerve block.

The pulps of lower incisor teeth may not be satisfactorily anaesthetized by inferior alveolar nerve or mental and incisive nerve block injections as a result of cross-over supply from the contralateral inferior alveolar nerve. A buccal infiltration adjacent to the tooth of interest is sufficient to deal with this supply. The method of choice for pulpal anaesthesia in the permanent lower incisors is a combination of buccal and lingual infiltrations.

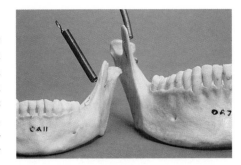

Fig. 5.4 The mental foramen faces anteriorly in children (left) compared with posteriorly in adults. (By kind permission of *Dental Update*.)

Maxillary block techniques

Regional block techniques are seldom required in a child's maxilla. Greater palatine and nasopalatine nerve blocks are avoided by infiltrating local anaesthetic solution through already anaesthetized buccal papillae and 'chasing' the anaesthetic through to the palatal mucosa (see further). This technique is equally effective in anaesthetizing lingual gingivae in the lower jaw if infiltration or mental block techniques have been used (it is obviously not needed if a lingual block has been administered with an inferior alveolar nerve block injection). The effects of an infraorbital block are often achieved by infiltration anaesthesia in the canine/maxillary first primary molar region in young children.

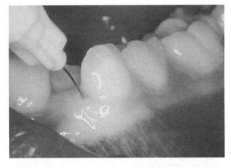

Fig. 5.5 Intraligamentary injection in a child.

5.5.3 Intraligamentary anaesthesia

Intraligamentary or periodontal ligament (pdl) anaesthesia is a very effective technique in children (Fig. 5.5). This is a method of intraosseous injection with local anaesthetic reaching the cancellous space in the bone via the periodontal ligament. This method allows the use of small amounts of local anaesthetic solution. The recommended dose per root is 0.2 ml. Although pulpal anaesthesia is not due to ischaemia, the technique is significantly more successful when a vasoconstrictor-containing solution is employed. The anaesthetic of choice is 2% lidocaine (lignocaine) with 1 : 80,000 epinephrine (adrenaline). Sensible dose limitations must be used, as entry into the circulation of intraosseously administered drugs is as rapid as by the intravenous route.

The technique involves inserting a 30-gauge needle at an angle of approximately 30° to the long axis of the tooth into the gingival sulcus at the mesiobuccal aspect of each root, and advancing the needle until firm resistance is met. It would seem sensible to have the bevel facing the bone when the solution is being expelled; however, it has never been demonstrated that the direction to which the bevel faces affects the efficacy of the technique. The needle will not advance far down the ligament, as even a 30-gauge needle is many times wider than a healthy periodontal ligament. The needle normally remains wedged at the alveolar crest. The solution is then injected under firm controlled pressure until 0.2 ml has been delivered. The application of the appropriate pressure is easier with specialized syringes (Figs 5.6 and 5.7) but the technique is equally effective with conventional dental syringes. Another advantage of the specialized syringes is that they deliver a set dose per depression of the trigger (0.06–0.2 ml depending on design). When using conventional syringes for intraligamentary injections the recommended dose of 0.2 ml for each root can be visualized as this is approximately the volume of the rubber bung in the cartridge.

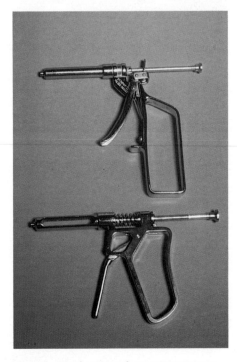

Fig. 5.6 Pistol-grip intraligamentary syringes.

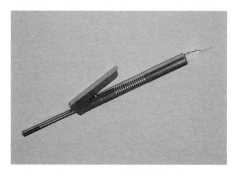

Fig. 5.7 A pen-grip intraligamentary syringe. This is a less-aggressive looking instrument than the pistol-grip type and is preferred in children.

It is important not to inject too quickly; about 15 s per depression of the specialized syringe lever is needed. Also, it is best to wait about 5 s after the injection before withdrawing the needle to allow the expressed solution to diffuse through the bone, otherwise it escapes via the gingival sulcus into the mouth. Intraligamentary anaesthesia reduces, but does not completely eliminate, the soft tissue anaesthesia which accompanies regional block anaesthesia in the mandible. This helps reduce the occurrence of self-mutilation of lip and tongue. Intraligamentary anaesthesia is often mistakenly considered a 'one tooth' anaesthetic. Adjacent teeth may exhibit anaesthesia and care must be used if this method is being used as a diagnostic tool in the location of a painful tooth. There are few indications for the use of the pdl technique in the maxilla because reliable pain-free anaesthesia should be possible in all regions of the upper jaw using infiltration techniques. In the maxilla, intraligamentary anaesthesia is best considered as a supplementary method of achieving pain control if conventional techniques have failed. The technique can be invaluable in the posterior mandible and can eliminate the need for uncomfortable regional block injections.

5.6 PAIN-FREE LOCAL ANAESTHESIA

The administration of pain-free local anaesthesia depends upon a number of factors which are within the control of the operator. These factors relate to: (1) equipment; (2) materials; (3) techniques.

5.6.1 Equipment

All components of the local anaesthetic delivery system can contribute to the discomfort of the injection. Needles should be sharp and the finest available gauge should be used. The narrowest needle used in dentistry is 30 gauge. A narrow gauge does not interfere with the ability to aspirate blood, but it is worth noting that narrow needles are more likely to penetrate blood vessels than their wider counterparts.

The choice of syringe used for conventional local anaesthetic injections in children must allow aspiration both before and during injection. There is evidence that inadvertent intravascular injection is more likely to occur in younger patients. Positive aspirate incidences of 20% of inferior alveolar nerve block injections in the 7–12 year age group have been reported.

One aspect of local anaesthetic delivery that can contribute to discomfort is the speed of injection. The use of computerized delivery systems such as 'The Wand' permits very slow delivery of solution (Fig. 5.8). This is particularly useful when injecting into tissue of low compliance such as the palatal mucosa and periodontal ligament. When using conventional syringes the choice of anaesthetic cartridge can also contribute to the discomfort experienced during injection. The type of cartridge used should be one that allows depression of the rubber bung at a constant rate with a constant force. Cartridges that produce a juddering action should not be employed.

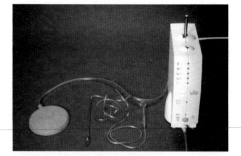

Fig. 5.8 The Wand computerized injection system, which permits slow delivery of solution.

5.6.2 Materials

In the past, heating the contents of local anaesthetic cartridges to body temperature prior to injection has been advised. There is no sound basis for this recommendation. There is ample evidence to suggest that patients cannot differentiate between local anaesthetics between room and body temperature. Indeed, storage of cartridges at higher temperatures can be detrimental to the solution as this can increase the chances of bacterial contamination, decrease the activity of epinephrine (adrenaline) in the solution due to increased oxidation, and finally decrease the pH of the solution (see further). Cartridges stored in a refrigerator should be allowed to reach room temperature before use. The pH of the injected solution may affect the discomfort of the injection. Local anaesthetic solutions vary in their pHs, those containing vasoconstrictors having lower values. For example, 2% plain lidocaine (lignocaine) has a pH of 6.8 compared with pH 3.2 for 2% lidocaine with 1 : 80,000 epinephrine (adrenaline). Thus if minimal sensation is to be produced it may be worthwhile using a small dose of a plain solution as an initial injection before using a vasoconstrictor-containing solution as the definitive local anaesthetic.

5.6.3 Techniques

Posterior maxillary buccal infiltrations

Assuming the proper materials and equipment have been chosen then the following technique can be used to reduce the discomfort of buccal infiltration injections in the maxilla posterior to the canine:

1. Dry the mucosa and apply a topical anaesthetic for 5 min.
2. Wipe off excess topical anaesthetic.
3. Stretch the mucosa.
4. Distract the patient (stretching the mucosa and gentle pressure on the lip between finger and thumb can achieve this).
5. Insert the needle—if bone is contacted withdraw slightly.
6. Aspirate, if positive reposition the needle without withdrawing from mucosa and when negative proceed.
7. Inject 0.5–1.0 ml supraperiosteally very slowly (15–30 s or via computerized system).

Anterior maxillary buccal infiltrations

Injection into the anterior aspect of the maxilla can be uncomfortable if some preparatory steps are not taken. Using the method described in steps 1–6 above, about 0.2 ml of local anaesthetic is deposited painlessly in the first primary molar buccal sulcus on the side to be treated (Fig. 5.9). The next injection is placed anteriorly to this a minute later when soft tissue anaesthesia has spread radially from the initial injection site, and further 0.2 ml increments are placed in the anterior aspect of the already anaesthetized area until the tooth of interest is reached. The buccal infiltration of 0.5–1.0 ml can now be delivered painlessly through the already anaesthetized soft tissue.

Palatal anaesthesia

Injection directly into the palatal mucosa is painful. In some individuals the deposition of the solution close to a cotton-wool bud coated with topical anaesthetic and applied with firm pressure may reduce discomfort, especially when the pressure on the bud is increased simultaneously with needle insertion and the child is warned of this pressure increase (Fig. 5.10). However, as mentioned earlier, conventional topical anaesthetics are not very effective on the attached mucosa of the hard palate and this method is not universally successful. The use of computerized delivery systems may reduce injection pain during palatal injections. When using conventional syringes a method of reducing the discomfort of palatal injections is to approach the palatal mucosa via already anaesthetized buccal interdental papillae. This is most readily achieved using ultra-short (12 mm) 30-gauge needles which are inserted into the base of the interdental papilla at an angle of approximately 90° to the surface. The needle is advanced palatally while injecting local anaesthetic into the papilla. This is performed through both the distal and mesial papillae. Blanching should be seen around the palatal gingival margin (Figs 5.11–5.13). With practice this technique can be used without the needle breaching the palatal mucosal surface, which prevents

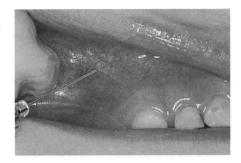

Fig. 5.9 Buccal infiltration injection in the upper primary molar region. (By kind permission of *Dental Update*.)

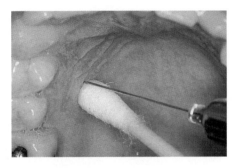

Fig. 5.10 Use of pressure and topical anaesthesia to lessen the discomfort of a palatal injection. (By kind permission of *Dental Update*.)

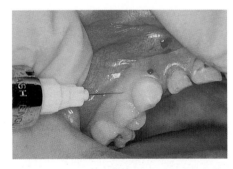

Fig. 5.11 Advancing local anaesthetic towards the palate via the buccal papilla. (By kind permission of *Dental Update*.)

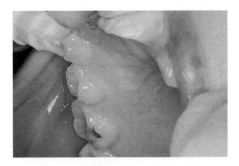

Fig. 5.12 Palatal view of Fig. 5.10 showing blanching of the palate. (By kind permission of *Dental update*.)

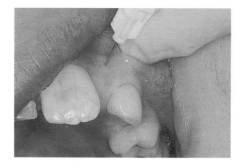

Fig. 5.13 It is simple to advance towards the palate when the teeth are spaced. (By kind permission of *Dental Update*.)

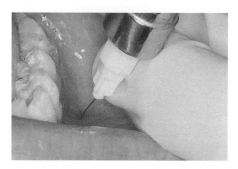

Fig. 5.14 Small-dose buccal infiltration in the lower premolar region for removal of a lower second molar.

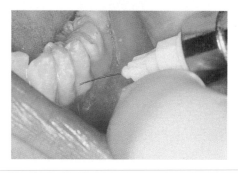

Fig. 5.15 Papillary injection after buccal infiltration.

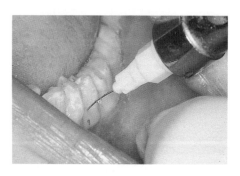

Fig. 5.16 Intraligamentary injection after papillary injection.

the unpleasant-tasting solution inadvertently appearing in the mouth. This method usually provides sufficient anaesthesia for extractions; however, it may be supplemented by a painless gingival sulcus injection on the palatal side.

Mandibular anaesthesia

Inferior alveolar nerve block injections can be uncomfortable, but infiltration anaesthesia is not successful in the posterior permanent dentition. Alternatively, intraligamental (pdl) injections may be employed to anaesthetize the posterior mandibular teeth. This technique is not very successful in the lower permanent incisors. This is probably due to a paucity of perforations in the cribriform plate of lower incisor sockets. As mentioned above infiltration anaesthesia is the method of choice for the incisor teeth. Lingual anaesthesia can be obtained by chasing through the buccal papillae as described for palatal injections above.

Studies in adults have suggested that pdl techniques are less unpleasant than conventional methods, but many children find delivery of anaesthetic solution via the pdl uncomfortable. The discomfort can be overcome by using the following methods. The mesial buccal papilla can be treated with topical anaesthetic applied with pressure. While pressure is still being applied, a papillary injection is administered followed by the intraligamental injection. As conventional topical local anaesthetics are not very effective on attached gingiva this method is not successful with all children. Alternatively, a small-dose buccal infiltration is given apical to the tooth (this can be given as one depression of the pdl syringe). This is followed by a papillary injection, which now should be painless, and finally by the intraligamental injection (Figs 5.14–5.16). Lingual gingival anaesthesia is obtained via the pdl by directing the needle through the interdental space (Fig. 5.17).

The techniques described should produce minimal discomfort during local anaesthetic administration in children. When these methods are combined with relative analgesia the production of injection pain is even less likely to arise. When pain-free reliable local anaesthesia is achieved in children confidence is gained both by the child and the operator, and a sound basis for a satisfactory professional relationship is established. This means that many of the treatments traditionally performed under general anaesthesia (such as multiple-quadrant extractions and minor oral surgery) can readily be performed in the conscious sedated child.

5.7 COMPLICATIONS OF LOCAL ANAESTHESIA

Complications can be classified as generalized and localized and divided into early and late.

5.7.1 Generalized complications

Psychogenic

The most common psychogenic complication of local anaesthesia is fainting. The chances of this happening are reduced by sympathetic management and administration of the anaesthetic to children in the semi-supine position.

Allergy

Allergy to local anaesthetics is a very rare occurrence, especially to the amide group to which most of the commonly used dental local anaesthetics (such as lidocaine (lignocaine) prilocaine, mepivacaine and articaine) belong. The only members of the ester group of local anaesthetics routinely used in the United Kingdom are benzocaine and tetracaine (amethocaine), which are available as topical anaesthetic preparations.

Allergy to other constituents of local anaesthetic cartridges may occur, for example, metabisulfite a reducing agent which prevents oxidation of epinephrine. Allergy can manifest in a variety of forms ranging from a minor localized reaction to the medical emergency of anaphylactic shock. If there is any suggestion that a child is allergic to a local anaesthetic they should be referred for allergy testing to the local dermatology or clinical pharmacology department. Such testing will confirm or refute the diagnosis, and in addition should determine which alternative local anaesthetic can safely be used on the child. The majority of referrals prove to have no local anaesthetic allergy.

Children who are allergic to latex merit consideration as this material is included in the rubber bungs of some cartridges. When treating such a child it is imperative to use a latex-free cartridge. Details of which cartridges are latex-free can be obtained from the manufacturers.

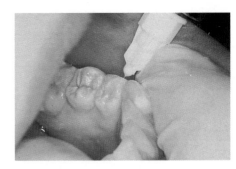

Fig. 5.17 Lingual view of showing blanching of the lingual gingiva.

Toxicity

Overdosage of local anaesthetics leading to toxicity is rarely a problem in adults but can readily occur in children. Children over 6 months of age absorb local anaesthetics more rapidly than adults; however, this is balanced by the fact that children have a relatively larger volume of distribution and elimination is also rapid due to a relatively large liver. Nevertheless, doses which are well below toxic levels in adults can produce problems in children, and fatalities attributable to dental local anaesthetic overdose have been reported. As with all drugs dosages should be related to body weight. The maximum dose of lidocaine (lignocaine) is 4.4 mg/kg. This is an easy dose to remember if one notes that the largest 2% (i.e. 20 mg/ml) lidocaine anaesthetic cartridges available in the United Kingdom are 2.2 ml, which means they contain 44 mg of lidocaine. Thus a safe maximum dose is one-tenth of the largest cartridge available per kilogram. If the 10th of a cartridge per kilogram rule is adhered to then overdose will not occur. Prilocaine, the other commonly used local anaesthetic drug in the United Kingdom, has a maximum dose of 6.0 mg/kg and as it is normally presented as a 3% solution the rule is one-eleventh of the cartridge per kilogram. When it is noted that a typical 5 year old weighs 20 kg it is easy to see that over-dose can easily occur unless care is exercised. The use of vasoconstrictor-containing local anaesthetics for definitive local anaesthesia is recommended in children, as agents such as epinephrine (adrenaline) might reduce the entry of local anaesthetic agents into the circulation. In addition, as vasoconstrictor-containing solutions are more effective, the need for multiple repeat injections is reduced.

CARDIOVASCULAR EFFECTS

Cardiovascular effects caused by the injection of a dental local anaesthetic solution will be due to the combined action of the anaesthetic agent and the vasoconstrictor. Local anaesthetics affect the cardiovascular system by their direct action on cardiac tissue and the peripheral vasculature. They also act indirectly via inhibition of the autonomic nerves that regulate cardiac and peripheral vascular function. Most local anaesthetic agents will decrease cardiac excitability, and indeed lidocaine (lignocaine) is used in the treatment of cardiac arrhythmias. Both vasoconstrictors commonly used in the United Kingdom, namely epinephrine (adrenaline) and felypressin, can influence cardiovascular function. In addition to the beneficial effect of peripheral vasoconstriction for surgical procedures, epinephrine has both direct and indirect effects on the heart and the doses used in clinical dentistry will increase cardiac output, although this is unlikely to be hazardous in healthy children. Felypressin at high doses causes coronary artery vasoconstriction, but the plasma levels that produce this are unlikely to be achieved during clinical dentistry.

CENTRAL NERVOUS SYSTEM EFFECTS

The fact that local anaesthetic agents influence activity in nerves other than peripheral sensory nerves is obvious to any practitioner who has inadvertently paralyzed the peripheral branches of the motor facial nerve during an inferior alveolar nerve block injection. Similarly, the central nervous system is not immune to the effects of local anaesthetic agents. Indeed, plasma concentrations of local anaesthetics that are incapable of influencing peripheral nerve function can profoundly affect the central nervous system. At low doses the effect is excitatory as central nervous system inhibitory fibres are blocked, at high doses the effect is depressant and can lead to unconsciousness and respiratory arrest. Fatalities due to local anaesthetic overdose in children are generally due to central nervous tissue depression.

METHAEMOGLOBINAEMIA

Some local anaesthetics cause specific adverse reactions when given in overdose. Prilocaine causes cyanosis due to methaemoglobinaemia.

In methaemoglobinaemia the ferrous iron of normal haemoglobin is converted to the ferric form which cannot combine with oxygen.

TREATMENT OF TOXICITY

The best treatment of toxicity is prevention. Prevention is aided by: (1) aspiration; (2) slow injection; (3) dose limitation. When a toxic reaction occurs then the procedure is: (1) Stop the dental treatment. (2) Provide basic life support. (3) Call for medical assistance. (4) Protect the patient from injury. (5) Monitor vital signs.

Drug interactions

Specialist advice from the appropriate physician should be requested in the treatment of children on significant long-term drug therapy. Apparently innocuous drug combinations can interact and cause significant problems in children, for example, an episode of methaemoglobinaemia has been reported in a 3-month-old child following the application of EMLA. It was concluded from that case that prilocaine (in the EMLA) had interacted with a sulfonamide (which can also produce methaemoglobinaemia) that the child was already receiving.

Infection

The introduction of agents capable of producing a generalized infection, such as human immunodeficiency virus (HIV) infection and hepatitis, is a complication which should not occur when appropriate cross-infection control measures are employed.

5.7.2 Early localized complications

Pain

Pain resulting from local anaesthetic injections can occur at the time of the injection due to the needle penetrating mucosa, too rapid an injection, or injection into an inappropriate site. The sites at which injection may be painful include: (1) intraepithelial; (2) subperiosteal; (3) into the nerve trunk; (4) intravascular. An intraepithelial injection is uncomfortable because at the start of the injection the solution does not disperse and this causes the tissues to balloon out. Subperiosteal injection may produce pain both at the time of injection and postoperatively. The initial pain is due to injection into a confined space, with the delivery of solution causing the periosteum to be stripped from the bone. Direct contact of the nerve trunk by the needle produces an electric-shock type of sensation and immediate anaesthesia. This is most likely to occur in the lingual and inferior alveolar nerves during inferior alveolar nerve blocks. Unfortunately, this complication is more common with experienced operators as it represents good location of the needle. When it does occur the solution should not be injected at that point but delivered after the needle has been withdrawn slightly, thus avoiding an intraneural injection. If the needle does contact the nerve then the patient and parent should be warned that anaesthesia of the nerve may be prolonged. Altered sensation may last up to a few weeks in some cases.

Intravascular injection

Accidental intravascular injections can occur in children if aspiration is not performed. Intravascular injections can cause local pain if the vessel penetrated is an artery and arterial spasm occurs. Intravenous injections can produce systemic effects such as tachycardia and palpitations. Intra-arterial injections are much rarer than intravenous injections, however the effects of an intra-arterial injection can be alarming. Such effects range from local pain and cutaneous blanching (Fig. 5.18) to severe intracranial problems. The reported, rare cases of hemiplegia following local anaesthetic injections can be accounted for by rapid intra-arterial injection. This can produce sufficient intracranial blood levels of the local anaesthetic to produce central nervous tissue depression.

Failure of local anaesthesia

The inability to complete the prescribed treatment due to failure of the local anaesthetic can be due to a number of causes, including: (1) anatomy; (2) pathology; (3) operator technique. Anatomical causes of failed local anaesthesia can result from either bony anatomy or accessory innervation. Bony anatomy can inhibit the diffusion of a solution to the apical region when infiltration techniques are used. This can occur in children in the upper first permanent molar region due to a low zygomatic buttress. To overcome this problem the anaesthetic is infiltrated both mesially and distally to the upper first molar/zygomatic buttress region. Accessory innervation may also produce failed local anaesthesia. In the upper molar region this may be due to pulpal supply from the greater palatine nerves, which can be blocked by supplementary palatal anaesthesia. In the mandible, accessory supply from the mylohyoid, auriculotemporal, and cervical nerves will not be blocked by inferior alveolar, lingual, and long buccal nerve blocks and may require supplementary injections. The commonest area of accessory supply occurs near the midline, where bilateral supply often necessitates supplemental injections when regional block techniques are employed.

The presence of acute infection interferes with the action of local anaesthetics. This is partly due to the reduction in tissue pH decreasing the number of unionized local anaesthetic molecules, which in turn inhibits their diffusion through lipid to the site of action (the number of ionized versus unionized molecules is governed by the pH and pK_a of the agent). More importantly, nerve endings stimulated by the presence of acute infection are hyperalgesic.

Regional block and intraligamental methods of local anaesthesia are technique dependent, and often failure of these forms of local anaesthesia are due to the operator. This cause of failure becomes less common with experience. Infiltration anaesthesia is a very simple method which is readily mastered by novices. When this injection fails reasons other than operator technique should be sought.

Motor nerve paralysis

Paralysis of the facial nerve can occur following deposition of local anaesthetic solution within the substance of the parotid gland due to malpositioning of the needle during inferior alveolar nerve block injections. The terminal branches of the facial nerve run through the parotid gland and will be paralyzed by the anaesthetic agent. The most dramatic manifestation of this complication is the loss of ability to close the eyelids on the affected side. An eye patch should be provided until the paralysis wears off. This side effect is probably more common in adults—the anatomy of the child's mandible is such that inability to successfully palpate the medial aspect of the mandible

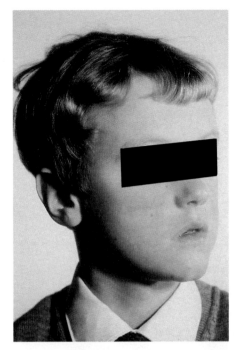

Fig. 5.18 Blanching of the cheek after an intra-arterial injection in a child.

with the needle is uncommon. Although paralysis of the eyelid is most often due to faulty technique during inferior alveolar nerve block anaesthesia, it can also result from the use of excessive amounts of solution in the maxillary buccal sulcus.

Interference with special senses

There have been reports of interference with vision and hearing after the intra-oral injection of local anaesthetics. Such occurrences most probably result from accidental intra-arterial injections.

Haematoma formation

Penetration of a blood vessel can occur during local anaesthetic administration. Haematoma formation is rarely a problem, however, unless it occurs in muscle following inferior alveolar nerve block techniques when it may lead to trismus (see further).

5.7.3 Late localized complications

Self-inflicted trauma

Self-inflicted trauma may occur after local anaesthetic injections in children. It may follow regional techniques in the mandible and infiltration anaesthesia in the maxilla. The commonest site is the lower lip (Fig. 5.19), but the tongue and upper lip can also be affected. It can be prevented by adequate explanation to the patient and parent by the clinician. The use of pdl techniques may reduce the frequency of this complication; however, it must be stressed that soft tissue anaesthesia is not completely avoided with this method in all cases.

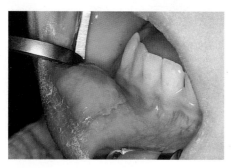

Fig. 5.19   Self-inflicted trauma following an inferior dental block injection. (By kind permission of *Dental Update*.)

Oral ulceration

Occasionally children will develop oral ulceration a few days following local anaesthetic injections. This is usually due to trauma initiating an aphthous ulcer. Needle trauma may activate a latent form of herpes simple on rare occasions.

Long-lasting anaesthesia

As mentioned above long-lasting anaesthesia can result from direct trauma to a nerve trunk from the needle, injection of solution into the nerve, or occasionally from the use of more concentrated anaesthetic solutions. This may occur after regional block techniques but it is a rare complication.

Trismus

Trismus may follow inferior alveolar nerve block injections and is usually the result of bleeding within muscle due to penetration of a blood vessel by the needle. Injection of a solution directly into muscle tissue may also result in trismus. The condition is self-resolving, although it may take a few weeks before normal opening is restored.

Infection

Localized infection due to the introduction of bacteria at the injection site is a complication that is rarely encountered.

Developmental defects

Local anaesthetic agents are cytotoxic to the cells of the enamel organ. It is possible that the incorporation of these agents into the developing tooth-germ could cause developmental defects. There is experimental evidence that such defects can arise following intraligamental injections in primary teeth in animal models. Such occurrences in humans have not been reported. In addition to cytotoxic effects of the anaesthetic agent, it is possible that physical damage caused by the needle to permanent successors could result from the overenthusiastic use of intraligamentary anaesthesia in the primary dentition.

5.8 CONTRAINDICATIONS TO LOCAL ANAESTHESIA

In certain children some local anaesthetic materials will be contraindicated, in others specific techniques are not advised.

5.8.1 General

Immaturity

Very young children are not suited to treatment under local anaesthesia as they will not provide the degree of cooperation required for completion of treatment. A child who cannot differentiate between painful and non-painful stimuli (such as pressure) is unsuitable for treatment under local anaesthesia.

Mental or physical handicap

Local anaesthesia is contraindicated where the degree of handicap prevents cooperation.

Treatment factors

Certain factors related to the proposed treatment may contraindicate the use of local anaesthesia. These factors include duration and access. Prolonged treatment sessions, especially if some discomfort may be produced such as during surgical procedures, cannot satisfactorily be completed under local anaesthesia. It is unreasonable to expect a child to cooperate for more than 30–40 min under such circumstances even when sedated. Similarly, where access proves difficult or uncomfortable, for example, during biopsies of the posterior part of the tongue or soft palate, satisfactory cooperation may be impossible under local anaesthesia.

Acute infection

As mentioned above, acute infection reduces the efficacy of local anaesthetic solutions.

5.8.2 Specific agents

Allergy

Allergy to a specific agent or group of agents is an absolute contraindication to the use of that local anaesthetic. Cartridges containing latex in their bung must be avoided in those allergic to this material.

Medical conditions

Some medical conditions present relative contraindications to the use of some agents. For example, in liver disease the dose of amide local anaesthetics should be reduced. Ester local anaesthetics should be avoided in children who have a deficiency of the enzyme pseudocholinesterase.

Poor blood supply

The use of vasoconstrictor-containing local anaesthetic solutions should be avoided in areas where the blood supply has been compromised, for example after therapeutic irradiation.

5.8.3 Specific techniques

Bleeding diatheses

Injection into deep tissues should be avoided in patients with bleeding diatheses such as haemophilia. Inferior alveolar nerve block techniques should not be used unless appropriate prophylaxis has been provided (e.g. Factor VIII for those with haemophilia). This can be overcome by the use of intraligamentary injections in the mandible in such patients for restorative dentistry.

Susceptibility to endocarditis

Intraligamentary anaesthesia will produce a bacteraemia. In patients susceptible to endocarditis this method should not be used for procedures in which gingival manipulation would not normally be involved. This is because it is unreasonable to provide antibiotic prophylaxis for the anaesthetic when other methods of local anaesthesia can be employed. When antibiotic prophylaxis has been provided to cover the operative procedure then intraligamental injections can be employed.

Incomplete root formation

The use of intraligamental techniques for restorative procedures on permanent teeth with poorly formed roots could lead to avulsion of the tooth if inappropriate force is applied during the injection.

Trismus

Trismus will preclude the usual direct approach to the inferior alveolar nerve block.

Epilepsy

As seizure disorders can be triggered by pulsing stimuli (such as pulses of light) it is perhaps unwise to use electroanalgesia in children with epilepsy.

5.9 SUMMARY

1. Surface anaesthesia is best achieved with a topical agent on a cotton bud applied to dry mucosa for 5 min.
2. Buccal infiltration anaesthesia is successful in the maxilla.
3. Regional block anaesthesia is successful in the mandible.
4. Intraligamentary anaesthesia is successful in children. This method may be the first choice in the posterior mandible and as a supplementary technique in the maxilla.
5. Pain-free local anaesthesia in the maxilla is possible with buccal infiltration and by anaesthetizing the palate via the buccal papillae.
6. In the mandible, intraligamental techniques may be used to avoid the discomfort of regional block injections.
7. Complications of local anaesthesia are reduced by careful technique and sensible dose limitations.
8. Contraindications to local anaesthesia may be related to certain agents or to specific techniques.

5.10 FURTHER READING

Malamed, S. F. (1997). *Handbook of local anesthesia* (4th edn). Mosby, St Louis. (*An excellent reference book.*)

Meechan, J. G. (2002). *Practical dental local anaesthesia.* Quintessence Publishing Co Ltd, London (*A practical guide to the administration of local anaesthesia.*)

Moore, P. A. (1992). Preventing local anesthetic toxicity. *J Am Dent Assoc*, **123**, 60. (*A salutary case report of a paediatric local anaesthetic fatality.*)

5.11 REFERENCES

Meechan, J. G., Cole, B., and Welbury, R. R. (2001). The influence of two different dental local anaesthetic solutions on the haemodynamic responses of children undergoing restorative dentistry: a randomised, single-blind, split-mouth study. *Br Dent J*, **190**, 502–4.

Primosch, R. E. and Brooks, R. (2002). Influence of flow rate delivered by the Wand Local Anesthetic System on pain responses to palatal injections. *Am J Dent*, **15**, 15–20.

6

Diagnosis and prevention of dental caries

6 Diagnosis and prevention of dental caries

C. Deery and K. J. Toumba

6.1 DEVELOPMENT OF DENTAL CARIES

Almost all research on the process of dental caries supports the chemoparasitic theory proposed by W. D. Miller in 1890. This is now more commonly known as the acidogenic theory of caries aetiology. The main features of the caries process are:

(1) fermentation of carbohydrate to organic acids by micro-organisms in plaque on the tooth surface;

(2) rapid acid formation, which lowers the pH at the enamel surface below the level (the critical pH) at which enamel will dissolve;

(3) when carbohydrate is no longer available to the plaque micro-organisms, the pH within plaque will rise due to the outward diffusion of acids and their metabolism and neutralization in plaque, so that remineralization of enamel can occur; and

(4) dental caries progresses only when demineralization is greater than remineralization. The realization that demineralization and remineralization is an equilibrium is key to understanding the dynamics of the carious lesion and its prevention.

One of the interesting features of an early carious lesion of the enamel is that the lesion is subsurface; that is, most of the mineral loss occurs beneath a relatively intact enamel surface. This contrasts strongly with the histological appearance of enamel after a clean tooth surface has been exposed to acid, where the surface is etched and there is no subsurface lesion. This dissolution of the surface of enamel, or etching, is a feature of enamel erosion caused, among other things, by dietary acids. The explanation for the intact surface layer in enamel caries seems to lie in diffusion dynamics: the layer of dental plaque on the tooth surface acting as a partial barrier to diffusion. Further erosion occurs at much lower pHs (<4) than caries.

Dental plaque forms on uncleaned tooth surfaces and is readily apparent if toothbrushing is stopped for 2–3 days. Contrary to popular opinion, plaque does not consist of food debris, but comprises 70% micro-organisms—about 100 million organisms per milligram of plaque. When plaque is young, cocci predominate but as plaque ages the proportions of filamentous organisms and veillonellae increase. Diet influences the composition of the plaque flora considerably, with mutans streptococci much more numerous when the diet is rich in sugar and other carbohydrates, and these organisms are particularly good at metabolizing sugars to acids.

Knowledge of the dental caries process increased considerably with the development of pH electrodes, particularly microelectrodes that could be inserted into plaque before, during, and after the ingestion of various foods. The pioneer of this area of research was Robert Stephan, and the plot of plaque pH against time (Fig. 6.1) has become known as the Stephan curve. Within 2–3 min of eating sugar or rinsing with a sugar solution, plaque pH falls from an average of about 6.8 to near pH 5, taking about 40 min to return to its original value. Below pH 5.5 demineralization of the enamel occurs, this is known as the critical pH.

The clinical appearance of these early lesions is now well recognized (Figs 6.2–6.5). They appear as a white area that coincides with the distribution of plaque. This might

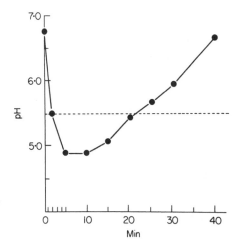

Fig. 6.1 Plot of the pH of dental plaque against time: this is commonly known as a Stephan curve. The curve was produced by rinsing with a 10% glucose solution. The dotted line represents a typical pH value below which enamel will dissolve (the critical pH). (Reproduced with permission from Jenkins 1978.).

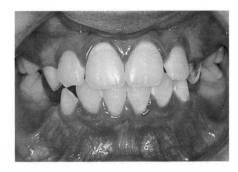

Fig. 6.2 Clinical appearance of precavitation carious lesions on the buccal surfaces of maxillary incisor teeth (white spot lesion).

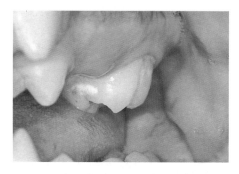

Fig. 6.3 Clinical appearance of a precavitation carious lesion on the mesial surface of a maxillary first molar tooth (brown spot lesion).

be around the gingival margin, as in Fig. 6.2, or between the teeth, as in Fig. 6.3. A histological section through a lesion such as that shown in Fig. 6.3 would look like Fig. 6.4 and a microradiograph like Fig. 6.5—in both the subsurface body of the lesion and surface zone can be seen clearly. If the process of dental caries continues, support for the surface layer will become so weak that it will crumble like an eggshell, creating a cavity. Once a cavity is formed, the process of dental caries continues in a more sheltered environment and the protein matrix of enamel and then dentine is removed by proteolytic enzymes produced by plaque organisms.

The progression of caries is traditionally described as enamel caries progressing through to the amelodentine junction at which the enamel breaks down and a cavity forms. Although it is now understood that the process is not this simple and cavitation can occur at an earlier stage—the enamel cavity and frequently at a much later stage when the caries has progressed significantly into dentine. Figure 6.6 shows the labial surface of a maxillary canine with a variety of stages of carious lesion ranging from white spot enamel caries to dentine cavity.

The ability of early carious lesions ('precavitation carious lesions') to remineralize is now well understood; periods of demineralization are interspersed with periods of remineralization, and the outcome—health or disease—is the result of a push in one direction or the other on this dynamic equilibrium. The shorter the time during which plaque-covered teeth are exposed to acid attack and the longer the time remineralization can occur, the greater is the opportunity for a carious lesion to heal. Satisfactory healing of the carious lesion can only occur if the surface layer is unbroken, and this is why the 'precavitation' stage in the process of dental caries is so relevant to preventive dentistry. Once the surface has been broken and a cavity has formed, it is usually necessary to restore the tooth surface with a filling. The carious process is driven by the plaque on the surface and therefore it is possible to arrest the caries by

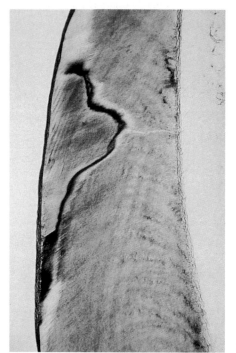

Fig. 6.4 Longitudinal ground section through a carious lesion of the type shown in Fig. 6.3 examined in water by polarized light: ×50. (Reproduced with permission from Soames and Southam, 1998.).

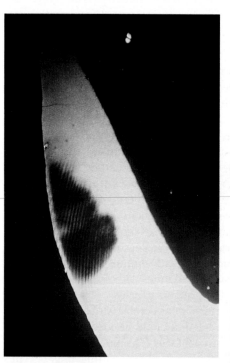

Fig. 6.5 Microradiograph of a longitudinal ground section through a lesion of the type shown in Figs 6.3 and 6.4. The body of the lesion shows marked radiolucency (loss of mineral) in contrast to sound enamel and the surface layer: ×70. (Reproduced with permission from Soames and Southam, 1998.).

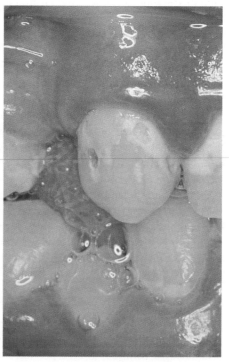

Fig. 6.6 Maxillary permanent canine tooth showing a variety of carious lesions ranging from white spot enamel caries to cavitated dentine caries.

effective removal of plaque even after cavitation has occurred. However, the lost tissue cannot be replaced.

The first stage of dental caries to be visible is the 'white spot' precavitation lesion stage. This can occur within a few weeks if conditions are favourable to its development. In the general population, though, it commonly takes 2–4 years for caries to progress through enamel into dentine at approximal sites.

The most important of the natural defences against dental caries is saliva. If salivary flow is impaired, dental caries can progress very rapidly. Saliva has many functions, which are listed in Table 6.1. The presence of food in the mouth is a powerful stimulus to salivation, with strong-tasting acid foods being the best stimulants. Saliva not only physically removes dietary substrates and acids produced by plaque from the mouth, but it has a most important role in buffering the pH in saliva and within plaque. Fast-flowing saliva is alkaline—reaching pH values of 7.5–8.0—and is vitally important in raising the pH of dental plaque previously lowered by exposure to sugar and carbohydrates. Because teeth consist largely of calcium and phosphate, the concentration of calcium and phosphate in saliva and plaque is thought to be important in determining the progression or regression of caries. Also, it is well known that fluoride aids the remineralization process. Although it may seem sensible to try to maximize the availability of calcium, phosphate, and fluoride in the environs of the tooth, in practice, fluoride is much the most important.

Table 6.1 The general functions of saliva

Digestive functions
  Assisting the mastication of food
  Forming a bolus
  Assisting in swallowing a bolus
  Taste perception
  Metabolism of starch

Protective functions
  Ensuring comfort through lubrication
  Preventing dessication of oral
    mucosa, gingivae, and lips
  Antimicrobial
    lavage
    bacteriostatic, bacteriocidal
    inhibiting adhesion of bacteria
    aggregation of bacteria
  Buffering
    within saliva
    within dental plaque
  Removal of toxins (including
    carcinogens)
  Aids speech

Key Points

Dental caries:

- occurs in plaque-covered areas frequently exposed to dietary carbohydrates;
- the initial lesion is subsurface before the thin surface layer collapses;
- the initial or pre-cavitation lesion is reversible;
- saliva plays an essential part in caries prevention;
- if all plaque is removed from the surface the carious process stops.

6.2 THE EPIDEMIOLOGY OF DENTAL CARIES

Dental caries is one of our most prevalent diseases and yet there is considerable variation in its occurrence between countries, regions within countries, areas within regions, and social and ethnic groups. One of the tasks of epidemiology is to record the level of disease and the variation between groups. A second task is to record changes in the levels of dental caries in populations over time, while a third task is to try to explain these variations.

The United Kingdom has one of the best series of national statistics on dental caries. The dental health of adults and children has been recorded every 10 years, beginning with the Adult Dental Health Survey of 1968 (Table 6.2).

The advantages of this series of surveys are:

1. They are national, using sound sampling methods to obtain representative samples of the populations.
2. They include both clinical and sociological data, giving the interaction between knowledge, attitude, behaviour, and disease.
3. The methods are well described and carefully standardized, resulting in meaningful longitudinal information.

Data on children at the ages of 5, 12, and 14 are also available through the annual studies conducted under the auspices of the British Association for the Study of Community Dentistry.

Table 6.2 National surveys of children's and adults' dental health in the United Kingdom

Children	
England and Wales	1973
United Kingdom*	1983
United Kingdom*	1993
United Kingdom*	2003
Adults	
England and Wales	1968
Scotland	1972
United Kingdom*	1978
United Kingdom*	1988
United Kingdom*	1998

* England, Wales, Scotland, and Northern Ireland.

The ravages of dental caries were so severe in the past that the extent of disease in a population was measured by the proportion of the population with no natural teeth or edentulousness. A marked decrease in the per cent edentulous between 1968 and 1998 was recorded, especially in adults aged 35–54 years. For younger people, it is common to record the prevalence (the proportion of people affected), the severity (number of teeth affected per person) of dental caries and the percentage of carious teeth restored (Care Index). The drastic improvement in these parameters in the UK between 1973 and 2003 is shown in Table 6.3. About half of all children are now clinically 'caries-free'. What is of concern is opinion that in the youngest age groups the improvement is not continuing, and indeed there are signs that caries experience is increasing in some areas. This is compounded by a decline in the Care Index in the UK.

A decline in caries, first noticed during the 1970s, has been recorded in a large number of industrialized countries. The dental health of older children continued to improve in the 1980s but caries experience in primary teeth, measured at ages 5 or 6 years, had stayed fairly constant. The Nordic countries used to have very high caries experience and the drastic improvement in all five Nordic countries can be seen in Fig. 6.7, although it occurred somewhat later in Iceland. One of the most dramatic improvements has been recorded in Switzerland where the mean DMFT (decayed, missing, filled teeth) in 12 year olds fell from 8.0 in 1964, to 5.1 in 1972, 3.0 in 1980, and to 1.1 in 1992. In 15 year olds it fell from 13.9 DMFT in 1964 to 2.2 DMFT in 1992. Caries experience in Australian children has been well recorded indicating a dramatic improvement in dental health (Fig. 6.8). Reports from North America indicate that caries prevalence and severity in the permanent dentition have continued to decline since 1982 in Canada and the United States, but that caries experience in the primary dentition may have stabilized since about 1986–7.

While dental surveys of schoolchildren have been quite common, there is much less information on the dental health of preschool children mainly because access to them is more difficult (Table 6.4). The prevalence and severity of dental caries in British preschool children was reviewed by Holt (1990), and in preschool children around the world by Holm (1990). In most European countries, North America, and Australia, caries experience has declined in parallel with the increasing use of fluoride toothpastes, although this decline appears to have stopped in the

Table 6.3 Decay experience of 5-year-old children (primary teeth), 12- and 14/15-year-old children (permanent teeth) in the UK (1973 England and Wales), as recorded in national surveys

	1973	1983	1993	2003
5 years olds				
Per cent affected	72	50	45	43
Mean dmft	4.0	1.8	1.7	1.6
Filled as a percentage of decay experience	–	28	17	15
12 years olds				
Per cent affected	93	81	52	34
Mean DMFT	4.8	3.1	1.4	0.8
Filled as a percentage of decay experience	–	70	58	69
14/15 year olds				
Per cent affected	96	93	63	49
Mean DMFT	7.4	5.9	2.5	1.6
Filled as a percentage of decay experience	–	74	57	77

dmft, DMFT: decayed, missing, and filled teeth.

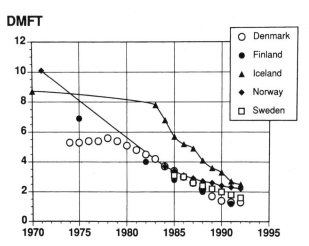

Fig. 6.7 Caries experience (DMFT) for 12-year-old children in Nordic countries (Reproduced from von der Fehr (1994) with kind permission of the *International Dental Journal*.).

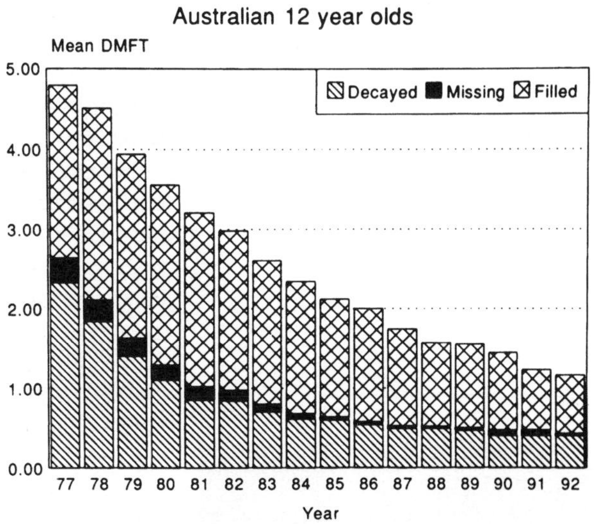

Fig. 6.8 Caries experience in Australian 12 year olds (Reproduced from Spencer *et al.* (1994) with kind permission of the *International Dental Journal*.).

United Kingdom. Caries experience of preschool children in South-East Asia, Central America, and parts of Africa is high and there are discernible trends of increasing prevalence in parallel with the rise in availability of sugar-containing snacks and drinks.

While the state of the permanent dentition in children has improved dramatically in many countries, caries in primary teeth is still a considerable problem in preschool and school-aged children. In industrialized countries, caries experience is highest in the more deprived groups of society and often in ethnic minority groups. In developing countries, the reverse social trend is observed, with the well-off, urban children having the most caries experience. Most of these variations in children's dental health can be explained in terms of the preventive role of fluoride and the caries-inducing role of sugary snacks. In adults, provision of dental services and patient preference for treatments can have a major effect on the state of the dentition, in addition to the aetiological and preventive roles of sugar, fermentable carbohydrates, and fluoride.

Table 6.4 Caries prevalence in UK preschool children in 1992/3

Age (years)	Prevalence (%)
1.5–2.5	4
2.5–3.5	14
3.5–4.5	30

Key Points

Dental caries

- Epidemiology indicates the size of the problem of caries and changes over time.
- Since 1968 there have been surveys every 10 years of adult's and children's dental health in the United Kingdom.
- Prevalence and extent have fallen markedly since the late 1970s in many countries, however, this decline appears to have ceased.
- Dental caries remains a significant problem.

6.3 CARIES DETECTION AND DIAGNOSIS

The presentation of caries has been described as resembling an iceberg with the clinically visual stages commencing with the white-spot lesion being above the waterline. Below the waterline lie the lesions which need the use of some form of additional aid to be identified. This can range from radiographs in the clinical situation to histopathology in the *in vitro* setting.

Caries diagnosis is difficult, it is a multi-stage process. Unfortunately, current training of undergraduate dental students and remuneration systems lead dentists frequently just to think of the diagnostic process as a treatment, that is, a dentinal carious lesion on the distal surface of a premolar being recorded as a DO amalgam.

The identification of caries depends on a systematic examination of clean dry teeth. The basic equipment consists of adequate lighting, compressed air for drying, dental mirror, and blunt or ball ended probe. The emphasis is on a visual examination, rather than a visual-tactile examination. Sharp probes which were traditionally used to aid diagnoses are contra-indicated for a number of reasons:

- The probe does not improve diagnosis—all a 'sticky' fissure means is that the probe fits the fissure.
- Probing a demineralized lesion will break the enamel matrix making remineralization impossible, thus creating an iatrogenic cavity.
- The probe may transfer cariogenic bacteria from one site to another, in effect inoculate caries free sites with cariogenic bacteria.

A ball-ended or blunt probe may be used gently to confirm the presence of cavitation, sealants, and restorations.

The first visible sign of caries is the white spot lesion, at first this can only be seen when the surface is dried (Fig. 6.9). This is because when demineralized enamel becomes porous, these pores contain water, if dried, the water in the pores is replaced with air and the lesion becomes more obvious. As the caries progresses the lesion will become obvious even when wet.

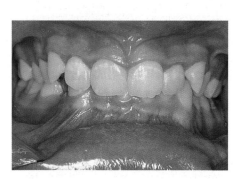

Fig. 6.9 Clinical appearance of white spot lesions on the labial and approximal surfaces of the upper permanent incisors.

Unfortunately active carious lesions are not the only causes of white areas on teeth; hypoplasia, fluorosis, and arrested hypermineralized carious lesions to name but a few can all mimic a white spot carious lesion. The decision as to the aetiology depends on factors such as site and surface characteristics. Caries tends to occur at predilection sites, therefore a white area at the gingival margin is much more likely to be caries than one of similar appearance at the incisal edge. Active carious lesions are matt white, while arrested lesions are glossy. A similar process is conducted for brown spot lesions.

Although large cavities are relatively easily identified dentine caries presents its own problems. On occlusal surfaces there may be no visible break in the surface, the evidence of caries being shadowing under the enamel. A similar picture is seen for approximal lesions.

Therefore as even the most thorough visual clinical examination will detect only some of the enamel and dentine carious lesions present, the clinician needs to be helped by diagnostic aids. The most commonly used of these are radiographs. The views which are of value for caries diagnosis are:

- bitewings,
- orthopantomogram (OPT),
- bimolars,
- periapicals.

Bitewings are the first choice view for caries diagnosis. These provide information on both occlusal dentine caries and approximal enamel and dentine caries. OPTs can detect the presence of an occlusal dentine carious lesion with a high degree of accuracy. OPTs have much less value in the detection of approximal lesions.

Bimolars are not as useful a view as bitewings because there is often overlap of structures. However, they are of use in the pre-cooperative child who will not cope with bitewings or an OPT. Periapicals are as accurate as bitewings for caries diagnosis but obviously less information is available on any one film.

As with the visual examination it is vital that the radiographs are viewed in a systematic way with appropriate illumination and ideal magnification.

Although not all children will tolerate them, bitewing radiographs should be considered for all children from the age of 4 years and above who are at risk of caries. The clinician should ask the question 'Why not take bitewings?' rather than 'Why take bitewings?'

The decision to take and the frequency of further radiographic examinations needs to be based on a thorough carious-risk assessment, the dentist having to balance the benefits of the additional diagnostic yield with the risks of exposure to ionizing radiation. Current guidelines from the Faculty of General Dental Practitioners UK (1998) suggest annually for the carious-active child and biennially for the child with controlled caries.

An interesting clinical phenomenon which may help the clinician decide if radiographs are warranted is the presence of a bleeding papilla, this suggesting the presence of an approximal cavity. This occurs because the cavity will be full of plaque, which together with driving the carious process on will cause gingivitis and thus the bleeding papilla.

Other diagnostic aids which may assist with approximal caries diagnosis include fibre-optic transillumination (FOTI) and temporary tooth separation (Fig. 6.10). FOTI consists of the placement of a 0.5 mm light source in the embrasure. If a carious lesion is present it will show as a dark shadow. Some studies have suggested that FOTI is as accurate as radiographs but the situation is confused by other studies which question the benefit of FOTI. Certainly if it is used FOTI provides the clinician with more information to base a decision on.

Temporary tooth separation consists of the placement of an orthodontic elastameric separator between the teeth (Fig. 6.11(a) and b)). The patient returns after 3–4 days, the teeth having separated allowing direct access for examination.

To assist with the diagnosis of occlusal carious lesions three adjuncts have been developed; FOTI as discussed above, laser fluorescence devices, and electronic caries meters.

Laser fluorescence devices measure the fluorescence of the tooth and of particular importance the fluorescence of bacterial by-products in the carious lesion (Fig. 6.12). This provides a digital reading indicating the status of the surface. Research on these devices is very promising but false readings are generated by staining, calculus, and hyperplasia. When used appropriately these provide a standardized, reproducible measure, which not only helps with the diagnostic decision but allows the possibility of monitoring over time.

Electronic caries meters also exist which measure the decrease in resistance of carious lesions compared to sound surfaces. When used meticulously these meters have shown good accuracy in clinical trials. The readings of electronic caries meters are confounded by areas of hyperplasia, immature teeth, and particularly moisture.

Key Points
The stages in caries diagnostic process

- Detect,
- Diagnose,
- Record.

6.4 PREVENTION OF DENTAL CARIES

The dramatic improvement in dental health, especially in children, in many developed countries during the past 20 years is proof that prevention works. Dental caries is not inevitable; the causes are well known, discouraging caries development and

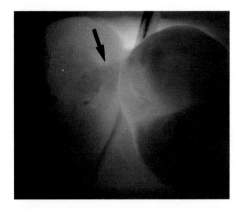

Fig. 6.10 FOTI of approximal surfaces of posterior permanent teeth. The arrow points to a shadow caused by an approximal carious lesion. (Illustration from Mitropoulos (1985) with kind permission of *Caries Research*.).

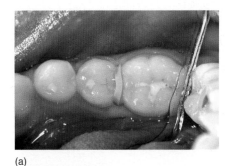

(a)

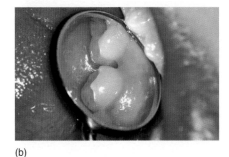

(b)

Fig. 6.11 (a) Temporary tooth separation, an elastomeric separator between a lower second premolar and first permanent molar. (b) The appearance after separation, showing access for examination of the approximal surfaces.

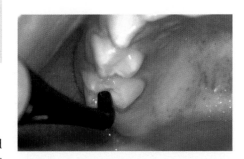

Fig. 6.12 The tip of a laser fluorescence device in place on the occlusal surface of a maxillary first permanent molar.

encouraging caries healing are realities to be grasped. Failure to do so is, at least, to provide second-class dental care.

There are four practical pillars to the prevention of dental caries: plaque control/toothbrushing, diet, fluoride, and fissure sealing. Each of these will be considered in turn before being brought together in treatment planning and in relation to caries-risk. Prevention of caries is so easy in theory but in practice involves many skills. The main reason for this is that control of the aetiological agents—plaque and fermentable carbohydrates—involve a change in behaviour. The value of fluoride is that it can be delivered in a variety of ways, some of which require minimal action by the patient. There is no 'magic bullet' that can be applied to teeth which will render them totally resistant to caries. Fissure sealants come close to this but they are expensive to apply, some fall off, and they only prevent caries of pits and fissures.

In dentistry there is no doubt that prevention is better than cure. Prevention of dental caries underpins all dental care provided to children. All children require preventive input. The type of input depends on the child and their caries risk. Forming a comprehensive treatment strategy, tailored to the needs of each individual child, is an essential component of all paediatric treatment planning.

Despite dental caries being a preventable disease epidemiological surveys in children in many countries have shown that the distribution of dental caries has become 'bimodal', with 80% of the disease present in only 20% of the child population. Consequently two approaches are required to improve dental health. This strategy will involve maintaining good dental health in those without dental decay, and secondly targeting resources to those that are at risk of developing decay. This means targeting the 'high caries-risk' groups comprising:

- the caries prone—especially early childhood caries (nursing bottle caries).
- the handicapped—medical and physical.
- the socially deprived, that is, low socio-economic groups.
- ethnic minority groups usually residing in inner city areas.

Low caries-risk children are those who are caries-free or have well-controlled caries, have good oral and dietary habits, are highly motivated and attend their dental appointments regularly.

It is thus important to institute effective preventive measures for children and advice for their patients. This is best achieved at treatment planning prior to commencing any restorative work (other than emergency and stabilizing procedures). It is also important to clarify what constitutes high and low caries-risk children (Chapter 3).

The mainstay of preventive measures are:

(1)   plaque control and regular toothbrushing with a fluoride toothpaste;
(2)   sensible dietary advice;
(3)   use of fluorides;
(4)   fissure sealants;
(5)   regular dental checks with appropriate radiographs.

All of these measures need to be co-ordinated and supervised by the dental team and reinforced with good patient and parental motivation.

6.4.1 Plaque control and toothbrushing

There are a number of plaque disclosing tablets and solutions available. Children need close supervision when using these agents and appropriate advice should be given to parents and guardians. Plaque charts can be used to monitor progress and to identify areas where cleaning is not ideal. It is customary to report the percentage number of clean surfaces so that patients aim to achieve as close to 100% clean as possible. After demonstrating the plaque disclosing procedure (Fig. 6.13) and performing the charting it is initially advisable to instruct patients to use the disclosing agent prior to toothbrushing. After 1 week it is advisable for patients to brush first and then disclose in order to identify areas that are being missed.

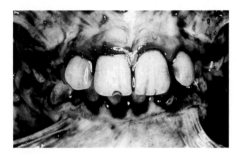

Fig. 6.13 Plaque disclosure of upper and lower dentition.

Toothbrushing

Advise regular toothbrushing with an appropriate concentration of fluoride toothpaste. Toothbrushing should become a routine and on at least two occasions every day. There are numerous types of brushes (manual and electric) and toothpastes available. Many brushes and pastes have cartoon characters etc., which can be good motivators for many children. Both manual (preferably with a small head) and electric brushes are equally effective for plaque removal. However, the cost of brushes and pastes can be prohibitive for some low socio-economic groups wherein reality toothbrushing has become a low priority. This is where community and school-based programmes are needed to ensure provision of oral health measures. Young children under 5 years need help with toothbrushing (Fig. 6.14). Children do not have the manual dexterity to brush their teeth effectively until they can tie their own shoelaces (about 7 years of age). However, even after this children should still be supervised to establish a regular routine and to ensure a good oral health practice. Only a small smear of fluoride toothpaste should be used up to 6 years of age. Fluoride is cleared quickly from the oral cavity that many advise to swish the toothpaste saliva slurry around the mouth and not to rinse with water in order to maintain elevated intra-oral fluoride levels for longer periods of time. A simple message for patients is 'brush your teeth first thing in the morning and last thing at night'.

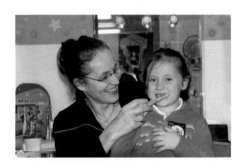

Fig. 6.14 Parent assisting toothbrushing of their young child's teeth.

As dental caries is caused by bacteria in plaque fermenting dietary carbohydrates to acids which dissolve enamel, it is logical to prevent caries by removing plaque from teeth, usually with a toothbrush. Unfortunately, many investigations indicate that caries reduction is not brought about by improved toothbrushing alone. However, it must be said straight away that, first, toothbrushing is a very important way of controlling gingivitis and periodontal disease and, second, that toothbrushing with toothpaste is a very important way of conveying fluoride to the tooth surface.

The results of the few studies to investigate the effect of flossing on dental caries are mixed. Daily flossing of the teeth of young children reduced caries in one study but no preventive effect was observed in older children who flossed their own teeth. Twenty-five years ago, in Kalstaad, Sweden, caries increments were virtually eliminated in children who had fortnightly prophylaxes and intensive preventive advice by dental hygienists. Other workers have tried to reproduce those sensational results (96% caries reduction compared with a control group) but have failed to do so, illustrating the difficulty of extrapolating findings of trials from one country to another.

Plaque growth can be prevented by twice-daily rinsing with chlorhexidine but because of the intra-oral side-effects of chlorhexidine (changed taste sensation, poor taste, and tooth staining), it is usually recommended for short-term use only to aid periodontal care.

6.4.2 Nutrition and diet in caries control

We are constantly eating and snacking and it is very important to be able to give sensible practical advice regarding diet and dental caries. Some consider that there are 'good foods' and 'bad foods' while others consider that there are 'good diets' and 'bad diets'. Further, some consider sugar to be the arch villain and enemy of dentistry. Caries has declined despite increased sales and consumption of sugars. However, the literature is controversial and there are many conflicting views and opinions regarding sugar consumption. The COMA report classified sugars as being either intrinsic

Table 6.5 Practical diet advice

- Confectionery and such foods should be used at mealtimes as a dessert rather than consumed between meals.
- Only milk or water should be given to children in a baby bottle.
- For the consumption of soft drinks the following recommendations should be followed:
  - Ideally serve only at meal times
  - Use a straw whenever possible
  - Never use on a dummy or as a comforter
  - Do not give at bedtime or during the night

(sugar within cell membrane, for example, fruits) or extrinsic (readily available sugars, for example, refined sugars). Are intrinsic sugars converted to extrinsic sugars on chewing? This is probably irrelevant, as bacteria need a fermentable source of carbohydrate to produce acid. The review paper of Burt and Pai (2001) summarizes the conflict in opinions on sugar. However, we should concentrate on giving sensible practical everyday advice to our patients as shown in Table 6.5. Advising parents to completely stop their children from eating sugary foods is not achievable! We should aim to ensure that our patients eat sensibly and safely. Baby drinks given in baby bottles led to 'nursing bottle' caries. Plaque pH responses of these drinks showed falls to below the critical pH of apatite (pH = 5.5). We should advise that only milk or water is given to children in a baby bottle. Many are not aware that no added sugar drinks contain natural sugar. We should promote that for young children drinks are consumed from trainer cups, beakers, and to use straws. 'Safer foods' have been recommended as alternatives for frequent snackers or nibblers. These alternatives include cheeses that have been shown to raise plaque pH. In addition to fruit and vegetables, crisps and peanuts have also been recommended as safer alternatives. However, citrus fruits have been implicated in the aetiology of dental erosion and peanuts are associated with inhalation risk in small children. The development of one 'safer' drink has been accredited by the British Dental Association (BDA) and showed that the plaque pH did not fall below the critical pH for enamel (Toumba and Duggal, 1999).

Frequency of eating

Frequency of eating has an important effect on teeth. However, is this anecdotal or based on scientific evidence? Eating meals leads to periods of acid attack when tooth mineral is lost. At the end of the meal or snack the acid is buffered by saliva and the mineral loss stops and reverses under favourable conditions. Frequent snackers have predominantly mineral loss and little if any remineralization. Duggal *et al.* (2001) demonstrated the importance of fluoride and frequency of sugar consumption in an *in situ* study using enamel slabs and transverse microradiography. When volunteers did not use a fluoride toothpaste mineral demineralization was observed with the frequency as low as three times per day. However, when fluoride toothpaste was used twice daily no significant mineral demineralization was observed up to a frequency of sugar consumption of seven times per day. Therefore, brushing twice per day with a fluoride toothpaste, subjects should safely be able to have five meal moments per day. This is a sensible and achievable dietary message for patients.

Non-sugar sweeteners

Those allowed for use in foods and drinks in the United Kingdom are given in Table 6.6. The list is very similar for most countries. There is much evidence that they are non-cariogenic or virtually so. The intense sweeteners and xylitol are non-cariogenic while the other bulk sweeteners can be metabolized by plaque bacteria but the

Table 6.6 Permitted sweeteners in foods (United Kingdom)

Bulk sweeteners
Sorbitol
Mannitol
Hydrogenated glucose syrup*
Isomalt*
Xylitol*
Lactitol[†]
Maltitol[‡]
Intense sweeteners
Saccharin
Acesulfame K*
Aspartame*
Thaumatin*

* Permitted 1982.
[†] Permitted 1988.
[‡] Permitted 1986.

rate is so slow that these sweeteners can be considered safe for teeth. The use of non-sugar sweeteners is growing rapidly particularly in confectionery and soft drinks. Confectionery products which have passed a well-established acidogenicity test can be labelled with the Mr Happy-Tooth logo (Fig. 6.15) which is a protected trademark, which informs the purchaser and consumer that these products are dentally safe. Tooth-friendly sweets are available in about 26 countries; in Switzerland about 20 per cent of confectionery sold carries the Tooth-friendly (or Mr Happy-Tooth) logo. There is good evidence that sugarless chewing gums are not only non-cariogenic but also positively prevent dental caries, by stimulating salivary flow. Indeed, xylitol gums are used in school-based preventive programmes in Finland. In the United Kingdom, the BDA accredits products which benefit oral health (Fig. 6.16). As an example, they have accredited dentrifices which have proven effectiveness, for many years. More recently, foods and drinks have been accredited—for example, a fruit-flavoured drink which demonstrated to have negligible cariogenic and erosive potential. The Tooth-friendly and BDA accreditation schemes help the consumer to make better choices. The bulk sweeteners can have a laxative effect and should not be given to children below 3 years of age. People vary in their sensitivity to these polyols as some adults in the Turku sugar studies were consuming up to 100 g of xylitol per day without effect.

Dietary advice for the prevention of dental caries

The basic advice is straightforward—reduce the frequency and amount of intake of fermentable carbohydrates. Dietary advice should be at two levels. First, every patient should receive basic advice. This especially applies to parents of young children who need to be given the correct advice at the appropriate age of the child. Dietary advice is often too negative; energy that has been provided by confectionery has to be replaced and it is very important to emphasize positive eating habits. The variety of foods available has increased enormously in most countries in recent years; we must use this increased choice to assist our patients to make better food choices. The second level of advice is a more thorough analysis of the diet of children with a caries problem. A well-accepted method is the 3-day diary record. One practical drawback of this method is that it requires at least three visits—an introductory visit where the patient is motivated and informed about the procedure and the diet diary given out, the diary collection visit, and a separate visit for advice and to agree targets. Each of these stages is important. At the first visit it is vital that the patient and parent appreciate that there is a dental problem and that you are offering your expert advice to help them overcome this problem. Once motivated they must understand how the diary is to be completed. Any requests by parents for advice at the first visit should be parried and delayed until the third visit. At the third visit, advice must be personal, practical, and positive—all three of these are important (Table 6.5). Food preference of children, cooking skills, food availability, and financial considerations vary enormously—advice must be personally tailored and practical for that patient. Positive advice has a much greater chance of acceptance than negative advice such as 'avoid this', 'don't eat that'—nagging is a de-motivator. Dietary changes are difficult, targets often have to be limited and constant reinforcement of advice and encouragement is essential. However, health gains can be considerable, to general as well as dental health and often to other members of the family, so that dietary advice is an essential part of care of children.

6.4.3 Fluoride and caries control

The use of fluorides date back to as early as 1874 when the German Erharde suggested the use of potassium fluoride tablets for expectant mothers and children in order to strengthen teeth. This recommendation was without any scientific evidence. What we

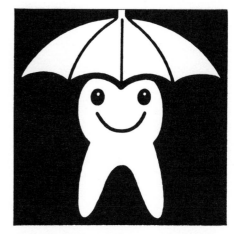

Fig. 6.15 Pictogram of Mr Happy-Tooth. This is the protected logo of the International Toothfriendly Association to be seen on products that have passed the internationally accepted toothfriendly test. (Reproduced by kind permission of the Association. Tooth friendly Sweets International, Hauptstrasse 63, CH-4102, Binningen 1, Switzerland.)

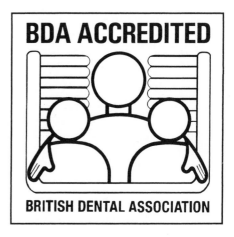

Fig. 6.16 BDA logo, which indicates that the product has been accredited by it (Reproduced by kind permission of the British Dental Association, Education and Science Department, British Dental Association, 64 Wimpole Street, London W1M 8YS.).

now know to be dental fluorosis (mottling) was noted by dentists long ago who reported on 'Colorado Stain' without the aetiology of the tooth defect being established.

Mode of action of fluoride and the caries process

The mineral of tooth tissues exists as a carbonated apatite, which contains calcium, phosphate, and hydroxyl ions, making it a hydroxyapatite $[Ca_{10} \cdot (PO_4)_6 \cdot (OH)_2]$. Carbonated portions weaken the structure and render the tissue susceptible to attack. Food remnants and debris mix with saliva and adhere to tooth surfaces as a slimy film known as dental plaque. Oral bacteria, and most importantly certain types of cariogenic bacteria (e.g. Mutans streptococci and Lactobacilli species), metabolize dental plaque and produce acid which lowers the pH of the oral environment. When the pH is below the critical pH for hydroxyapatite (<5.5), demineralization occurs with a net outward flow of calcium and phosphorous ions from the enamel surface into plaque and saliva. When the pH returns to 7.0, remineralization occurs with a net inward flow of ions into the enamel surface. If fluoride is present during remineralization, it is incorporated to form fluorapatite $[Ca_{10} \cdot (PO_4)_6 \cdot F_2]$, which is more stable and resistant to further acid attacks. The process of demineralization and remineralization is an ongoing one and frequently referred to as 'the ionic see-saw' or 'tug-of-war'. This is now widely believed to be the most important preventive action of fluoride, and a constant post-eruptive supply of ionic fluoride is thought to be most effective.

A number of mechanisms have been proposed to explain the action of fluoride (Table 6.7). The first is that fluoride has an effect during tooth formation by substitution of hydroxyl ions for fluoride ions, thereby reducing the solubility of the tooth tissues. Second, fluoride can inhibit plaque bacterial growth and glycolysis. At pH 7.0, fluoride ions are precluded from entering bacteria. However, at pH 5.0, fluoride exists as hydrofluoric acid, which crosses the bacterial cell membrane to interfere with its metabolism, by specifically inhibiting the enzyme enolase in the glycolytic pathway. Third fluoride inhibits the demineralization of tooth mineral when present in solution at the tooth surface. Fourth, fluoride enhances remineralization by combining with calcium and phosphate to form fluorapatite. Fluoride enhances crystal growth, stabilizes and makes the tissue resistant to further acid attack. Enamel apatite demineralizes when the pH drops to pH 5.5. However, when fluorapatite is formed during remineralization, it is even more resistant to demineralization as the critical pH for fluorapatite is pH 3.5. Therefore, it is most important to have an intraoral source of fluoride when remineralization is taking place. Lastly, fluoride affects the morphology of the crown of the tooth, making the coronal pits and fissures shallower. Such shallower pits and fissures will be less likely to collect food debris, allow stagnation and become decayed. The most important of these mechanisms is that when fluoride is present in the oral environment at the time of the acid attack it inhibits demineralization and promotes remineralization.

As early as 1890, Miller drew attention to the dissolutive process of dental caries and directed efforts to inhibit dissolution. The clinical findings of the anti-caries activity of drinking water with fluoride caused researchers to seek reasons for this. The finding

Table 6.7   Mechanisms of action of fluoride

1. It has an effect during tooth formation making the enamel crystals larger and more stable.
2. It inhibits plaque bacteria by blocking the enzyme enolase during glycolysis.
3. It inhibits demineralization when in solution.
4. It enhances remineralization by forming fluorapatite when in solution.
5. It affects the crown morphology making the pits and fissures shallower and hence less likely to create stagnation areas.

that fluoride-treated enamel had a lower solubility led many to consider this as a cause and effect relationship. The anti-caries action of fluoride was thought to be one of preventing dissolution of enamel, and efforts were made to incorporate more and more amounts of fluoride into surface enamel. The first topical agent used, after water fluoridation, was a 2% sodium fluoride solution and there was a greater uptake of fluoride into enamel from acidified solutions. Numerous fluoride preparations with varying concentrations of fluoride were employed for topical application and used as anticaries agents. It was noted that there was not much difference in the caries reductions reported from the topical fluoride studies despite great variations in the fluoride concentrations used. In addition, the difference in the levels of fluoride in surface enamel of residents of fluoridated and non-fluoridated areas was limited. Therefore, it is difficult to explain the 50% reduction of caries observed, on the basis of the fluoride level in the surface enamel. Furthermore, there has been no study to show any clear-cut inverse relationship between fluoride content of surface enamel and dental caries.

All the available evidence is that caries results from the presence of an acidogenic plaque on elements of the tooth mineral. The diffusion of acidic components into the tooth mineral is accompanied by the reverse diffusion of components of the mineral. During the carious process there is a preferential loss of calcium, accompanied by dissolution of magnesium and carbonate. The first clinical sign of enamel caries is the so-called 'white spot' lesion, where an apparently sound surface overlies an area of decalcification. The remineralization effect of fluoride has since come into favour. It has been reported that attacked enamel could re-harden on exposure to saliva and that softened enamel could be re-hardened by solutions of calcium phosphates *in vitro*. However, it is now known that it is the presence of fluoride in the oral cavity, and in particular, its presence in the liquid phase at the enamel-plaque interface, that is of most importance.

In the past it was thought that the systemic action of fluoride was important for caries prevention. This view has completely changed and it is now known that it is the topical action of fluoride that is essential for caries prevention. It is the presence of fluoride in the liquid phase at the plaque-enamel interface that is of most importance. Studies have shown that even low levels of fluoride (0.10 ppm) were effective in preventing the dissolution of enamel. It has been stated that the activity of the fluoride ion in the oral fluid that is important in reducing the solubility of the enamel rather than a high content of fluoride in the enamel. Saliva, the fluid that bathes the teeth has been extensively studied. The level of fluoride in saliva is thought to be important for caries prevention and it has been shown that caries susceptible subjects had salivary fluoride levels of <0.02 ppm, whereas caries resistant subjects had levels of >0.04 ppm.

Key Points

Fluorides

- It is the activity of the fluoride ion in the oral fluid that is of most importance in reducing enamel solubility rather than having a high content of fluoride in surface enamel.
- A constant supply of low levels of intraoral fluoride, particularly at the saliva/plaque/enamel interface, is of most benefit in preventing dental caries.

There are a vast number of fluoride products that are available for systemic and topical use. They can be applied professionally by the dental team or by the patient at home.

Water fluoridation

This is a systemic method of providing fluoride on a community basis. Over 300 million people worldwide receive naturally or artificially fluoridated water. 1.0 ppm fluoride was shown by Dean to be the optimum level in 1942. This was in a pre-fluoride era and perhaps the optimum level needs to be reviewed. There have been 113 studies in 23 countries over the last 60 years showing that dental caries is reduced by 50%. It is cheap and cost-effective but there are opponents to its use.

Fluoride supplements

These are in the form of tablets and drops. Caries reductions vary from 20% to 80%. There is usually very poor patient compliance especially for high-caries risk groups. A 'Catch 22' situation is the case in that those patients that are compliant do not need supplements whereas those that will benefit will not take them. The doses vary worldwide and are being increasingly held responsible for the rise in fluorosis. The fluoride supplement doses depend on the age of the patient and the level of fluoride in the drinking water. No supplements should be prescribed if the water fluoride level is greater than 0.7 ppm. The European view on supplements is that they have no role as a public health measure, and when they are prescribed 0.5 mg per day should be the maximum dose. The tablets should be allowed to dissolve slowly in the mouth, thus providing a topical application of fluoride to the teeth.

Other methods for providing systemic fluoride

There are of course other systemic methods for providing fluoride to the community. These are:

(1)   salt—50% caries reductions in Switzerland and Hungary;
(2)   milk—15–65% caries reductions;
(3)   mineral Water—46% caries reductions in Bulgaria.

Are we therefore receiving more than the optimum daily amount of fluoride and therefore at increased risk of fluorosis? Are there other hidden sources of fluoride? Mineral waters are used extensively as the main source of household drinking water. The fluoride levels of bottled waters vary considerably from 0.0 to 2.0 ppm mainly, but can be as high as 10.0–13.0 ppm in some countries. Therefore, before prescribing fluoride supplements we must first determine the fluoride level of the patient's drinking water, be that tap or bottled water. In addition some baby milk formulas have high amounts of fluoride themselves, and if made up with a high fluoride bottled water the infant may be at increased risk of developing dental fluorosis. The maxillary permanent central incisors are most susceptible to fluorosis at about 2 years of age. On the continent fluoride chewing gum is available providing 0.25 mg fluoride per stick of gum. Some foods, for example, fish and tea have high fluoride contents. We also ingest fluoride from sources without realizing it. The 'Halo Effect' is the term used to describe the ingestion of fluoride from hidden sources. For example, fizzy drinks like 'pepsi' or 'coca-cola' may contain fluoride if the bottling plant is in a fluoridated area and therefore uses fluoridated water. The 'fluoridated' drinks may be transported to non-fluoridated areas. The same applies to foods that are processed and canned or packaged in plants using fluoridated water.

Toothpastes

A dramatic decrease in worldwide caries levels has been seen since their introduction in the early 1970s. They usually contain 1000 or 1450 ppm fluoride. The fluoride is either sodium fluoride or sodium monofluorophosphate (MFP) or a combination of both. There are many different brands to suit all tastes. Child formulations contain up to 550 ppm fluoride to limit fluoride ingestion and therefore reduce the risk of fluorosis. There are limited studies on the efficacy of child formulations on caries. A systematic review of low fluoride toothpastes showed a reduced efficacy of 250 ppm fluoride in comparison to 1000 ppm fluoride. Therefore, it is advisable to recommend toothpastes for children containing at least 500 ppm fluoride to ensure caries preventive efficacy. It is sometimes difficult to decide which concentration of fluoride toothpaste is to be recommended to parents for their children. There is a balance between caries-risk and fluorosis-risk. If the child is caries-free, low fluoride (500 ppm F) children's pastes can be recommended to minimize the risk of fluorosis. However, if a young child under 6 years presents with caries, a fluoride toothpaste of at least 1000 ppm is indicated as these have been proven to be more efficacious for caries prevention.

Fluoride gels

These can be applied in trays or by brush and 26% caries reductions have been reported. They are high in fluoride (1.23% = 12,300 ppm) for professional use and lower (1000 ppm) for home use. There is a risk of toxicity with the high fluoride containing gels and the following safety recommendations should be followed:

(1) no more than 2 ml per tray;
(2) sit patient upright with head inclined forward;
(3) use a saliva ejector;
(4) instruct the patient to spit out for 30 s after the procedure (usually 4 mins but newer types are for 1 min).
(5) Do not use for children under 6 years.

Home use gels contain 1000–5000 ppm fluoride for use by patients at home at bedtime in addition to toothbrushing. Thirty-six percent caries reductions have been reported.

Fluoride mouth rinses

These can be either daily rinses containing 0.05% (225 ppm) or weekly rinses 0.20% (900 ppm) of sodium fluoride. It is best to advise patients to use their fluoride rinses at a different time to toothbrushing so that the number of fluoride exposures increases. Caries reductions of 20–50% have been reported for fluoride rinse studies. The effect of toothbrushing and rinsing with fluoride has been shown to be additive. All orthodontic patients should be using a daily fluoride rinse to minimize the risk of demineralization and white spot lesions. Children under the age of 6 years should not be recommended to use fluoride mouth rinses due to the increased risk of swallowing the product.

Varnishes

Duraphat 5% by wt fluoride = 22,600 ppm fluoride is the main fluoride varnish. This has a very high fluoride concentration. It is supplied in a small tube, but used lavishly by most dentists as if it were toothpaste. Again there is the possibility of toxicity with young children. It should be used sparingly with a cotton bud, a small pea-size amount is sufficient for a full mouth application in children up to 6 years. Caries reductions of 50–70% have been reported in Scandinavian studies.

Slow-release fluoride devices

Many dental materials like amalgam, composites, cements, acrylics, and fissure sealants have had fluoride added, but the fluoride release was either short term or the properties of the materials were adversely affected, to make them of any use to provide a long-term source of intraoral fluoride. Glass ionomer cements are a group of materials that have fluoride, but long-term release is debatable. Some researchers have reported that these materials have a fluoride 'recharging' capacity. That is when the fluoride is released from the material it later takes up fluoride from other dental products that are used by the patient, for example, fluoride toothpaste or mouth rinse, and this fluoride is released at a later time. The very latest fluoride

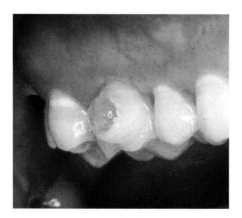

Fig. 6.17 A fluoride slow-release glass device attached to the buccal surface of the upper right first permanent molar tooth.

research is with slow-release devices. The objective is to develop an intraoral device that will release a constant supply of fluoride over a period of at least a year. The fluoride glass slow-release devices (Fig. 6.17) were developed at Leeds and shown to release fluoride for at least 2 years. Studies in Leeds demonstrated that there were 67% fewer new carious teeth and 76% fewer new carious surfaces in high caries-risk children after 2 years in a clinical caries trial for children with the fluoride devices in comparison to the control group with placebo devices. There were 55% fewer new occlusal fissure carious cavities showing that occlusal surfaces were also protected by the fluoride released from the devices. The fluoride glass devices release low levels of fluoride for at least 2 years and have great potential for use in preventing dental caries in high 'caries-risk' groups and irregular dental attenders. The fluoride glass devices have been patented and commercial development is now under progress. The provision of fluoride for each individual must be tailor-made to suit varying social and working circumstances. Slow-release fluoride devices seem ideal for targeting the high caries-risk groups who are notoriously bad dental attenders with very poor oral hygiene and motivation. This is a very promising development with application for use in numerous high-risk groups including the medically compromised.

Deciding which fluoride preparation to use for differing clinical situations:

This will depend on:

(1)   Which groups of children?
(2)   Which fluoride preparation?
(3)   Daily or weekly use?
(4)   Topical or systemic application?

In addition, the expected patient/parent motivation and compliance is very important in deciding what to use. Each individual patient will require a 'tailor-made' fluoride regime, and the dentist will need to use his expertise and knowledge of each patient in formulating individual fluoride regimes and preventive treatment plans. Table 6.8 gives some suggestions for some different clinical situations.

Table 6.8   Suggestions for fluoride use in some different clinical situations

Caries 0–6yrs:
   F toothpaste (1000+ ppm F)
   F supplements (0.5 mg/day)
   F varnish every 6 months.
	Caries 6+yrs:
	   F toothpaste (1000+ ppm F)
	   F supplements (1.0 mg/day)
	   APF gels or F varnish every 6 months.
	   Home use fluoride gels or fluoride daily rinse

Rampant caries 0–6yrs:
   F toothpaste (1000+ ppm F)
   F supplements (0.5 mg/day)
   F varnish every 3 months
	Rampant caries 6+yrs:
	   F toothpaste (1000+ ppm F)
	   F supplements (1.0 mg/day)
	   APF gels or F varnish every 3 months
	   Home use fluoride gels or fluoride daily rinse

Caries free 0–6yrs:
   Low fluoride toothpaste (500 ppm F)
	Caries free 6+yrs:
	   F toothpaste (1000+ ppm F)
	   Home use fluoride gels or fluoride daily rinse

Orthodontic cases:
   F toothpaste
   Daily fluoride rinse
	Erosion cases:
	   F toothpaste
	   F varnish
	   Daily fluoride rinse

6.4.4 Fissure sealing

Pit and fissure sealants (sealants) have been described as materials which are applied in order to obliterate the fissures and remove the sheltered environment in which caries may thrive. Initially developed to prevent caries their use has been developed further and they now have a place in the treatment of caries.

The decline in caries observed in industrialized countries over recent decades has affected all tooth surfaces but has been greatest on smooth surfaces. Therefore the pit and fissured surfaces, particularly of the molars have the greatest disease susceptibility. This means that the potential benefits of effectively used sealants continue to increase.

The technique for placement of sealants is relatively simple but is technique sensitive. Salivary contamination of as little as half a second can affect the bond and therefore the retention of the sealant.

Several sealant materials are available but the most effective is bis-GMA resin. Current resin materials are either autopolymerizing or photo-initiated, and most operators prefer the advantages of demand set offered by photo-initiation. Although there are theoretical advantages to chemically cured materials in terms of retention, as these materials have longer resin tags extending into the etched surface. Filled and unfilled resins are available, the filled materials being produced to provide greater wear resistance. However, this is not clinically relevant and clinical trials demonstrate superior efficacy for unfilled materials. Irrespective of the presence of fillers some materials are opaque or tinted to aid evaluation. This is an advantage but means the clinician is unable to view the enamel surface to assist with caries detection and to detect the presence of restorations such as sealant restorations.

Key Points

Fissure sealing technique

- Prophylaxis before etching does not enhance retention but is advisable if abundant plaque is present. A dry brush should be used rather than paste as these are retained in the depths of the fissures preventing penetration of the resin.
- Isolate the tooth surface,
- Etch for 20–30 s with 37% phosphoric acid,
- Wash and dry the surface maintaining isolation,
- Apply the resin,
- Cure,
- Check for adequacy.

Isolation is critical to successful sealant application. Operator and assistant must act as a team as it is impossible for single operators to apply sealant effectively. The vast majority of trials have demonstrated cotton wool and suction to be an effective means of isolation. Rubber dam is advocated by some because of the superior isolation offered by this material. This is probably true but its use is frequently not possible because of the stage of eruption of the tooth or level of co-operation of the patient. It would be inappropriate to delay sealant application to allow further eruption to permit the application of rubber dam. The application of sealant is a relatively non-invasive technique, frequently used to acclimatize a patient. It is difficult to justify the use of rubber dam with the associated use of local anaesthetic and clamps for the majority of patients, on both clinical and economic grounds.

Glass ionomers have also been used as sealants, the application technique is less sensitive, than that for resins. Unfortunately glass ionomer sealants have poor retention. It is suggested that the fluoride release from glass ionomers provides additional protection but the clinical relevance of this remains doubtful. The addition of fluoride to resin sealants has been demonstrated to provide no additional benefit. Glass ionomer sealants only have a place as temporary sealants during tooth eruption, when adequate isolation to permit the application of resin is not possible or in patients whose level of anxiety or co-operation similarly prevent placement of resin. Glass ionomers have been developed specifically for this role but clinical evidence of their effectiveness is not yet available.

Key Points

Application of glass ionomer sealants

- Clean the surface
- Isolate the tooth
- Run the glass ionomer into the fissures
- Protect the material during initial setting
- Apply unfilled resin, petroleum jelly, or fluoride varnish to protect the material.

For anxious patients application can be done with a gloved finger until the material is set.

Resin fissure sealants are effective; a recent systematic review has demonstrated 57% caries reductions at 4 years, with retention of 71–85% at 2 years falling to 52% at 4 years (Ahovuo-Saloranta *et al.*, 2004). To gain the full caries preventive benefit sealants should be maintained, that is, sealants with less than optimal coverage identified and additional resin applied.

Since the development of sealants there has been a question regarding the effect of sealing over caries, the concern being that caries will progress unidentified under the sealant. Given the difficulty in diagnosing caries this must be a frequent occurrence in daily practice. A number of trials have examined this by actively sealing over caries, and all have shown that sealants arrest or slow the rate of caries progression. We are not at the point where sealing of active caries is recommended by most authorities but the maxim if in doubt seal is good advice. The surface should then be monitored clinically and radiographically at regular intervals until its status is confirmed. One instance where actively sealing over caries is to be recommended is in the pre-cooperative patient where the placement of sealant may help acclimatization of the patient, with the added benefit of controlling the caries, until a definitive restoration can be placed.

Sealants are also effective at preventing pit and fissure caries in primary teeth. Primary teeth have more aprismatic enamel than permanent teeth, and doubt about the effectiveness of etching deciduous enamel lead to a belief that they required prolonged etching times. This has been demonstrated not to be the case and the technique for sealant application to primary teeth is identical to that employed with permanent teeth.

Although the effectiveness of fissure sealants is beyond doubt, to be used cost effectively their use should be targeted. Guidelines for patient selection and tooth selection have been published by the British Society for Paediatric Dentistry, and these are summarized below.

Patient selection

1. Children with special needs. Fissure sealing of all occlusal surfaces of permanent teeth should be considered for those who are medically compromised, physically or mentally disabled, or have learning difficulties, or for those from a disadvantaged social background.
2. Children with extensive caries in their primary teeth should have all permanent molars sealed soon after their eruption.
3. Children with carious-free primary dentitions do not need to have first permanent molars sealed routinely; rather these teeth should be reviewed at regular intervals.

Tooth selection

1. Fissure sealants have the greatest benefit on the occlusal surfaces of permanent molar teeth. Other surfaces should not be neglected, in particular the cingulum pits of upper incisors, the buccal pits of lower molars, and the palatal pits of upper molars.

2. Sealants should normally be applied as soon as the selected tooth has erupted sufficiently to permit moisture control.

3. Any child with occlusal caries in one first permanent molar should have the fissures of the sound first permanent molars sealed.

4. Occlusal caries affecting one or more first permanent molars indicates a need to seal the second permanent molars as soon as they have erupted sufficiently.

Since their development in the mid-1960s there have been a number of advances in sealant technology. We are possibly at another time of change with the development of non-rinse bonding. There is evidence that the use of bonding agents during sealant placement helps reduce the effect on retention of slight salivary contamination. There is also one small trial showing that sealants placed with non-rinse bonding are as retentive as those placed following traditional acid etching. Further larger trials are required to confirm this but the advantages in ease of placement are obvious if this proves to be the case (Fig. 6.18).

6.5 TREATMENT PLANNING FOR CARIES PREVENTION

The above summaries of the various methods of preventing dental caries have highlighted the advantages and disadvantages of the four practical methods of caries prevention: diet, fluoride, fissure sealing, and plaque control. Each is capable of preventing caries, but achieving changes in diet and toothbrushing, undertaking fissure sealing, and applying fluoride in the dental chair are all time-consuming. It is unrealistic to attempt to use each method to its maximum potential and it is necessary to agree an overall philosophy. Everyone should receive some advice in caries prevention and those perceived to be at greater risk of and from dental caries should receive a more thorough investigation and preventive treatment plan.

Four clear preventive messages are promoted by the Health Education Authority (HEA) in England (Table 6.9). This is the minimum advice. Parents of infants and young children should be advised on sensible eating habits; the abuse of sugar-containing fruit-flavoured drinks and the need for meals which will reduce the demand for snacks. Toothbrushing should be observed in the surgery giving an opportunity to discuss the type of toothbrush and toothpaste. Some patients are more likely to develop dental caries than others, and these patients need more aggressive preventive advice and therapy. Effective toothbrushing with an appropriate fluoride toothpaste is an essential first goal. Other forms of fluoride therapy should be considered, as outlined above: drops/tablets (if the drinking water is fluoride deficient), mouth rinses,

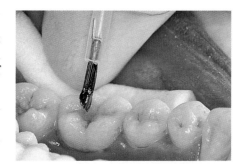

(a)

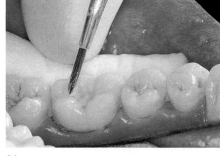

(b)

Fig. 6.18 Fissure sealant placement on a first permanent molar tooth. (a) Etching gel applied with a brush; (b) fissure sealant application after washing and drying.

Table 6.9 The scientific basis of dental health education

Summary

1. Reduce the consumption, and especially the frequency of intake, of sugar-containing food and drink and very acid drinks.
2. Clean the teeth thoroughly every day with a fluoride toothpaste.
3. Request your local water company to supply water with the optimum fluoride level.
4. Have an oral examination every year.

Health Education Authority (1996).

and topical applications of solutions, gel or varnish. Dietary habits should be investigated using a 3-day diet diary and appropriate advice given that is personal, practical, and positive. As toothbrushing, rinsing, and dietary control all require changes in life-style especially at home, continuous encouragement is essential. Fissure sealing is likely to be sensible, in line with the guidelines set out above.

The order in which the various carious preventive measures are scheduled in the treatment plan is of some importance. It is sensible to investigate toothbrushing early, as it is a good bridge between the home and the dental surgery and it gives proper emphasis to this vital preventive measure. If done first, it allows you to work on clean teeth. As investigation of diet and dietary advice requires at least three visits, it is sensible to introduce this at an early appointment. Fissure sealing can be commenced early in the treatment plan as a relatively easy procedure giving emphasis to prevention rather than restoration, while topical fluoride therapy could be carried out after fissure sealing. If fluoride dietary supplements and/or mouth rinses are going to be recommended, it is sensible to introduce them on the first or second appointment so that continuous encouragement in their use might be given at later appointments. The above intensive preventive therapy is for patients 'at risk' of developing caries. This begs the question on how to predict future caries development. There has been much work on this topic with many risk factors or markers of caries risk proposed. Overall, the findings are not encouraging. The most successful are: past caries experience, saliva properties (flow rate, buffering power, and microbiological content), and social status. These can be used in combination to increase discriminatory power. Despite much work, one large American investigation showed that the best predictor of future caries increment in children was 'intuition of the dentist'.

6.6 SUMMARY

1. Dental caries is caused by dietary carbohydrates being fermented by plaque bacteria to acid.
2. Caries detection and diagnosis requires a meticulous systematic approach.
3. The pre-cavitation lesion is a danger sign indicating the need for prevention.
4. The four practical pillars to caries prevention are: toothbrushing, diet, fluoride, and fissure sealing.
5. Preventive advice must be to parent and child and should be appropriate to the age and circumstances of the child.
6. Motivation and continuous encouragement is essential if prevention is to be successful.

6.7 ACKNOWLEDGEMENT

Some parts of this text have been reproduced from Dental Update, by permission of George Warman Publications.

6.8 FURTHER READING

Ashley, P. F., Blinkhorn, A. S., and Davies, R. M. (1998). Occlusal caries diagnosis: an in vitro histological validation of the Electronic Caries Monitor (ECM) and other methods. *Journal of Dentistry*, **26**, 83–8.

British Society of Paediatric Dentistry. (2000). A policy document on fissure sealants. *International Journal of Paediatric Dentistry*, **10**, 174–7.

Ekstrand, K. R., Ricketts, D. N., and Kidd, E. A. (2001). Occlusal caries: pathology, diagnosis and logical management. *Dental Update*, **28**, 380–7.

Feigal, R. J. (2002). The use of pit and fissure sealants. *Pediatric Dentistry*, **24**, 415–22.

Kidd, E. A. M. and Joyston-Bechal, S. (1996). *Essentials of dental caries*. (2nd edn.) Oxford University Press, Oxford.

Lussi, A., Imwinkelried, S., Pitts, N. B., Longbottom, C., and Reich, E. (1999). Performance and reproducibility of a laser fluorescence system for detection of occlusal caries in vitro. *Caries Research*, **33**, 261–6.

Marinho, V. C. C., Higgins, J. P. T., Sheiham, A., and Logan, S. (2004). Combinations of topical fluoride (toothpastes, mouthrinses, gels, varnishes) versus single topical fluoride for preventing dental caries in children and adolescents. *The Cochrane Database of Systematic Reviews* 2004, Issue 1. Art. No.: CD002781.pub2.DOI:10.1002/14651858.CD002781.pub2.

Naylor, M. N. (1994). Second international conference on declining caries. *International Dental Journal*, **44** (Suppl. 1), 363–458.

Nyvad, B., ten Cate, J. M., Robinson, C., (eds.) (2004). Cariology in the 21st Century. *Caries Research*, **38**, 167–329.

Rugg-Gunn, A. J., Nunn, J. H. (1999). Nutrition, diet and dental health. Oxford University Press, Oxford.

Scottish Intercollegiate Guidelines Network National Guideline 47. (2000). *Preventing dental caries in high risk children*. Royal College of Physicians, Edinburgh.

Scottish Intercollegiate Guidelines Network National Guideline. (2005). *Preventing dental caries in the pre-school child*. Royal College of Physicians, Edinburgh: 2005 (in press).

Selection Criteria for Dental Radiography. Produced by the Faculty of General Dental Practitioners (UK) 1998.

6.9 REFERENCES

Ahovuo-Saloranta, A., Hiirri, A., Nordblad, A., Worthington, H., and Makela, M. (2004). Pit and fissure sealants for preventing dental decay in the permanent teeth of children and adolescents. *The Cochrane Database of Systematic Reviews* 2004, Issue 3. Art. No.: CD001830.pub2.DOI:10.1002/14651858.CD001830.pub2.

Axelsson, P., Lindhe, J., and Waseby, J. (1976). The effect of various plaque control measures on gingivitis and caries in schoolchildren. *Community Dentistry Oral epidemiology*, **4**, 232–9.

Burt, B. A., Pai, S. (2001). Sugar consumption and caries risk: A systematic review. *Journal of Detal Education*, **65**, 1017–23.

Duggal, M. S., Toumba, K. J., Amaechi, B. T., Kowash, M. B., and Higham, S. M. (2001). Enamel demineralisation *in situ* with various frequencies of carbohydrate consumption with and without fluoride toothpaste. *Journal of Detal Research*, **80**, 1721–4.

Ekstrand, K. R., Bruun, G., and Bruun, M. (1998). Plaque and gingival status as indicators for caries progression on approximal surfaces. *Caries Research*, **32**, 41–5.

Holm, A. K. (1990). Caries in the preschool child; international trends. *Journal of Dentistry*, **18**, 291–5.

Holt, R. D. (1990). Caries in the pre-school child: British trends. *Journal of Dentistry*, **18**, 296–9.

Jenkins, G. N. (1978). *The physiology and biochemistry of the mouth*. (4th edn). Blackwell, Oxford.

Soames, J. V. and Southam, J. C. (1998). *Oral pathology* (3rd edn). Oxford University Press, Oxford.

Spencer, A. J., Davies, M., Slade, G., and Brennan, D. (1994). Caries prevalence in Australasia. *International Dental Journal*, **44**, 415–23.

Toumba, K. J. and Duggal, M. S. (1999). Effect on plaque pH of fruit drinks with reduced carbohydrate content. *British Dental Journal*, **186**, 626–9.

Toumba, K. J. (2001). Slow-release devices for fluoride delivery to high-risk individuals. *Caries Research*, **35** (Suppl. 1), 10–13.

von der Fehr, F. R. (1994). Caries prevalence in the Nordic countries. *International Dental Journal*, **44**, 371–8.

7

Treatment of dental caries in the preschool child

7 Treatment of dental caries in the preschool child

S. A. Fayle

7.1 INTRODUCTION

Dental caries is still one of the most prevalent pathological conditions in the child population of most Western countries. A UK study of 1.5–4.5-year-old children demonstrated that 17% have decay, and in many parts of the UK up to 50% of the child population has experience of decay by the time they are 5 years of age. Successfully managing decay in very young children presents the dentist with a number of significant challenges. This chapter will outline approaches to the management of the preschool child with dental caries.

> **Key Points**
> - Dental caries is one of the most prevalent diseases in the preschool child population of Western countries.
> - By 5 years of age up to 50% of the child population have experienced dental decay.

7.2 PATTERNS OF DENTAL DISEASE SEEN IN PRESCHOOL CHILDREN

7.2.1 Early childhood caries

Early childhood caries (ECC) is a term used to describe dental caries presenting in the primary dentition of young children. Terms such as 'nursing bottle mouth', 'bottle mouth caries', or 'nursing caries' are used to describe a particular pattern of dental caries in which the upper primary incisors and upper first primary molars are usually most severely affected. The lower first primary molars are also often carious, but the lower incisors are usually spared—being either entirely caries-free or only mildly affected (Fig. 7.1). Some children present with extensive caries that does not follow the 'nursing caries' pattern. Such children often have multiple carious teeth and may be slightly older (3 or 4 years of age) at initial presentation (Fig. 7.2). This presentation of caries is sometimes called 'rampant caries'. There is, however, no clear distinction between rampant caries and nursing caries, and the term 'early childhood caries' has been suggested as a suitable, all-encompassing term.

In many cases, early childhood caries is related to the frequent consumption of a drink containing sugars from a bottle or 'dinky' type comforters (these have a small reservoir that can be filled with a drink) (Fig. 7.3). Fruit-based drinks are most commonly associated with nursing caries. Even many of those claiming to have 'low sugar' or 'no added sugar' appear to be capable of causing caries. The sparing of the lower incisors seen in nursing caries is thought to result from the shielding of the lower incisors by the tongue during suckling, whilst at the same time they are being bathed in saliva from the sublingual and submandibular ducts. The upper incisors, on the other hand, are bathed in fluid from the bottle/feeder.

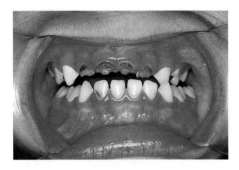

Fig. 7.1 Early childhood caries presenting as nursing caries in a 2-year-old child.

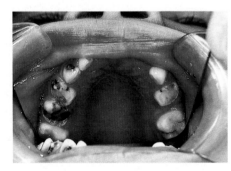

Fig. 7.2 Extensive caries affecting primary molars in a 4-year-old child.

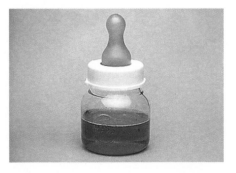

Fig. 7.3 Dinky type comforter with a small reservoir that can be filled with something to drink.

Frequency of consumption is a key factor. Affected children often have a history of taking a bottle to bed as a comforter, or using a bottle as a constant comforter during the daytime. Research has shown that children who tend to fall asleep with the bottle in their mouths are most likely to get ECC, and this is probably a reflection of the dramatic reduction in salivary flow that occurs as a child falls asleep. However, the link between bottle habits and ECC is not absolute and studies have suggested that other factors, such as linear enamel defects and malnutrition, may play an important role in the aetiology of this condition.

There is some circumstantial evidence that, in a few cases, ECC may be associated with prolonged, on-demand breast-feeding. Breast milk contains 7% lactose and, again, frequent, prolonged, on-demand consumption appears to be an important aetiological factor. Most affected children sleep with their parents, suckle during the night, and are often still being breast-fed at 2 or more years of age. It is important to appreciate that this does not imply that normal breast-feeding up to around 1 year of age is bad for teeth, but that prolonging on-demand feeding beyond that age possibly carries a risk of causing dental caries. Experiments in animal models suggest that cows' milk (which contains 4% lactose) is not cariogenic, although some clinical studies have suggested that the night-time consumption of cows' milk from a bottle might be associated with early childhood caries in some children. Whether or not cows' milk has the potential to contribute to caries is currently uncertain.

Key Points

- Early childhood caries (ECC) is an all-encompassing term that can be used to describe dental caries presenting in preschool children.
- The most commonly presenting pattern of ECC is often called 'nursing caries' or 'bottle mouth caries', where the upper anterior primary teeth are carious but the lower anterior teeth are usually spared.
- A prime aetiological factor is frequent consumption of a sweetened or fruit-based drink from a bottle or dinky feeder.
- Enamel defects and malnutrition may also play a role in the causation of ECC.

7.3 IDENTIFYING PRESCHOOL CHILDREN IN NEED OF DENTAL CARE

Identification of dental caries at an early stage is highly desirable if preventive measures and restorative care are to be successful. Yet, at 5 years of age a significant number of children will still not have had their first check-up visit to a dentist. In the UK, the Community Dental Service often identifies untreated caries in children of 5 years and over at school dental screenings. However, the large-scale screening of preschool children is fraught with logistical difficulties. In addition, many parents are under the misconception that they do not need to take their child for a dental check-up visit until they are 4 or 5 years of age.

Parents should be encouraged to bring their child for a dental check as soon as the child has teeth, usually around 6 months of age. This allows appropriate preventive advice regarding tooth cleaning, fluoride toothpastes, and the avoidance of bottle habits. It also allows the child to be become familiar with the dental environment and enables the dentist to identify any carious deterioration of the teeth at an early stage. Other health professionals, such as health visitors, can also be valuable in delivering key preventive advice and helping to identify young children with possible decay. Hence, making contact with local health visitors and delivering dental health messages via mother and toddler groups can be useful strategies.

Key Points
- Parents should be encouraged to bring their children for a dental check-up as soon as the child has teeth (around 6 months of age).
- Making contact with local health visitors, baby clinics, and mother-and-baby groups can be effective ways of getting dental information to the parents of preschool children.

7.4 MANAGEMENT OF PAIN AT FIRST ATTENDANCE

Unfortunately, the preschool child with caries is often already in pain when they first attend a dental surgery. Not only does this present the immediate problem of having to consider active treatment in a very young, inexperienced patient, but these problems are often compounded by the child's lack of sleep and time constraints on the dentist.

Pulpitis can sometimes be effectively managed, in the short term, by gentle excavation of caries and dressing with a zinc oxide and eugenol-based material, such as IRM (intermediate restorative material). Polyantibiotic and steroid pastes (e.g. Ledermix) may be useful beneath such dressings, and over exposures/near-exposures of the pulp.

The pulp chamber of abscessed teeth can sometimes be accessed by careful hand excavation, in which case placing a dressing of dilute formocresol on cotton wool within the pulp chamber will frequently lead to resolution of the swelling and symptoms. An acute and/or spreading infection or swelling may require the prescription of systemic antibiotics, although there is little rationale for the use of antibiotics in cases of toothache without associated soft tissue infection/inflammation.

Dental infection causing significant swelling of the face, especially where the child is febrile or unwell, constitutes a dental emergency and consideration should be given to referral to a specialized centre for immediate management.

Key Points
- Pain is a common presenting feature in preschool children.
- Appropriate dressing of teeth will usually help to temporarily manage pain and localized infection.
- Antibiotics should be prescribed where acute soft tissue swelling or signs of systemic involvement (e.g. pyrexia) are present.
- Children with increasing facial swelling and/or serious systemic involvement should be referred to a specialized centre for urgent management.

7.5 PRINCIPLES OF DIAGNOSIS AND TREATMENT PLANNING FOR PRESCHOOL CHILDREN

When planning dental treatment for preschool children, it is important to appreciate that dental caries of enamel is essentially a childhood disease and that progression of caries in the primary dentition can be rapid. Therefore, early diagnosis and prompt instigation of appropriate treatment is important. Preschool children should be routinely examined for dental caries relatively frequently (at least 2–3 times per year). More frequent examination (e.g. every 3 months) may be justified for children

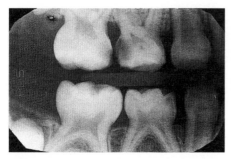

(a)

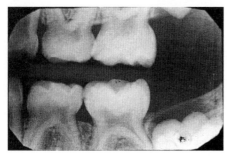

(b)

Fig. 7.4 Bitewing radiographs of a 4-year-old child. The caries in the upper right molars would be clinically obvious but the early approximal lesions in the lower left molars would not. Bitewing radiographs not only enable an accurate diagnosis, but early lesions can be compared on successive radiographs to enable a judgement to made about caries activity and progression.

in high-risk groups (Chapter 6). Approximal caries is common in primary molars so, in children considered to be at increased risk of developing dental caries and where posterior contacts are closed, a first set of bitewing radiographs should be taken at 4 years of age, or as soon as practically possible after that (Fig. 7.4). In such children consideration should be given to repeating bitewings at least annually.

Key Points

- Coronal enamel caries is essentially a childhood disease.
- In children deemed to be at increased risk of developing caries, bitewing radiographs should be obtained at 4 years of age, or as soon as practically possible after that, and consideration should be given to repeating such radiographs at least annually.

7.6 PREVENTIVE CARE

Preventive measures are the cornerstone to the management of dental caries in children. There is often a failure to appreciate that those aspects of care we refer to as prevention are actually a fundamental part of the treatment of dental caries. Repairing the damage caused by dental caries is also important, but this will only be successful if the causes of that damage have been addressed. A good analogy is that of a burning house. Repairing the house (new windows, roof, furniture, etc.) is important, but all this will be of little benefit in the long term if the fire has not been put out! A structured approach to prevention should form a key part of the management of every preschool child.

Key Point

- Preventive measures are the cornerstone to the successful treatment of dental caries in children.

7.6.1 Fluorides

Self-administered

FLUORIDE TOOTHPASTE

Parents should be advised to start brushing their child's teeth with a fluoride toothpaste as soon as the first tooth erupts, at around 6 months of age. For children considered to be at low risk of developing caries a toothpaste containing 450–600 p.p.m. fluoride may be used. Toothpastes with a lower fluoride concentration are available, but there is some question about their efficacy. Many authorities now support the prescribing of toothpastes containing higher concentrations of fluoride (around 1000 p.p.m.) to preschool children deemed to be at higher risk of developing caries, irrespective of their age. In children at highest risk, toothpastes with higher concentrations (i.e. 1400–1500 p.p.m. F^-) may even be justified, especially in children aged 6 and above. Where higher concentration toothpastes are prescribed for preschool children, parents should be counselled to ensure that brushing is supervised (see Section 7.6.4), small amounts of toothpaste are applied to the brush ('small pea size blob' or 'thin smear'), and that children spit out as well as possible after brushing.

Key Point

- In areas without optimum levels of fluoride in the water supply, fluoride toothpaste is the most important method of delivering fluoride to preschool children.

Table 7.1 Dosage schedule for fluoride supplements in areas where the water supply contains up to less than 0.3 p.p.m. as currently advised by the British Society of Paediatric Dentistry

Age	mg fluoride per day
6 months up to 3 years	0.25
3 up to 6 years	0.50
6 years and over	1.00

In areas with water supplies containing more than 0.3 ppm but less than 0.7 ppm of fluoride dentists should consider a lower dosage. ie 6 months–3 years no supplementation, 3–6 years 0.25 mg and 6 years and over 0.5 mg.

FLUORIDE SUPPLEMENTS

Supplementary fluoride, in the form of either drops or tablets, should be considered in those at high risk of caries and in children in whom dental disease would pose a serious risk to general health (e.g. children at increased risk of endocarditis). Such supplementation is only maximally effective if given long term and regularly. Unfortunately, studies have shown that long-term compliance with daily fluoride supplement protocols is poor. Parental motivation and regular reinforcement are essential for such measures to be effective. Dosage should follow the protocol advised by the British Society of Paediatric Dentistry (Table 7.1). No supplements should be prescribed if the water fluoride level is greater than 0.7 ppm. The European view on supplements is that the maximum dose should be 0.5 mg/day.

FLUORIDE MOUTHRINSES

Fluoride mouthrinses are contraindicated in children less than 6 years of age, because of the risk of excessive ingestion.

Professionally applied fluorides

Site-specific application of fluoride varnish can be valuable in the management of early, smooth surface and approximal carious lesions (Fig. 7.5). However, the most popularly used varnishes contain 5% sodium fluoride (i.e. 22, 600 p.p.m. of fluoride). Hence, when using these products in young children great care should be taken to avoid overdosage (see below).

Fluoride overdosage

A dose of 1 mg of F/kg body weight can be enough to produce symptoms of toxicity and a dose of 5 mg of F/kg is considered to be potentially fatal. Symptoms of toxicity include nausea, vomiting, hypersalivation, abdominal pain (production of hydrogen fluoride, HF), and diarrhoea. Subsequently, depression of plasma calcium levels results in convulsions, and cardiac and respiratory failure. The appropriate management of fluoride overdosage is detailed in Table 7.2.

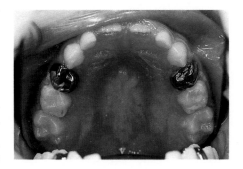

Fig. 7.5 Site-specific application of fluoride varnish.

Some of the terms used when describing fluoride toxicity are given in Table 7.3. In a 10-kg, 18-month-old child, the ingestion of 0.5 ml of a 2.26% fluoride varnish can produce toxicity, and slightly more than 2 ml may be a potentially lethal dose (PLD). In this 10-kg child the STD (safely tolerated dose) would be 10 mg of F, the PLD 50 mg, and the CLD (certain lethal dose) 320–640 mg of F.

Toothpaste containing 1000 p.p.m. F will contain 1 mg of F in a gram or 1 inch (25 mm) of paste. Toothpaste tubes vary from 25 g to 140 g. Even if the larger tube was completely swallowed the amount of F (140 mg of F) would still be less than the CLD for the 10-kg child, but would exceed the PLD. A container of 120 tablets, each of 1 mg , would contain 120 mg of fluoride. Again, this would be within the CLD but exceed the PLD. All containers with fluoride tablets should have childproof tops and be kept out of reach of young children.

Table 7.2 Management of accidental fluoride overdosage

Amount swallowed (mg F/kg of body weight)	Management
Less than 5 mg F/kg	Give milk to slow the absorption of fluoride.
5–15 mg F/kg	The stomach contents need to be emptied unless other poisons were simultaneously swallowed. Ipecacuanha emetic mixture, Paediatric BP (Ipecac syrup), at a dose of 10 ml for a 6–18-month-old child, 15 ml for older children, and 30 ml for adults should be given. In addition, milk, epsom salts, or aluminium hydroxide antacid mixture will help to slow the absorption of any remaining fluoride.
More than 15 mg F/kg	Urgent admission to a paediatric intensive care unit for neurological, cardiological, and respiratory support.

Table 7.3 Terms used in relation to fluoride toxicity

Safely tolerated dose (STD)	Dose below which symptoms of toxicity are unlikely to occur. Usually considered to be 1 mg/kg of body weight
Potentially lethal dose (PLD)	Lowest dose associated with a fatality, i.e. 5 mg/kg body weight
Certainly lethal dose (CLD)	Survival after consuming this amount of fluoride is unlikely. Considered to be 32–64 mg/kg body weight

Acidulated phosphate-fluoride (APF) gels and foams are contraindicated in preschool children.

7.6.2 Chlorhexidine gels

Clinical research in very young children is limited, but there is substantial agreement that daily professional applications of chlorhexidine followed by applications every few months can be significant in controlling caries. This probably results from chlorhexidine's ability to reduce the levels of mutans streptococci in both saliva and plaque.

7.6.3 Fissure sealants

Although not used routinely in the primary dentition, fissure sealants may be of value on primary molars (especially second primary molars) where one or more primary molars has already developed occlusal caries.

7.6.4 Toothbrushing

Plaque removal with a soft, small-headed toothbrush in combination with a suitable fluoride toothpaste should start as soon as the child's first tooth erupts. Preschool children need help from their parents if effective oral hygiene is to be maintained, so parental involvement in oral hygiene instruction is essential. Some toddlers can be resistant to parental (and professional!) attempts to brush their teeth. Parents should be encouraged to persevere through such difficulties, ensuring that their child's teeth are thoroughly cleaned at least once daily. Standing or kneeling behind the child in front of the sink or mirror is often the easiest way to effectively brush a young toddler's teeth (Fig. 7.6). Supervision of toothbrushing is also important to avoid overingestion of toothpaste.

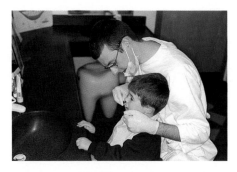

Fig. 7.6 Standing or kneeling behind the child in front of the sink or mirror is often the easiest way to effectively brush a young toddler's teeth.

> **Key Points**
> - Preschool children need help with toothbrushing.
> - Parents should help with brushing to ensure effective cleaning and avoid overingestion of fluoride toothpaste.

7.6.5 Diet

Frequent consumption of drinks and food containing sugars is a key aetiological feature in many preschool children who present with caries. Hence, reducing the frequency of sugar-containing food and drinks is a key dietary message to deliver to parents. However, for such advice to be effective, it must be delivered in an understanding way and should take into account some of the difficulties parents may face in making such changes to their child's diet. Young children have a high metabolic rate and their dietary calorific requirements are high. Many young children with early childhood caries are also 'poor eaters', their parents often reporting that the child does not eat well at meal times. Such children often make up the calories missed at meal times by consuming fruit-based drinks between meals, which are high in calories. As well as helping to meet the child's nutritional requirements this also suppresses the appetite so that when the next mealtime approaches the child is not very hungry. Parents frequently misinterpret this, and think the child asks for drinks because of thirst. A history of poor sleeping is also common, with parents relating that the child 'will not sleep without the bottle'.

Once established, such cycles of behaviour can be difficult to break and many parents have a sense of guilt that their child has dental decay, feeling that they must have done something wrong. For counselling to be effective it is essential to avoid making the parent feel excessively guilty, but to concentrate on the aetiology of the condition and practical strategies to deal with these problems. Stopping a night-time bottle habit can be achieved quickly by some parents, but can prove difficult for others. The idea of leaving the child to cry rather than giving it a bottle might seem a good idea whilst in the dental surgery, but is a more challenging proposition at three o'clock in the morning! Weaning children from a night or daytime bottle of juice can often be achieved by gradually making the juice in the bottle more dilute over a period of a few weeks until the contents become just water. At this point the child will either discard the bottle or will continue to suckle on water alone, which is, of course, non-cariogenic. Thirsty children will always drink water.

> **Key Points**
> - Children have a high calorific requirement.
> - Children who are poor eaters at mealtimes and snack and drink frequently between meals are more likely to get decay.

7.7 MANAGING BEHAVIOUR

7.7.1 Managing the preschool child's behaviour in the dental setting

The importance of establishing effective communication and adopting strategies which help to alleviate anxiety, in both child and parent, have already been fully discussed

(Chapter 2). Where possible, restorative treatment should be carried out under local analgesia alone, but strategies such as sedation, by either the inhalation or oral route, or general anaesthesia are sometimes indicated, especially in young children with extensive disease who are in acute pain, or where a non-pharmacological approach to behaviour management has failed (Chapter 4). Whichever strategy is chosen, it is essential to involve the parent in the decision and to obtain written consent.

The fundamental principles of effectively managing child behaviour in the surgery are fully covered in Chapter 2. However, there are some specific aspects that relate particularly to very young children.

7.7.2 Parental presence

This has been a topic of great controversy for many years. Dentistry for children is complicated by the fact that the dentist must establish a working relationship and communicate effectively with both child and parent. Virtually all studies designed to investigate the effect of parental presence in the surgery on the child's co-operation with dental treatment have failed to demonstrate any difference between behaviour with or without the parent present. Only one reasonably well-designed study, by Frankl in 1962 (from which came the useful Frankl scale), has ever suggested that parental presence might affect child behaviour. Frankl's results indicated that children of around 4 years old and younger behave more positively when parents were present. However, no difference was demonstrated in older children.

In most of the aforementioned studies, parents were carefully instructed to sit quietly in the surgery and not to interfere with dentist-child communication, so as to avoid the introduction of inconsistent variables. Frankl commented upon this in his concluding comments:

the presence of a passively observing mother can be an aid to the child. This can be accomplished if the mother is motivated positively, is instructed explicitly and co-operates willingly in the role of a 'silent helper'.

Certainly having the parent present in the surgery when treating young children facilitates effective communication and helps to fulfil the requirements of informed consent. It also has the advantage that should any problems arise, or the child becomes upset during treatment, the parent is fully aware of the circumstances and of the dentist's approach to management. If a parent is sat outside and hears their 3-year-old child start to cry in the surgery, events associated with the child's distress can easily be misinterpreted. Also, studies have shown that many parents would wish to be present during dental treatment, especially at the child's first visit. Having said this, in the absence of any convincing evidence one way or the other, having the parent present during the treatment of preschool children remains a matter of individual choice.

7.7.3 Sedation

Sedation will not necessarily convert an uncooperative child into a co-operative one. However, it can help to alleviate anxiety, improve a child's tolerance of invasive procedures, and increase the child's ability to cope with prolonged treatment. Several routes of administration are available and of these, two are generally suitable for outpatient use: inhalation and oral. Intravenous sedation is unsuitable for preschool children.

Key Points
- Whether or not the parent is present does not seem to have a great effect on the child's behaviour in the surgery.
- Very young children are probably more settled when the parent is present.
- Parents should be encouraged to adopt the role of 'silent helper'.

Inhalation sedation with nitrous oxide and oxygen produces both sedation and analgesia. The reader is referred to Chapter 4 for a full review of this technique. The technique works most effectively on children who wish to co-operate, but are too anxious to do so. Its use for preschool children is limited to those who are able to tolerate the nasal hood, but where this can be achieved, the technique is often effective.

Orally administered sedation has the advantage that, once administered, no further active co-operation of the child is required for the drug to take effect. However, unlike inhalation or intravenous sedation, it is impossible to titrate the dose of the drug to the patient's response, which results in some variation in effect from one patient to another.

Over the years, many agents have been advocated for use in dentistry as oral sedative agents, and none of these are ideal. In studies, most of the more popular agents produce a successful outcome in 60–70% of cases. For this reason, some workers, especially in the United States of America, advocate combinations of oral drugs, sometimes supplemented with inhaled nitrous oxide and oxygen, in order to achieve a more reliable result. However, administering multiple sedation drugs does not fall within the definition of 'simple dental sedation', where only a single sedative drug should be used. Many authorities consider such 'poly-pharmacy' to carry an increased risk and discourage the practice.

Of the orally administered sedation agents available, the most useful for preschool children are the chloral derivatives and some of the benzodiazepines.

Chloral derivatives

Chloral hydrate is a long-standing and effective sedative hypnotic. Its use in children's dentistry has been well researched, it has a good margin of safety, causes little or no respiratory depression at therapeutic levels, and has few serious side-effects. The optimum dosage is 30–50 mg/kg, up to a maximum of 1.0 g. However, its bitter taste makes it unpleasant to take and it is a potent gastric irritant, producing vomiting in many children. This not only has the potential to increase the child's distress, but also reduces the efficacy of the drug. Trichlofos, a derivative of chloral hydrate, causes less gastric irritation, but otherwise appears to produce similar results, although there has been little research to confirm this.

Benzodiazepines

Many benzodiazepines have been investigated as potential sedation agents for use in children's dentistry. They have a wide therapeutic index and can be reversed by flumazenil. Diazepam can be used for oral sedation, but produces prolonged sedation and has proved somewhat unpredictable in young children. Temazepam was popular some years ago, especially as its duration of action is shorter than diazepam. However, idiosyncratic reactions in some children have caused temazepam to fall from favour. In the UK, temazepam also has the disadvantage of being a Schedule 3 controlled drug.

Recent studies using midazolam, another short-acting benzodiazepine, have reported good results. Midazolam is easy to take orally and seems to offer safe and reliable sedation, with far fewer idiosyncratic reactions than with temazepam. Onset of sedation is rapid (around 20 minutes) and recovery is also relatively quick. The optimum dose is 0.3–0.5 mg/kg when given orally. The preparation designed for intravenous administration is used, often mixed into a small volume of a suitable fruit drink. Some studies report successful delivery via the nasal mucosa, where doses of 0.2–0.3 mg/kg have been advocated. However, midazolam is not yet available as an oral or nasal preparation and is not yet licensed for oral sedation. Practitioners are therefore advised to seek specific training before prescribing midazolam for oral sedation.

When using any sedative agent in children it is essential that suitable precautions are taken and that appropriate emergency drugs and equipment are available. These important aspects are detailed fully in Chapter 4 and, hence, will not be further rehearsed here.

7.7.4 General anaesthesia

Dental extraction under general anaesthesia has been used widely in the UK as a strategy for the treatment of dental caries in preschool children. Recently, the justification for such extensive use has been questioned, and it is now widely agreed that general anaesthesia should only take place in hospital and should only be employed where other behaviour management strategies have failed or are inappropriate. General anaesthesia is, however, indicated for some child patients. Comprehensive full mouth care under intubated general anaesthesia enables children with multiple carious teeth to be expediently rendered caries-free in one procedure (Fig. 7.7). This approach does have a place in the management of young, anxious, or handicapped children with extensive caries, and in some medical conditions where multiple treatment episodes over a prolonged period increase the risks of systemic complications. Extractions under general anaesthesia may be preferable to no treatment at all in the management of extensive caries in young children, especially when facilities for restorative care under general anaesthesia are not available or parental motivation is poor and reatten-dance for multiple visits is unlikely to occur. In addition, general anaesthesia may be the only practical approach for children with acute infection.

Where general anaesthesia is employed in the dental treatment of the preschool child, the emphasis must be on avoiding the need for repeated general anaesthesia. Hence, each procedure needs careful planning with consideration being given to the management of all disease present in the child's mouth, while also considering the effect of premature extractions on the developing dentition. This may require the extraction plan to be quite radical, especially where facilities for restorative care under general anaesthesia are not available.

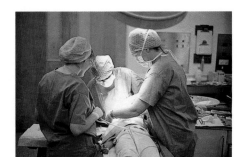

Fig. 7.7 Comprehensive full mouth care under intubated general anaesthesia enables children with multiple carious teeth to be expediently rendered caries-free in one procedure.

Key Points
- Sedation can be a useful adjunct for anxious preschool children.
- General anaesthesia should only be used where other management strategies have failed or are deemed inappropriate.

7.8 TREATMENT OF DENTAL CARIES

7.8.1 Temporization of open cavities

As an initial step in the management of caries, open cavities should be hand-excavated and temporized with a suitable material such as a reinforced zinc oxide and eugenol cement, or, better still, a packable glass ionomer cement (Fig. 7.8). Carious exposures of vital or non-vital teeth can be dressed with a small amount of a polyantibiotic steroid paste (Ledermix) on cotton wool covered by a suitable dressing material.

Dressing open cavities has a number of advantages. It serves as a simple and straightforward introduction for the child to dental procedures. By removing soft caries and temporarily occluding cavities, the oral loading of mutans streptococci is significantly reduced. It helps to reduce sensitivity, making toothbrushing and eating more comfortable, and also makes inadvertent toothache less likely. If a suitable material is used, it can produce a source for low-level fluoride release within the mouth.

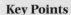

(a)

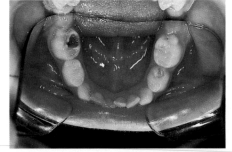

(b)

Fig. 7.8 The large cavity in the lower right, second primary molar has been hand excavated and temporized with a packable glass ionomer cement.

Key Points

Temporization of teeth:

- helps to reduce dental sensitivity and prevent toothache occurring before definitive care is complete;
- reduces the oral mutans streptococci load;
- serves as an introduction to dental treatment; and
- provides a source for fluoride release if a glass ionomer-based material is used.

7.8.2 Definitive restoration of teeth

The highly active nature of dental caries in the young primary dentition should be borne in mind when planning restorative care, but it is also important to plan to carry out such care in a way that the child can successfully accept. Approaches such as 'tell–show–do' (Chapter 2) and behaviour shaping utilizing positive reinforcement to encourage appropriate behaviours are important. Communicating in terms the child can understand, and using vocabulary that avoids negative associations, is also important. For example, the term 'local anaesthetic' will mean nothing to most children and words such as 'injection' and 'needle' may convey the suggestion of pain or discomfort. Suitable alternative terms might be 'sleepy juice' or 'jungle juice'. Such 'childrenese' can be developed for most routine dental equipment and procedures (Table 7.4)

The pace of treatment should take into account the preschool child's need to be familiarized with the dental environment and equipment. Starting treatment by temporizing any open cavities as described above serves as an easy introduction to operative care.

From that point on, planning to include both a preventive and a restorative component at each visit allows effective treatment to progress at a reasonable pace. Table 7.5

Table 7.4 Common terms used for introducing dental equipment to children

Item of equipment	Suitable term for children
Slow handpiece	Buzzy Bee Buzzy brush
Airotor	Wizzy brush Tooth shower
Air/water syringe	Water spray
Local anaesthetic	Jungle juice Sleepy juice
Dental mirror	Spoon (with a mirror on the end)
Dental probe	Tickling stick
Rubber dam	Rubber raincoat
Inhalation sedation	Magic wind

Table 7.5 A typical visit-by-visit treatment plan for a young child with caries

	Preventive/other	Restorative
Visit 1	History and examination Bitewing radiographs Give diet sheet Baseline plaque score and OHI	Temporization of open cavities
Visit 2	Repeat plaque score plus reinforce OHI and discuss fluoride toothpaste Collect diet sheet Apply Duraphat 55 m, 65 m 75 m	Restoration of 63b GIC (no LA/Rdam)
Visit 3	Diet counseling Fluoride supplements-discuss	LA, Rdam intro Restn 64 pulpot and SSC Fissure seal 65
Visit 4	Duraphat 55 m, 65 m, 75 m	Restn 54 do Fissure seal 55
Visit 5	Repeat plaque score	Restn 74 do Restn 75 o
Visit 6	Review diet/fluorides Duraphat 55 m, 65 m, 75 m	Restn 84 o Fissure seal 85
Recall period Next bitewings	4 months 8 months	

Table 7.6 Maximum dosage in children of commonly used local anaesthetic agents

Solution	Max. dose	Max. dose by age of child		
		1 year (10 kg)	3 year (15 kg)	5 year (20 kg)
2% lidocaine/1 : 80 000 epinephrine (20 mg/ml lidocaine)	4.4 mg/kg	2.2 ml	3.6 ml	4.4 ml
3% prilocaine/felypressin (30 mg/ml prilocaine)	6.6 mg/kg	2.2 ml	3.3 ml	4.4 ml
4% prilocaine (40 mg/ml prilocaine)	5 mg/kg	1.2 ml	1.8 ml	2.5 ml

The size of the cartridge of LA in the UK is commonly 2.2 ml.

shows one way of constructing a treatment plan for a typical young child with caries. It is customary to start with treatment in the upper arch first, as this is usually easier for both the child and the dentist, although this approach may need to be modified if there are lower teeth in urgent need of attention. Appropriate use of local analgesia (Chapter 5) and rubber dam (Chapter 8) cannot be overemphasized and any dentist treating young children needs to be proficient at both. Many preschool children are far more accepting of carefully delivered local analgesia than most dentists realize. Using techniques to deliver local analgesia painlessly are crucial (Chapter 5, Section 5.6) and care should be taken to avoid overdosage with local analgesics (Table 7.6). It is also important to explain to the child the unusual feelings associated with soft tissue analgesia, and to warn both the child and parent of the need to avoid lip biting/sucking whilst these effects persist (Chapter 5, Section 5.7.3).

Placement of rubber dam using a trough technique, where the clamp is placed on the tooth first, then the dam is stretched over (as described in Chapter 8) is, in the author's experience, the most straightforward approach in the young child. Careful attention to obtaining adequate analgesia of the gingival tissues, both buccally and lingually, ensures comfortable clamp placement. Intrapapillary injections are very useful for this (Chapter 5, Section 5.6.3). Encouraging the child to watch in a hand mirror helps to distract the child's attention from the intraoral manipulations during actual placement of the dam (Fig. 7.9).

The techniques employed for definitive restoration in young children should take into account the often active nature of the disease in this age group. The use of plastic restorative materials should be limited to occlusal and small approximal lesions. Extensive caries, teeth with caries affecting more than two surfaces, and teeth requiring pulpotomy or pulpectomy should be restored with stainless-steel crowns. Amalgam is still widely used as a restorative material, but materials including newer glass ionomer cements, resin-modified glass ionomers, polyacid-modified resins (compomers), and composite resins may be preferred. However, all the latter mentioned materials are far more sensitive to moisture contamination and technique than amalgam, so adequate isolation, preferably with rubber dam, is essential. Cermet restorations perform poorly in primary teeth and are best avoided. A fuller discussion on material selection for the restoration of primary molars is given in Chapter 8.

Composite strip crown restorations are the most effective way of repairing carious anterior teeth (Chapter 8).

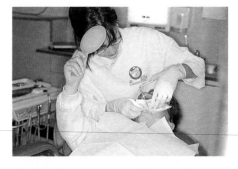

Fig. 7.9 Encouraging the child to watch in a hand mirror helps to distract the child's attention from the intraoral manipulations during rubber dam placement.

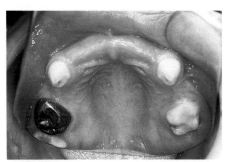

Fig. 7.10 Extraction of first primary molars with maintenance and restoration of the second primary molars.

7.8.3 Extraction of teeth

Extraction is indicated for teeth that are unrestorable, and it may also be enforced by acute pain or infection. In preschool children the extraction of one or two teeth can often be accomplished under local analgesia—inhalation or oral sedation being a useful adjunct for anxious children. If more extractions are needed, these can sometimes be carried out at the same time as restoring adjacent teeth. However, general anaesthesia is the only practical strategy for some children, in which case referral to an appropriate dental general anaesthesia facility is mandatory.

When planning extractions, it is important to consider the need for balancing (Chapter 14). Factors such as the likelihood of continued future attendance and co-operation of the child should also be borne in mind. In preschool children with extensive caries, extraction of first primary molars with maintenance and restoration of the second primary molars where possible is often a good plan (Fig. 7.10). Not only does this limit the risk of further decay by eliminating posterior primary contact areas, but it also minimizes the deleterious effect of early extraction on the developing dentition.

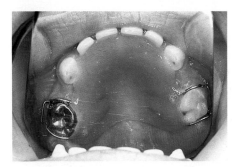

(a)

7.8.4 Replacing missing teeth

Where the child is motivated, dentures are suprisingly well tolerated. A simple removable acrylic denture with gum-fitted primary prosthetic teeth and clasps on the second molars can effectively restore aesthetics (Fig. 7.11). Even full dentures can be highly successful in cases where the child is keen to have teeth replaced. The methods of constructing dentures are essentially the same as those in adults. It is important that careful attention is given to cleaning such appliances to avoid them contributing to further disease.

(b)

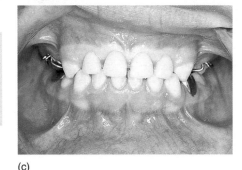

7.9 SUMMARY

1. Dental caries is a prevalent disease in the preschool population.
2. Nursing caries and rampant caries are common patterns of caries in preschool children.

(c)

Fig. 7.11 Extracted primary incisors can be easily and effectively replaced by providing a removable acrylic denture with gum-fitted primary prosthetic teeth and clasps on the second molars.

3. Parents should be encouraged to bring their children for a dental check-up as soon as the child's first tooth has erupted.

4. Prevention is a cornerstone of the management of caries in the preschool child.

5. Planned treatment should be carried out at a pace the child can accept.

6. Preschool children need careful introduction to dental equipment and procedures.

7. Inhalation or oral sedation can be effective strategies for anxious preschool children.

8. General anaesthesia should be reserved for those cases where other approaches to management have either failed or are deemed inappropriate.

9. Local analgesia is advisable for definitive restoration of all but small cavities, but care should be exercised to avoid overdosage in the small child.

10. Rubber dam makes good quality treatment easier to achieve for both the child and dentist.

11. Choice of restorative materials should reflect the high risk of further caries in the young child.

12. Stainless-steel crowns are the most effective restoration for primary molars with caries on more than two surfaces.

7.10 FURTHER READING

British Society of Paediatric Dentistry (1997). A policy document on the dental needs of children. *International Journal of Paediatric Dentistry*, **7**, 203–7. (*BSPD consensus view document which reviews current standards of UK child dental care and suggests how these might be improved.*)

British Society of Paediatric Dentistry (2003). A policy document on oral health care in preschool children. *International Journal of Paediatric Dentistry*, **13**, 279–85. (*BSPD concensus document giving guidance for the delivery of oral health care to preschool children.*)

Duggal, M. S., Curzon, M. E. J., Fayle, S. A., Pollard, M. A., and Robertson, A. J. (2002). *Restorative techniques in paediatric dentistry.* (2nd edn). Taylor & Francis, London. (*A practical guide to the restoration of carious primary teeth.*)

Seow, W. K. (1998). Biological mechanisms of early childhood caries. *Community Dentistry and Oral Epidemiology*, **26**, (Suppl. 1), 8–27. (*An excellent review of the various aetiological factors involved in early childhood caries.*)

7.11 REFERENCE

Frankl, S. N., Shiere, F. R., Fogels, S. H. R. (1962). Should the parent remain with the child in the dental operatory? *Journal of Dentistry for Children*, **29**, 150–63.

8

Operative treatment of dental caries in the primary dentition

8 Operative treatment of dental caries in the primary dentition

M. S. Duggal and P. F. Day

8.1 INTRODUCTION

While there is no doubt that the best way to tackle the problem of dental caries is through an effective programme of prevention as outlined in the previous chapters, it is unfortunate that many children still suffer from the disease and its consequences. Hence there is a need to consider operative treatment to prevent the breakdown of the dentition.

Over the years the treatment of dental caries in children has been discussed and many attempts made to rationalize the management of the disease. Writing more than 150 years ago, Harris (1939) was one of the first to address the problem of restoring the primary dentition. Even in those days he was emphasizing the importance of prevention by good toothbrushing. Caries could be arrested by 'plugging', but from his description he obviously found treatment for the young patient difficult and not as successful as in adults. However, he did emphasize the importance of looking after the teeth of children: 'If parents and guardians would pay more attention to the teeth of their children, the services of the dentist would much less frequently be required', and, 'Many persons suppose that the teeth, in the early periods of childhood, require no attention, and thus are guilty of the most culpable neglect of the future well-being of those entrusted to their care'. Unfortunately, this statement still applies today.

The huge number of different techniques and materials that have been advocated over the years since Harris wrote those words testify to the fact that no ideal solutions have so far been found. Unfortunately, most treatments are advocated on the basis of dentists' clinical impressions and there have been very few objective studies that have attempted to discover which treatments succeed and which do not.

Treatment can be a stressful experience for the child, the parent, and the dentist. It is important that there is a positive health gain from any treatment that is provided.

It is impossible to cover the whole field of operative treatment for children in one chapter and the reader is directed to other texts for a fuller account of available techniques. However, it is possible to outline the rationale for providing operative treatment, to give advice on the selection of appropriate ways of providing care, and to describe a few of the more useful treatment methods.

8.2 PHILOSOPHY OF CARE

Children are the future dental patients and, therefore, the dental care that they receive should promote positive dental experiences, which in turn would promote positive dental attitudes. When faced with a tooth that has caries, the first decision has to be whether it does in fact require treatment or not. It may be felt that the caries is so minor and prevention so effective that further progress of the lesion is unlikely. Less rationally it may be felt that a carious tooth with a non-vital pulp is unlikely to cause great problems and may be left to its own devices. Recently there has been

Table 8.1   The five-point treatment philosophy for the provision of high quality dental care for children

1. Gain co-operation and trust of the child and parent.
2. Make an accurate diagnosis and devise a treatment plan appropriate to the child's need.
3. Comprehensive preventive care.
4. Deliver care in a manner the child finds acceptable.
5. Use treatment methods and restorative techniques, which produce a cost-effective, long-lasting result.

much discussion in the United Kingdom on whether most carious primary molars need to be restored at all! In the authors view there is no doubt that untreated caries in the primary dentition causes abscesses, pain, and suffering in children. This can then need hospital admission and invasive treatment, sometimes under general anaesthesia, whereas a simple restoration, at the time when the caries was diagnosed, would have prevented this extremely distressing episode for the child. It is therefore essential for all dentists involved in the care of young children to learn restorative techniques that give the best results in primary teeth and this should always be alongside excellent preventive programmes, and this chapter is devoted to the discussion of such techniques. Good quality restorative care (Fig. 8.1(a) and (b)), as and when caries is diagnosed, would also obviate the need for extractions of primary teeth under general anaesthesia for thousands of children, particularly in the United Kingdom. A treatment philosophy which the authors believe is effective in the management of caries in children is shown in Table 8.1.

8.3 REMOVE, RESTORE, OR LEAVE

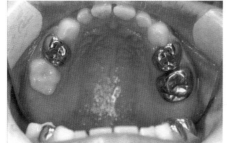

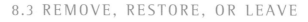

There are certain situations where the clinician might decide not to carry out invasive restorative procedures in primary teeth and instead use a rigorous preventive approach. Such an approach can be justified where it is likely that remineralization would occur or the tooth maintained in a state, free from pain or infection until exfoliation. Recently (Pitts and Longbottom, 1995) it has been proposed that it should be possible to divide lesions into those for which preventive care is advised (PCA) and those for which operative care is advised (OCA). More work is required on this concept but the following sections discuss conflicting reasons to treat or not to treat particular carious lesions.

(a)

8.3.1 Reasons not to treat

These can be divided into several distinct categories.

1. *The damage done by treatment to:*

    (a) *The affected tooth.* However conservative the technique it is inevitable that some sound tooth tissue has to be removed when operative treatment is undertaken. This weakens the tooth and makes it more likely that problems such as cracking of the tooth or loss of vitality of the pulp may occur in the future.

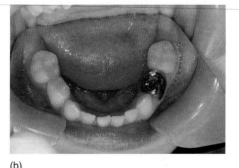

(b)

Fig. 8.1 A well-restored primary dentition (a) upper arch and (b) lower arch in a child. High quality restorative care is supplemented with prevention in the form of sealants placed in other molars deemed to be susceptible to future carious attack.

Key Point

• Every time that a restoration is replaced more sound tissue has to be removed, putting the tooth at further risk.

(b) *The adjacent tooth.* It is almost inevitable when treating an approximal lesion that the adjacent tooth will be damaged. The outer surface has a far higher fluoride content than the rest of the enamel so that even a slight nick of the intact surface will remove this reservoir of fluoride. Additionally, it has been shown that early lesions that remineralize are less susceptible to caries than intact surfaces and these areas of the tooth are all too easily removed when preparing an adjacent tooth.

Key Point
- Early lesions that remineralize are less susceptible to caries.

(c) *The periodontal tissues.* Dental treatment can cause both acute and long-term damage to the periodontium. It is virtually impossible to avoid damaging the interdental papillae when treating approximal caries. The papillae can be protected by using rubber dam and/or wedges and if well-fitting restorations are placed the tissues will heal fairly rapidly, but long-term damage can be more critical. Many adults can be seen to be suffering from overenthusiastic treatment of approximal caries in their youth; and while the relative importance of poor margins compared to bacterial plaque can be debated, the potential damage from approximal restorations is sufficient reason to avoid treatment unless a definite indication is present.

(d) *The occlusion.* Poor restoration of the teeth can, over time, lead to considerable alteration of the occlusion. It is tempting when restoring occlusal surfaces to leave the material well clear of the opposing teeth to avoid difficulties, or to be unconcerned if the filling is slightly 'high'. However, this can allow the teeth to erupt into contact again or the interocclusal position to change and alter the occlusion. Often this is felt to be of little concern, but there are a large number of adults where the cumulative effect of many poorly restored teeth has severely disturbed the occlusion, thus making further treatment difficult, time consuming, and expensive.

2. *The difficulty of diagnosis.* It is well known that it is difficult to diagnose dental caries accurately. Even when coarse criteria such as those developed for the United Kingdom Child Dental Health Surveys are used, there is wide variation between examiners. It is not just variations between examiners that need to be considered as there is also a marked difference between the same examiner on different occasions. The implications need to be considered in relation to the decision to treat or not.

3. *The slow rate of caries attack.* Caries usually progresses relatively slowly, although some individuals will show more rapid development than others. The majority of children and adolescents will have a low level of caries and progress of carious lesions will be slow. In general, the older the child at the time that the caries is first diagnosed the slower the progression of the lesion. However, a substantial group of children will have caries that develops rapidly.

4. *The fact that remineralization can arrest and repair enamel caries.* It has long been known that early, smooth surface lesions are reversible. In addition, it is now accepted that the chief mechanism whereby fluoride reduces caries is by encouraging remineralization, and that the remineralized early lesion is more resistant to caries than intact enamel. Although it is difficult to show reversal of lesions on radiographs, many studies have demonstrated that a substantial proportion of early enamel lesions do not progress over many years.

5. *The short life of dental restorations.* Surveys of dental treatment have often shown a rather disappointing level of success. In general, 50% of amalgam restorations

in permanent teeth can be expected to fail during the 10 years following placement. Some studies have shown an even poorer success rate when looking at primary teeth, and this has been put forward as a reason for not treating these teeth.

8.3.2 Reasons to treat

1. *Adverse effects of neglect.* The fact that the treatment of approximal caries can cause damage to the affected tooth, the adjacent tooth, the periodontium, and the occlusion is a valid reason to think twice before putting bur to tooth. But, of course, a case could equally well be made that the neglect of treatment will cause as much or more damage. Lack of treatment can, and all too often does, lead to loss of contact with adjacent and opposing teeth, exposure of the pulp resulting in the development of periapical infection, and/or loss of the tooth. At worst, the child may end up having a general anaesthetic for the removal of one or more teeth. A procedure which has a significant morbidity and mortality.

2. *Unpredictability of the speed of attack.* While it is true that the rate of attack is usually slow, it is quite possible for the rate in any one individual to be rapid so that any delay in treatment would not then be in the best interests of the child.

3. *Difficulty in assessing if a lesion is arrested or not.* Because of the normally slow rate of attack it is difficult to be sure if a lesion is arrested or merely developing very slowly. It is true that remineralization will arrest and repair early enamel lesions, but there is, in fact, little evidence that remineralization of the dentine or the late enamel lesion is common.

4. *Success when careful treatment is provided.* The majority of published studies show that class II amalgam restorations in primary teeth have a poor life expectancy, but this is not the experience of the careful dentist. Some of these dentists have published their results, which show that the great majority of their restorations in primary teeth survive without further attention until they exfoliate. The treatment procedures used are not particularly difficult in comparison to others that dentists attempt on adults, and it is difficult to avoid the conclusion that the reasons for poor results in some studies are due to poor patient management and lack of attention to detail. It should be the aim of the profession to develop better and more effective ways of treating the disease rather than throwing our hands up in surrender.

5. *Early treatment is more successful than late.* Small restorations are more successful than large, and therefore if a carious lesion is going to need treatment it is better treated early rather than late. This was the rationale behind the early suggestions of Hyatt of a 'prophylactic filling' for pits and fissures and for the modern versions in the form of fissure sealants and preventive resin restorations. The fact that small restorations are often more successful makes for difficult decisions when the management of caries involves preventive procedures, which need both time to work and time to assess whether they have been effective.

8.3.3 Remove or restore

Once a decision has been made to treat a carious tooth a further decision has to be made as to whether to remove or restore it. This decision should take into account the following:

1. *The child.* Each child is an individual and treatment should be planned to provide the best that is possible for that individual. Too often treatment is given which is the most convenient for the parent or, more likely, the dentist. Is it really in the

best interest of the child to remove a tooth which could be saved? In the United Kingdom, general anaesthesia is still widely used for removing the teeth of young children despite the risks of death, its unpleasantness, and the cost involved.

Key Point

- Treat the child—not the convenience of parents or dentist.

---

2. *The tooth.* It is not usually in a child's interest for a permanent tooth to be removed. However, if the pulp of a carious permanent tooth is exposed then a considerable amount of treatment may be required to retain it, and the prognosis for the tooth would still be poor. It may therefore be in the child's long-term interest to lose it and to allow another tooth to take its place, either by natural drift or with orthodontic assistance.

   Primary teeth are often considered by parents and some dentists as being disposable items because there comes a time when they will be exfoliated naturally. However, it is an unusual child who thinks the same way! Loss of a tooth before its time has a considerable significance in a child's life. Losing a tooth early gives a message to the child that teeth are not valuable and not worth looking after. It can then be difficult to persuade a child to care for their teeth. A well-restored primary dentition can be a source of pride to young children and an encouragement for them to look after the succeeding teeth.

   It is usually more important and fortunately rather easier to save and restore a second primary molar than a first. While anterior teeth might be less important for the maintenance of space, their premature loss can cause low esteem in both child and parent.

3. *The stage of the disease.* It is easier for both child and dentist to restore teeth at an early stage of decay. Later the pulp may become involved and subsequent restoration difficult, making loss of the tooth more likely.

4. *The extent of the disease.* A large number of teeth requiring treatment may put a strain on a young child and, less importantly, on the parent and dentist.

Caries in children is significantly less than it was 20 years ago, and it would be good to think that the dental profession would be able to restore the reduced number of decayed teeth that now present.

8.4 DIAGNOSIS AND TREATMENT PLANNING

This was discussed in Chapter 3 and will be only briefly outlined here. As stated above the treatment of carious teeth should be based on the needs of the child. The long-term objective should be to help the child reach adulthood with an intact permanent dentition, with no active caries, as few restored teeth as possible, and a positive attitude to their future dental health. If restoration is required it should be carried out to the highest standard possible in order to maximize longevity of the restoration and avoid re-treatment.

8.4.1 Diagnosis

An accurate diagnosis of dental caries is important in the management of the primary dentition. Enamel of the primary tooth is thin compared with that of the permanent teeth, and caries progresses quickly through the enamel into the dentine, especially

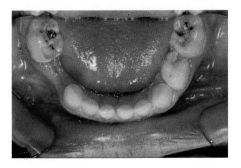

Fig. 8.2 The marginal ridges of both the lower left first and lower right second primary molar have been involved in the carious process, the pulp in these teeth is likely to be inflamed.

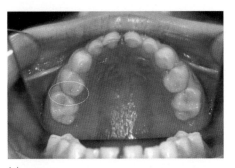

(a)

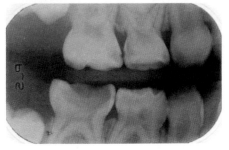

(b)

Fig. 8.3 (a) A clinical examination in the upper arch gives a little clue to the presence of proximal carious lesions on both the upper right first and second primary molars. (b) However, extensive caries is evident when these were examined with BW radiographs.

at the proximal area below the contact point making an early diagnosis paramount. When caries is still confined to the enamel then preventive measures stand a chance of halting and reversing the lesion as discussed in Chapter 6.

Pulpal involvement

Once the caries is into the dentine then removal of the carious tissue and restoration of the tooth is required. Caries progresses very rapidly through the primary dentine with early pulp involvement. When this stage of the process is reached the marginal ridge becomes undermined and collapses. The diagnosis of the integrity of the marginal ridge in primary molars is important in treatment planning for children. Research has shown that once the marginal ridge of a primary molar has broken away the pulp of the tooth is affected and irreversible changes have commenced (Fig. 8.2).

Radiographs

The importance of radiographs for the diagnosis of caries in children cannot be over-emphasized, as clinical examination alone would mean that many proximal lesions could be missed (Fig. 8.3). As mentioned earlier many early lesions may be halted or reversed by a rigorous preventive programme. But this depends on adequate early diagnosis. While several techniques for caries diagnosis have been introduced recently, most notable of which is Diagnodent (KAVO), bitewing (BW) radiography is by far the most acceptable and widely available for use in general practice. Radiographs should form a routine part of any dental examination and it is necessary to repeat radiographs for dental caries diagnosis at suitable intervals. The intervals that are appropriate to children vary according to the level of caries that a child presents with. After an initial examination and BW radiographs a second series should be taken within 1 year if the child is caries free but at 6 months if this is active caries. Once it has been established that a child remains caries free, then, the interval between BWs can be increased to 24 months or even longer. However, if active caries remains a problem, then 6 monthly intervals between BWs are necessary.

> **Key Point**
> Destruction by caries of the marginal ridge of a primary molar indicates likely pulpal involvement.

8.4.2 Treatment planning

Following diagnosis of the extent of caries in each tooth and the probable state of the pulp, a logical treatment plan should be made which would usually involve treating a quadrant of the mouth at a time. It used to be felt that multiple short visits placed least stress on a child particularly if they were under 6 years of age. However, the most important aspect of child management is to gain the confidence of the child and make sure that there is as little discomfort as possible. Restorative care must be conducted with good pain control and management of a child's behaviour. Local analgesia is therefore mandatory and is easily performed these days with topical analgesia, fine gauge needles, and short-acting local analgesia agents. Due consideration should be given to the use of a rubber dam that ensures a much higher quality of restorations that last for the duration of a tooth as well as being an aid in behaviour management. Once the tissues have been anaesthetized and the child is confident that there will be no pain, it is usually best to complete treatment on a whole quadrant. The number of visits can then be kept to a minimum and a reservoir of co-operation maintained. If a child is in pain then it matters little if an appointment is 5 or 45 min. Where there is pulpal involvement of primary teeth then pulpotomies or pulpectomies are essential. Such teeth also need restoration with preformed metal crowns, which have repeatedly been shown to have one of the highest success rates of any restoration for children's teeth. No doubt, the least interventionist approach can be the correct one for some children, but integrated within a treatment plan which is best in the long-term interest of the child and not an easy way out for the dentist. If this predisposes the child to repetitive treatment, and worse still pain, abscesses, and extractions under general anaesthesia, then it should be rejected in favour of comprehensive care using restorative techniques, such as described in this chapter.

8.5 DURABILITY OF RESTORATIONS

In contrast to the amount of useful research that has been carried out with regard to the diagnosis and prevention of dental caries, methods of treatment are still empirical. Treatment decisions ought to be based on sound scientific evidence but, unfortunately, despite the great effort that has been spent providing treatment over many years, little in the way of resources has been spent on clinical research into the success or otherwise of dental treatment methods. This is especially true with regard to the primary dentition. There are few reports in the literature on the relative success in the primary dentition of different treatment methods or materials. The majority of those reports are retrospective and therefore need to be treated with caution.

The choice of restoration for primary teeth is based upon the degree of carious involvement, whether the marginal ridge is intact or not and the length of time that will elapse before exfoliation. The decision regarding the type of restoration to be used is therefore based on the diagnosis of the extent of the dental caries. Here again if the marginal ridge has broken away then simple Class II type restoration will fail as the pulp involvement has possibly occurred already.

8.5.1 Conventional restorative materials

Many different materials have been advocated over the years, but, as indicated above, very little research has been carried out to find out which ones might be the most useful. Therefore the popularity of any particular material has depended on clinical impression and fashion. This section provides a brief overview of those materials that are both currently widely available and have been subject to some clinical research.

Silver amalgam

Silver amalgam has been used for restoring teeth for over 150 years and, despite the fact that it is not tooth coloured and that there have been repeated concerns about its safety (largely unfounded), it is still widely used. This is probably because it is relatively easy to use, is tolerant of operator error, and has yet to be bettered as a material for economically restoring posterior teeth. Modern, non-gamma 2 alloy restorations have been shown to have extended lifetimes in permanent teeth when placed under good conditions, and have also been shown to be much less sensitive to poor handling than tooth-coloured materials.

In clinical trials and retrospective studies, no intracoronal material has so far performed more successfully than amalgam.

Stainless-steel crowns

These were introduced in 1950 and have gained wide acceptance in North America. In Europe they have been less popular, being seen by most dentists as too difficult to use, although in reality they are often easier to place than some intracoronal restorations (Fig. 8.4).

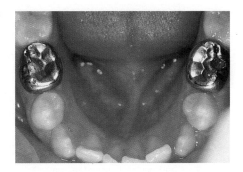

Fig. 8.4 Restoration of lower second primary molars with stainless-steel crowns 7 years after placement.

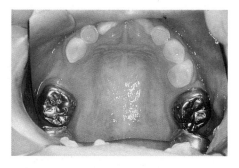

Fig. 8.5 Temporary restoration of carious upper first permanent molars with stainless-steel crowns in an 8-year-old child with a high caries rate.

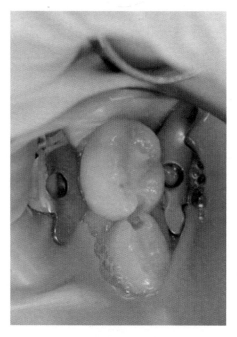

Fig. 8.6 Rubber dam placement prior to restoration of approximal lesions with composite resin.

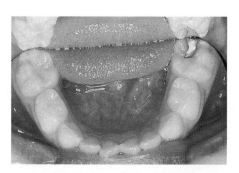

Fig. 8.7 Distal–occlusal restorations on both lower second primary molars after 3 years—one restored with conventional amalgam, the other with glass ionomer cement.

All published studies have shown stainless-steel crowns to have a higher success rate in primary teeth than all other restorative materials. They are certainly the preferred treatment option for first primary molars with anything other than minimal caries.

Stainless-steel crowns are also advocated for hypoplastic or very carious first permanent molars, where they act as provisional restorations prior either to strategic removal at age 9–12 years or later restoration with a cast crown (Fig. 8.5). Etched retained castings may now be used for the definitive restoration of permanent hypoplastic teeth without involvement of the approximal surface; more conservative provisional restorations than stainless-steel crowns should be considered if this is intended.

Composite resin

Composite resins came on the market in the early 1970s and have been modified since then in an attempt to improve their properties. Current materials are still best applied to anterior teeth and small restorations in posterior teeth. The development of acid etching at the time that these materials were introduced has ensured that they have performed reasonably well in terms of marginal seal. They are sensitive to variations in technique and take longer to place than equivalent amalgam restorations. They must be placed in a dry field (Fig. 8.6).

The long-term success of composite resins is jeopardized by their instability in water. The best materials have maximum inorganic filler levels and low water absorption, but will deteriorate over time.

> **Key Point**
> * All composite resin and glass ionomer restorations must be placed in a dry field.

Glass ionomer

Glass ionomer cements came on to the market in the late 1970s and have also been modified since then in order to enhance their properties. Current materials are much improved and have some advantages over composite resins. Being made from glasses with a high fluoride content they not only provide a sustained release over an extended period but also act as a rechargeable reservoir of fluoride, which may protect adjacent surfaces from caries progression.

They adhere to enamel and dentine without the need for acid etching, do not suffer from polymerization shrinkage, and, once set, are dimensionally stable in conditions of high humidity such as exist in the mouth (Fig. 8.7). Similarly to composite resins it is imperative that they are placed in a dry field.

8.5.2 New restorative materials

Recently, a number of new materials have come on to the market which aim to maximize the best qualities of both composite resins and glass ionomers. Some of these show promise and should be considered for the restoration of children's teeth. None of them have had more than 3–4 year clinical trials so it is still unclear how valuable they are compared to conventional materials.

They can be classified according to whether they retain the essential acid–base reaction of the glass ionomers or not.

Resin-modified glass ionomer

These consist of a glass ionomer cement to which has been added a resin system that will allow the material to set quickly using light or chemical catalysts (or both) while allowing the acid–base reaction of the glass ionomer to take place. Thus, the materials will set, albeit rather slowly, without the need for the resin system and the essential qualities of a glass ionomer cement should be retained (Fig. 8.8).

Polyacid-modified composite resin (Compomer)

In contrast, these materials have a much higher content of resin and the acid–base reaction of the glass ionomers does not take place. Therefore although they are easier to use (being premixed in capsules), there is some doubt as to the longer term benefits over conventional composite resins (Fig. 8.9). However, recently published work has shown compomer to be as durable as amalgam after 3 years in approximal cavities in primary molars (Marks *et al.* 1999; Welbury *et al.* 2000).

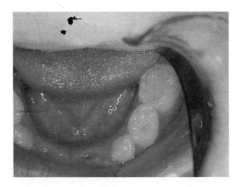

Fig. 8.8 Resin-modified glass polymer restoration after 2 years in a lower second primary molar.

8.6 RUBBER DAM

Most texts that discuss operative treatment for children advocate the use of rubber dam, but it is used very little in practice despite many sound reasons for its adoption. In the United Kingdom less than 2% of dentists use it routinely. It is perceived as a difficult technique that is expensive in time and arduous for the patient.

In fact, once mastered, the technique makes dental care for children easier and a higher standard of care can be achieved in less time than would otherwise be required. In addition, it isolates the child from the operative field making treatment less invasive of their personal space.

The benefits can be divided into three main categories as shown below.

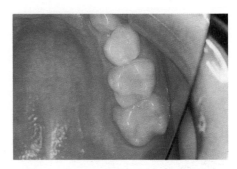

Fig. 8.9 Mesial-occlusal restoration after 1 year in an upper second primary molar with polyacid-modified composite resin.

8.6.1 Safety

Damage of soft tissues

The risks of operative treatment include damage to the soft tissues of the mouth from rotary and hand instruments and the medicaments used in the provision of endodontic and other care. Rubber dam will go a long way to preventing damage of this type.

Risk of swallowing or inhalation

There is also the risk that these items may be lost in the patient's mouth and swallowed or even inhaled and there are reports in the literature to substantiate this risk.

Risk of cross-infection

In addition, there is considerable risk that the use of high-speed rotary instruments distribute an aerosol of the patients' saliva around the operating room, putting the dentist and staff at risk of infection. Again, a risk that has been substantiated in the literature.

Nitrous oxide sedation

If this is used it is quite likely that mouth breathing by the child will increase the level of the gas in the environment, again putting dentist and staff at risk. The use of rubber dam in this situation will make sure that exhaled gas is routed via the scavenging system attached to the nose piece. Usually less nitrous oxide will be required for a sedative effect, increasing the safety and effectiveness of the procedure.

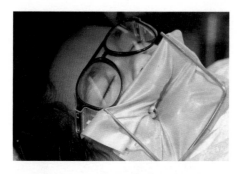

Fig. 8.10 Shows rubber dam placed in the a child and with the comfort it provides it is not unusual for children to fall asleep in the dental chair during treatment under rubber dam.

8.6.2 Benefits to the child

Isolation

One of the reasons that dental treatment causes anxiety in patients is that the operative area is very close to and involved with all the most vital functions of the body such as sight, hearing, breathing, and swallowing. When operative treatment is being performed, all these vital functions are put at risk and any sensible child would be concerned. It is useful to discuss these fears with child patients and explain how the risks can be reduced or eliminated.

Glasses should be used to protect the eyes and rubber dam to protect the airways and the oesophagus. By doing this, and provided that good local analgesia has been obtained, the child can feel themselves distanced from the operation. Sometimes it is even helpful to show the child their isolated teeth in a mirror. The view is so different from what they normally see in the mirror that they can divorce themselves from the reality of the situation.

Relaxation

The isolation of the operative area from the child will very often cause the child to become considerably relaxed—always provided that there is good pain control. It is common for both adult and child patients to fall asleep while undergoing treatment involving the use of rubber dam—a situation that rarely occurs without (Fig 8.10). This is a function of the safety perceived by the patient and the relaxed way in which the dental team can work with its assistance.

8.6.3 Benefits to the dentist

Reduced stress

As noted above, once rubber dam has been placed the child will be at less risk from the procedures that will be used to restore their teeth. This reduces the effort required by the operator to protect the soft tissues of the mouth and the airways. Treatment can be carried out in a more relaxed and controlled manner, therefore lessening the stress of the procedure on the dental team.

Retraction of tongue and cheeks

Correctly placed rubber dam will gently pull the cheeks and tongue away from the operative area allowing the operator a better view of the area to be treated.

Retraction of gingival tissue

Rubber dam will gently pull the gingival tissues away from the cervical margin of the tooth, making it much easier to see the extent of any caries close to the margin and often bringing the cervical margin of a prepared cavity above the level of the gingival margin thus making restoration considerably easier. Interdentally, this retraction should be assisted by placing a wedge firmly between the adjacent teeth as soon as the dam has been placed. This wedge is placed horizontally below the contact area and above the dam, thus compressing the interdental gingivae against the underlying bone. Approximal cavities can then be prepared, any damage from rotary instruments being inflicted on the wedge rather than the child's gingival tissue.

Quite often it can be difficult and time consuming to take the rubber dam between the contacts because of dental caries or broken restorations. It is possible to make life easier by using a 'trough technique', which involves snipping the rubber dam between the punched holes. All the benefits of rubber dam are retained except for the retraction and protection of the gingival tissues (Fig. 8.11).

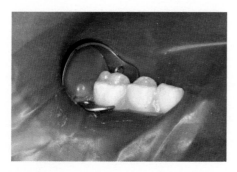

Fig. 8.11 'Trough technique' of rubber dam placement.

Moisture control

As mentioned previously, silver amalgam is probably the only restorative material that has any tolerance to being placed in a damp environment, and there is no doubt that it and all other materials will perform much more satisfactorily if placed in a dry field. Rubber dam is the only technique that readily ensures a dry field.

8.6.4 Technique

Most texts on operative dentistry demonstrate techniques for the use of rubber dam. It is not intended to duplicate this effort, but it would seem useful to point out features of the technique that have made life easier for the authors when using rubber dam with children.

Analgesia

Placement of rubber dam can be uncomfortable especially if a clamp is needed to retain it. Even if a clamp is not required the sharp cut edge of the dam can cause mild pain. Soft tissue analgesia can be obtained using infiltration in the buccal sulcus followed by an interpapillary injection. This will usually give sufficient analgesia to remove any discomfort from the dam. However, more profound analgesia may be required for the particular operative procedure that has to be performed.

Method of application

There are at least four different methods of placing the dam, but most authorities recommend a method whereby the clamp is first placed on the tooth, the dam stretched over the clamp and then over the remaining teeth that are to be isolated. Because of the risk of the patient swallowing or inhaling a dropped or broken clamp before the dam is applied, it is imperative that the clamp be restrained with a piece of floss tied or wrapped around the bow. This adds considerable inconvenience to the technique and the authors favour a simpler method whereby the clamp, dam, and frame are assembled together before application and taken to the tooth in one movement. Because the clamp is always on the outside of the dam relative to the patient there is no need to use floss to secure the clamp.

A 5-inch (about 12.5 cm) square of medium dam is stretched over an Ivory frame and a single hole punched in the middle of the square. This hole is for the tooth on which the clamp is going to be placed and further holes should be punched for any other teeth that need to be isolated. A winged clamp is placed in the first hole and the whole assembly carried to the tooth by the clamp forceps. The tooth that is going to be clamped can be seen through the hole and the clamp applied to it. The dam is then teased off the wings using either the fingers or a hand instrument. It can then be carried forward over the other teeth with the interdental dam being 'knifed' through the contact areas. It may need to be stabilized at the front using either floss, a small piece of rubber dam, a 'Wedjet' (Figs 8.6 and 8.11), or a wooden wedge.

8.7 OPERATIVE TREATMENT OF PRIMARY TEETH

8.7.1 Pit and fissure caries

Pit and fissure caries is less of a problem in primary teeth than in permanent ones. The fissures are usually much shallower and less susceptible to decay, so the presence of a cavity in the occlusal surface of a primary molar is a sign of high caries activity. Because of this it is quite likely that the children who require treatment of these surfaces will be young. However, treatment is not difficult and can usually be accomplished without problem. Infiltration analgesia should be given together with supplemental intrapapillary injection. Caries is removed using a 330 bur in a high-speed handpiece. For restoration—although, as indicated above, silver amalgam has not so far been bettered in clinical trial—because occlusal caries in the primary dentition indicates high caries activity, the material of choice may be a resin-modified glass ionomer cement with its possible caries preventive properties (Fig. 8.8).

8.7.2 Approximal caries

Silver amalgam

Failure of amalgam itself as well as faults in the cavity design have been the most commonly reported causes of failure of approximal restorations in primary teeth. Attempts to overcome these deficiencies and to improve durability have come through alteration in cavity design and the choice of material used. A reduction in the size of the occlusal lock, rounded line angles, and minimum extension for prevention all result in less destruction of sound tooth tissue. In addition, the 'minimal' approximal cavity with no occlusal 'dovetail' has been described for both amalgam and adhesive restorations, and incorporates some mechanical retention in the form of small internal resistance grooves placed with a very small round bur just inside the enamel–dentine junction. Figure 8.12(a)–(f) demonstrate the clinical stages in the placement of two-surface amalgam restorations in the primary dentition.

It is unlikely that the 'perfect cavity design' exists for an amalgam restoration in primary molars due to certain anatomical features:

1. Widened contact areas make a narrow box difficult to achieve.
2. Thin enamel means that cracking and fracture of parts of the crown are more common.
3. Primary teeth may undergo considerable wear under occlusal stress themselves and this in turn will affect the restorations.

It is therefore necessary to investigate other materials for use in restoring the primary dentition.

Fig. 8.12 (a)–(f) Technique sequence for the placement of two-surface amalgam restorations in lower primary molars. The first molar could have been restored with a stainless-steel crown.

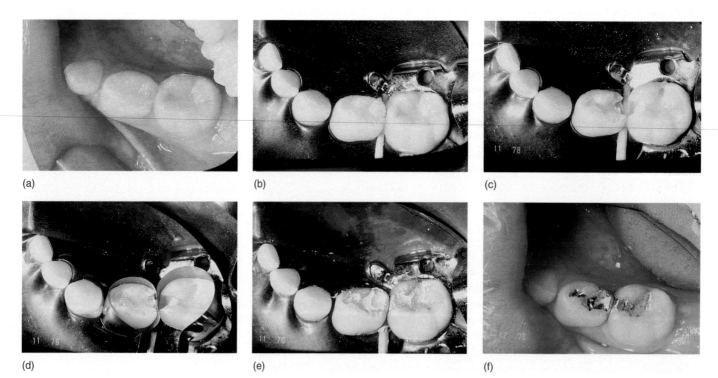

(a)　(b)　(c)

(d)　(e)　(f)

Composite resin

Composite resin has been used quite widely to restore primary teeth and results are generally acceptable. Cavity design is usually a modified approximal design with bevelling of the margins to increase the amount of enamel available for etching and bonding.

The use of rubber dam is essential if a dry field is to be achieved. This fact together with the material's relative expense probably reflects the lack of widespread use of composite resin in many countries.

Glass ionomer cement

More studies have been conducted using glass ionomer cements than composite resins. However, the cavity designs used in the different studies vary considerably and it is difficult to draw firm conclusions. Certainly, glass ionomer cement will undergo significantly more loss of anatomical form than amalgam in the approximal area, and as such conventional glass ionomers have not been shown to be as durable as amalgam. However, the operator will need to balance this fact with the obvious mechanical and chemical advantages of the cement—namely its ability to bond to enamel and dentine, thus requiring a more conservative preparation, and its ability to act as a reservoir of fluoride.

Compomers

Compomers are now widely used in general dental practice for the restoration of approximal lesions in primary teeth. After good initial results, longer follow-up periods have shown that this material indeed lived up to its early promise and good survival rates have been reported for restorations in primary molars. However, it must be placed in cavities prepared to the usual principles of cavity design for a most favourable outcome.

8.7.3 Stainless-steel crowns

Stainless-steel crowns should be considered whenever posterior primary teeth (especially first molars) require restoration. They were originally developed to provide a 'restoration of last resort' for those teeth that were not salvageable by any other means. At the time that they were introduced in the early 1950s the only alternatives were silver or copper amalgam or a selection of cements, materials completely unsuited to the restoration of grossly carious teeth or those that had been weakened by pulp treatment. Over the years, it has become apparent that the life expectancy of these crowns is far better than any other restoration for primary posterior teeth and that they come close to the ideal of never having to be replaced prior to exfoliation. In addition, they are less demanding technically than intracoronal restorations in primary teeth.

They should therefore now be considered for any tooth where the dentist cannot be sure that an alternative would survive until the tooth is lost. It is unfair to put a child through more treatment situations than necessary because a less successful material, which needs frequent replacement, was chosen.

The *indications* for stainless-steel crowns are shown in Table 8.2.

Table 8.2 Indications for stainless-steel crowns

1. Restoration of primary molars needing large multisurface restorations.
2. Restoration of primary molars in children with rampant caries.
3. Restoration of teeth after pulp therapy.
4. Restoration of teeth with developmental defects, for example, amelogenesis imperfecta.
5. Abutment for space maintainers.
6. Restoration of fractured primary molars.
7. Protection of molars in children with bruxism.
8. Restoration of hypomineralized young permanent molars.

The technique

Wherever possible local anaesthesia should be given, although in certain situations, for example, while preparing a non-vital tooth, this is not always necessary. Nevertheless, even in these teeth there will need to be some tooth preparation involving the gingival margin, which can cause some discomfort for which local anaesthesia is advisable. It is sometimes possible to use only a topical anaesthesia, such as a benzocaine ointment on the gingival cuff. In other instances, when the preparation for a crown is carried out at the same visit as a pulpotomy, local analgesia would already have been administered. Where crowns are being fitted because of extensive cavities or decalcification, a rubber dam is advisable, even though the authors acknowledge that the use of rubber dam for restorations in children in general dental practice is quite low.

Prior to preparation, all caries is removed and any pulp treatment that may be required carried out. A recent preoperative radiograph must be available to make sure that the periapical and interradicular tissues are healthy and that the tooth is unlikely to be exfoliated in the near future.

Preparation and fitting is easier if rubber dam is in place but even if this is not the case it is advisable to place wedges mesially and distally, gingival to the contact area (Fig. 8.13(a)). These wedges should be placed firmly using the applicator supplied with them or a pair of flat-beaked pliers. It is essential that good soft tissue anaesthesia be obtained so that this procedure is not painful, although the wedges should compress the gingivae away from the contact area and not be driven into the tissue. The use of wedges in this manner protects the tissues and reduces the contamination of the operating field as well as making the margins of the preparation easier to see. The mesial and distal surfaces of the tooth are removed using a 330 bur or a fine tapered fissure bur or diamond (Fig. 8.13(b)). It is important to cut through the tooth, away from the contact area, to avoid damage to the adjacent tooth. The bur should be angled away from the vertical so that a shoulder is not created at the gingival margin. The same bur may be used for the whole preparation, although it can be quicker to use a larger diamond for the next stage, which is to reduce the occlusal surface to allow 1.5–2 mm of space between the prepared tooth and its opposite number.

Fig. 8.13 (a) Rubber dam and wedges in place, pulpotomy and coronal reduction completed. (b) Mesial and distal surfaces reduced. (c) Crown 'try-in'. (d) Cementation of crown. (e) Excess cement removed prior to rubber dam removal and occlusal analysis. (f) Approximal hole in stainless-steel crown prior to placement.

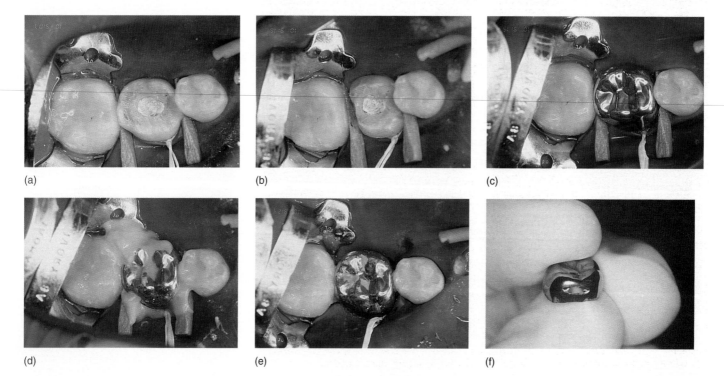

(a)   (b)   (c)

(d)   (e)   (f)

Many authorities advocate doing no more preparation than this but it takes little further time to reduce the buccal and lingual surfaces sufficiently to remove any undercuts above the gingival margin. Any sharp line angles are rounded off to avoid interferences that might prevent the crown seating.

The mesial and distal preparation might seem rather radical in comparison to that required when a cast crown is constructed for a permanent tooth, but the principles of retention and resistance of the two types of crown are different. A cast crown is retained by friction between the walls of the prepared tooth and the internal surface of the crown. It is, therefore, important to have near parallel walls of adequate height. A stainless-steel metal crown is retained by contact between the margins of the crown and the undercut portion of the tooth below the gingiva. The shape of the preparation above the gingiva is relatively unimportant and difficulty in fitting these crowns is most often because of under-preparation. However, it is most important that a shoulder is not formed at the gingival margin as this would make the seating of a well-adapted crown impossible.

Try the crown on and check to feel that it is within the gingival crevice (Fig. 8.13(c)) by probing. If it rests on the gingival crevice then crimp in with some pliers. Again seat the crown. If it is over-extended, cut down in that area with a stone or scissors and smooth off before retrying. Check contacts with adjacent teeth and finally polish the margins with a stone or rubber wheel. Wash and dry the tooth before cementation with a glass ionomer cement. Seat the crown from lingual to buccal pressing down firmly (Fig. 8.13(d)). Remove excess cement when set with a probe and dental floss (Fig. 8.13(e)), before removing rubber dam and checking the occlusion. Although not proven statistically beneficial, some operators favour making small holes in the approximal surfaces of the stainless-steel crown, to confer the benefits of fluoride release from the glass ionomer cement to the adjacent teeth (Fig. 8.13(f)).

Figure 8.14(a)–(d) shows how the restoration of heavily carious primary molars with stainless-steel crowns has maintained arch space and allowed permanent premolars to erupt into ideal occlusion.

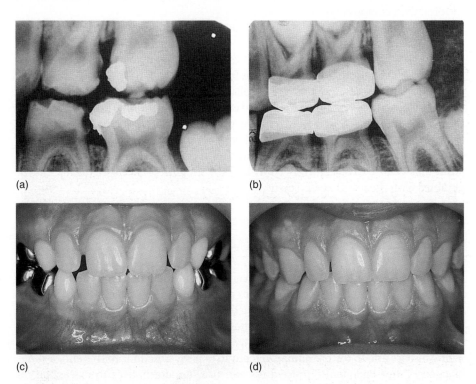

(a)   (b)

(c)   (d)

Fig. 8.14   (a) Carious upper and lower primary molars. (b) After placement of stainless-steel crowns. (c) Occlusion in the mixed dentition. (d) 'Ideal' final occlusion in the permanent dentition.

Success rates of stainless-steel crown restoration

Over the last 20–30 years authors have consistently recorded and reported higher success rates for stainless-steel crowns as compared with other restorations in primary molars. In a recently published meta-analysis, it was clear that stainless-steel crowns were by far the most durable restorations for primary molars, and the most remarkable fact was that once placed they seldom needed replacing.

8.7.4 Anterior teeth

The treatment of decayed primary incisors depends on the stage of decay and the age and co-operation of the patient. In the preschool child, caries of the upper primary incisors is usually as a result of 'nursing caries syndrome' due to the frequent or prolonged consumption of fluids containing fermentable carbohydrate from a bottle or feeder cup (Chapter 6). The lower incisors are rarely affected as they are protected during suckling by the tongue and directly bathed in secretions from the sub-mandibular and sublingual glands. In 'nursing caries' the progression of decay is rapid, commencing on the labial surfaces and quickly encircling the teeth. It is impossible to prepare satisfactory cavities for restoration and after a comprehensive preventive programme the most suitable form of restoration is the 'strip crown technique'. This utilizes celluloid crown forms and a light-cured composite resin to restore crown morphology. Either calcium hydroxide or glass ionomer cement can be used as a lining and the high polishability of modern hybrid composites make them aesthetically, as well as physically, suitable for this task.

In older children over 3 or 4 years of age new lesions of primary incisors, although not usually associated with the use of pacifiers, do indicate high caries activity (Fig. 8.15). Such lesions do not progress so rapidly and usually appear on the mesial and distal surfaces, here a glass ionomer cement or composite resin can be used for restoration. Glass ionomer lacks the translucency of composite resin but has the useful advantages of being adhesive and releasing fluoride.

Fractures of the incisal edges in primary teeth, as in permanent teeth, should be restored with composite resin.

Strip Crowns (3M ESPEE) are a useful aid in the restoration of primary incisors. Unfortunately, owing to their low sales in the United Kingdom and the rest of Europe, the company has discontinued the sale of these crowns and now they are only available on special request. They are however, freely available in the United States. In the authors opinion, these crowns are excellent for building primary incisors where extensive tooth tissue has been lost due to either caries or trauma. The technique for their use is similar to that of such crowns used in permanent teeth; the crowns are easily trimmed with sharp scissors, filled with composite, and seated on a prepared and conditioned tooth. The celluloid crown form can be stripped off after the composite has been cured. Figure 8.16(a) and (b) show that excellent results can be obtained with the use of strip crowns.

8.8 PULP THERAPY IN PRIMARY TEETH

Contemporary advances in primary prevention have reduced dental disease in the developed world. But there is no room for complacency. Dental caries and traumatic dental injuries are still prevalent and treatment of the damage they cause is still a major component of paediatric dental practice.

The principal goals of paediatric operative dentistry are to prevent the extension of dental disease and to restore damaged teeth to healthy function. To this end, a range of conservative endodontic procedures can provide alternatives to extraction for

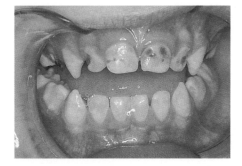

Fig. 8.15 Labial and approximal caries in upper anterior primary teeth.

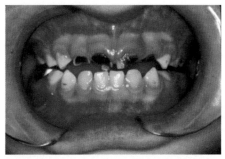

(a)

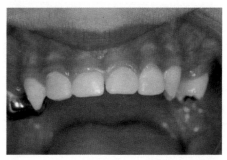

(b)

Fig. 8.16 The figure shows (a) carious primary incisors that were restored (b) using strip crowns, and composite resins to give an aesthetically pleasing result.

many pulpally compromised primary teeth. They are within the grasp of all practitioners and are central to the practice of paediatric dentistry.

While many of the general principles and operative procedures in paediatric endodontics are shared with adult endodontics, a number of important differences exist which justify the special coverage given in this chapter.

Key Points

Disadvantages of unplanned extractions in the primary and mixed dentitions:

- loss of space, promoting malocclusion;
- reduced masticatory function (especially posterior teeth);
- impaired speech development (especially anterior teeth);
- psychological disturbance (especially anterior teeth);
- anaesthetic and surgical traumas.

8.8.1 The dental pulp

Dental pulp is the living, soft tissue structure which resides in the coronal pulp chamber and root canals of primary and permanent teeth.

Histologically, it is composed of loose connective tissue, surrounded on its periphery by a continuous layer of specialized secretory cells, the odontoblasts. Odontoblasts are unique to the dental pulp and are responsible for dentine deposition.

Blood vessels and nerves enter the pulp through the apical foramen and occasionally through lateral or accessory root canals. The pulps of primary and young permanent teeth, especially those with incomplete apices, have a very rich blood supply.

The most important function of the pulp is to lay down dentine which forms the basic structure of teeth, defines their general morphology, and provides them with mechanical strength and toughness.

Dentine deposition commences many months (primary teeth) or years (permanent teeth) before tooth eruption and while the crown of a newly erupted tooth has a mature external form, the pulp within still has considerable work to do in completing tooth development. Newly erupted teeth have short roots, their apices are wide and often diverging, and the dentine walls of the entire tooth are thin and relatively weak.

Provided the pulp remains healthy, dentine deposition will continue during the posteruptive year for primary teeth. One of the key goals of paediatric dentistry is therefore to protect and preserve the pulps of teeth in a healthy state *at least* until this critical phase of tooth development is complete.

8.8.2 Diagnosis of pulp pathosis and rationale

Studies in the early 1970s had shown that in over 50% of the primary molars where the loss of the marginal ridge had occurred, pulp inflammation was irreversible. Research carried out recently in the Department of Paediatric Dentistry of the Leeds Dental Institute (Duggal *et al.*, 2002), has corroborated these findings. In this study, it was shown that most teeth had pulp inflammation involving the pulp horn adjacent to the proximal carious lesion, even when caries had involved less than half the marginal ridge, studied by measuring the inter-cuspal distance (bucco-lingual) involved in the carious process. This suggests that inflammation of the pulp in primary molars develops at an early stage of proximal carious attack and by the time most proximal caries is manifest clinically, the pulp inflammation is quite advanced. These findings have important clinical implications, the most important being that restoration carried out without pulp therapy in most primary molars, where proximal caries has manifest clinically with the involvement of the marginal ridge, will fail. Once the breakdown of marginal ridge is evident pulp therapy is invariably required. It also reiterates the importance of early diagnosis of proximal caries with the use of BW radiographs. Because of this early onset of inflammation in primary molars direct pulp capping is also contraindicated.

8.8.3 Indirect pulp capping

In the majority of circumstances, carious lesions can and should be fully excavated before tooth restoration. A clinical dilemma is presented by a deep lesion in a vital, symptom-free tooth where complete removal of softened dentine on the pulpal floor is likely to result in frank exposure. The advancing front of a carious lesion contains very few cariogenic bacteria. Provided the bulk of infected overlying dentine is removed, a small amount of softened dentine may often be left in the deepest part of the preparation without endangering the pulp. This is the basis of indirect pulp capping.

All caries is first cleared from the cavity margins with a steel round bur running at slow speed. Gentle excavation then follows on the pulpal floor, removing as much of the softened dentine as possible without exposing the pulp. Precisely how much dentine should be removed becomes a matter of experience and clinical judgement, although some have advocated the use of indicator dyes (e.g. 0.5% basic fuchsin) to show when all infected dentine has been eliminated. A thin layer of setting calcium hydroxide cement is then placed on the cavity floor to destroy any remaining micro-organisms and to promote the deposition of reparative secondary dentine.

In its classical application, the indirect pulp cap was covered with zinc oxide–eugenol cement, and following several weeks' observation, the cavity was re-entered to remove all remaining softened dentine. More commonly, the calcium hydroxide pulp cap is simply covered with a layer of hard setting cement and the tooth permanently restored at the same visit. Periodic clinical and radiographic review is then undertaken to monitor the pulp response.

If, as has been discussed in the previous sections, the pulp is deemed to be inflamed, pulp therapy should be considered even in the absence of a clinical exposure. Direct pulp capping should not be carried out if an exposure is found on removal of caries, as placing a medicament, such as calcium hydroxide on an inflamed pulp will lead to failure.

8.8.4 The vital pulpotomy

Pulp therapy usually refers to two terms; pulpotomy and pulpectomy. A pulpotomy involves the coronal removal of the pulp tissue that is diagnosed to be inflamed or infected as a result of deep caries. This usually leaves an intact radicular pulp tissue upon which a medicament is applied before placing a coronal restoration.

Indications for a pulpotomy

The indications for a pulpotomy that are of direct relevance to general dental practitioners are given in Table 8.3.

There are certain conditions such as congenital heart defects, history of heart surgery where pulpotomy is not usually performed due to the risk of precipitating bacterial endocarditis. Also, in immuno-compromised (e.g. leukaemia) or deficient conditions, pulpotomy is contraindicated and extraction with the relevant essential precautions is usually preferred.

The pulpotomy technique

The various steps involved in carrying out a pulpotomy in a primary molar are shown in Fig. 8.17.

Table 8.3 Indications for pulpotomy

1. Large proximal carious lesion with the involvement of the marginal ridge (one-third or more) in an otherwise restorable tooth.

2. Tooth free from radicular pulpitis diagnosed by:
   (a) no history of spontaneous pain;
   (b) haemorrhage from the radicular tissue, which is easy to control.

3. Absence of an abscess or a fistula.

4. Instances where extraction is contraindicated, for example, haemophilia.

Administer local analgesia and apply rubber dam wherever possible.

Remove caries and identify the site of pulp exposure (Fig. 8.18). If there is no pulp exposure, then access to the pulp chamber is made from the base of the cavity.

Remove roof of the pulp chamber. When the bur passes through the roof of the chamber a 'dip' is felt. Once this is felt the bur is not taken any deeper but moved sideways to remove the roof of the pulp chamber.

Remove coronal pulp with a large round bur or large excavators (Fig. 8.19(a)). Excavators are safer to avoid perforation in the furcation region (Fig. 8.20).

Apply medicament to the radicular pulp on a cotton pledget (Fig. 8.19(b)).

Remove the cotton pledget and check that there is no excessive haemorrhage from the remaining pupal tissue (Fig. 8.19(c)).

Fill chamber with zinc oxide eugenol cement, pressing on the zinc oxide with a damp pledget to make sure that it is well condensed in the pulp chamber (Fig. 8.19(d)).

Place coronal restoration, preferably a stainless-steel crown.

Fig. 8.17 The pulpotomy technique.

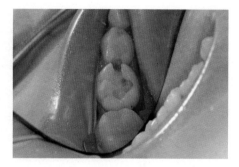

Fig. 8.18 On removal of caries an exposure of the pulp below the mesio-lingual cusp is clearly evident.

Pulpotomy medicament

Formocresol has traditionally been used and widely recognized within the profession, as a medication that has delivered the best long-term results. A one-fifth dilution of original Buckleys formulation has been shown to be as effective as the full strength concentrate. Formocresol is not easily available in the United Kingdom and there have been some concerns about its toxicity, both locally and systemically. These concerns have grown recently with formaldehyde, one of the important components of formocresol linked to certain forms of cancer. Attempts have been ongoing for the last few years to find a suitable replacement and one material that has generated a lot of interest recently as a suitable alternative to formocresol is ferric sulfate. Ferric sulfate has been widely used to control gingival bleeding, prior

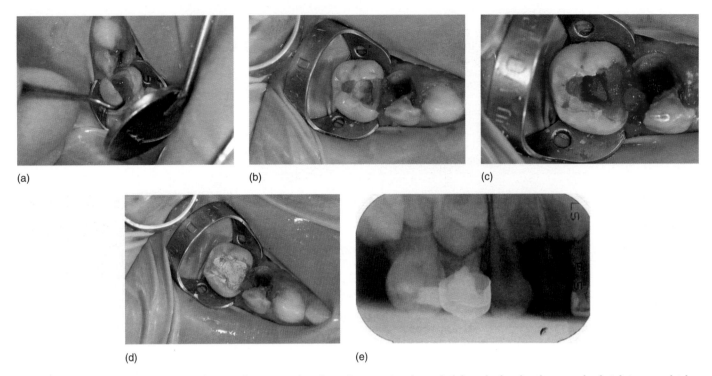

(a)   (b)   (c)

(d)   (e)

Fig. 8.19 (a) The figure shows a lower right second primary molar where after removing the roof of the pulp chamber the coronal pulp is being completely removed using excavators. (b) Cotton pledget with the medicament placed over the radicular pulp tissue to control the bleeding. (c) On removal of the cotton pledget bleeding from the amputation sites has stopped. (d) Kalzinol (or any other zinc oxide eugenol preparation) placed in the pulp chamber prior to placing the coronal restoration. (e) Periapical radiograph of right upper first primary molar showing a completed pulpotomy. Note excellent condensation of cement in the pulp chamber and coronal restoration with stainless-steel crown.

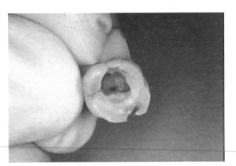

Fig. 8.20 Shows perforation in the floor of the pulp chamber in a second primary molar. If this happens extraction is usually indicated.

to impression taking and also in endodontics. It is an excellent haemostatic agent, forming a ferric ion–protein complex on contact with blood, which then stops further bleeding by sealing the vessels (Fig. 8.21(a)–(c)). It has also now been shown to be as effective as formocresol in medium-and long-term studies when used in a concentration of 15.5%. This is available commercially as Astringident. The authors view is that ferric sulfate will emerge as the most suitable alternative to formocresol in the next few years. In light of recent evidence, ferric sulfate can be used as a suitable alternative for those concerned about the toxicity of formocresol or have difficulty obtaining it in the United Kingdom. However, it must be remembered that ferric sulfate has no "fixative" effect. For this reason, an accurate diagnosis of the state of the pulp tissue being left behind and on which ferric sulfate is being applied will need to be made.

> **Key Points**
>
> - Ferric Sulfate is a suitable medicament for pulpotomy in primary molars when the inflammation is diagnosed to be restricted only to the coronal pulp.
> - Though it stops bleeding at the site of amputation of the coronal pulp, it should be applied, almost immediately, for about 1 min.

Follow-up

Teeth that have undergone pulpotomy should be reviewed clinically and if possible radiographically, though the authors accept that routine radiographic follow-up is not possible in general dental practice. Clinically, the following criteria indicate success:

- absence of symptoms;
- absence of any abscess or draining sinus;
- no excessive mobility or tenderness.

Radiographically there should be:

1. Either no further bone loss in the furcation region or regeneration of bone in this area. Figure 8.19(e) demonstrates good bone condition in the bifurcation region 6 months after the pulpotomy was performed.
2. No evidence of internal resorption. Internal resorption usually indicates chronic inflammation and the activity of giant cells causing resorption of the dentine. It creates few symptoms, and is usually detected as an incidental finding on radiographic examination. It should be considered as a form of irreversible pulpitis (Fig. 8.22).

Key Points

- Direct pulp capping has a poor prognosis in carious primary molars.
- Pulpotomy has a better prognosis than pulp capping.
- A pulpotomy should only be performed when the pulp inflammation is thought to be limited to the coronal pulp.
- Ferric sulfate (15.5%), available as Astringident is emerging as a good alternative to formocresol for use as a pulp medicament.

8.8.5 Management of non-vital and abscessed primary molars—the pulpectomy technique

Primary molars with abscesses are usually indicated for extractions. Persistent and chronic infection in primary molars can cause damage to the developing permanent tooth germs and such foci of infection should be removed.

In some cases the non-vital primary molars (Fig. 8.23) or ones with a chronic discharging sinus might need to be retained. Some of the reasons for this could be:

- orthodontic,
- medical, where extraction is not appropriate, such as in severe haemophiliacs,
- parents refusal to accept extraction.

In such cases these teeth can be retained by carrying out the *Pulpectomy* procedure. In the United Kingdom, there is reluctance among many dentists to carry out a pulpectomy as it is perceived to be difficult in a young child, with extraction being preferred. The authors feel that this is a misconception. This technique should be learnt by all paediatric dentists, as it can often save the child from the trauma of a GA for extraction of primary teeth. Pulpectomy involves accessing the root canal system of primary molars, cleaning them as best as is possible, and then using an appropriate material, usually pure zinc oxide eugenol, to obturate the root canals. Pure zinc oxide eugenol is preferred as it is entirely resorbable and is easily removed as the roots of the primary teeth undergo resorption. Also, if it is extruded through the apices, it gets completely resorbed by the apical tissues. Other materials such as Iodoform paste, and even calcium hydroxide are also sometimes used.

The root canal morphology of primary molars is quite similar to that of permanent molars with either three of the four root canals present. In the lower primary molars there are always two mesial root canals—mesio-buccal and mesio-lingual, with one or sometimes two distal root canals. In upper primary molars there are three root canals—mesio-buccal, disto-buccal, and palatal (Fig. 8.24 (a)–(c)).

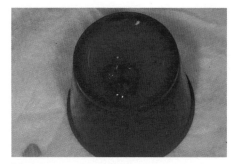

(a)

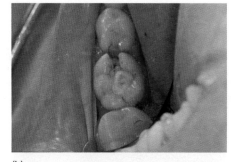

(b)

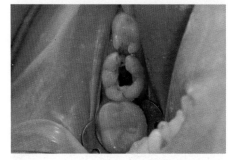

(c)

Fig. 8.21 (a) Ferric sulfate in a concentration of 15.5% solution is available commercially as Astringident (Ultradent, USA). (b) Ferric sulfate being applied on the root canal tissue after the amputation of coronal pulp in the upper right second primary molar. (c) Bleeding stops almost immediately on application of ferric sulfate.

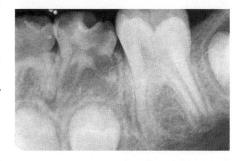

Fig. 8.22 Internal inflammatory resorption, identified as an incidental finding on routine radiographic examination.

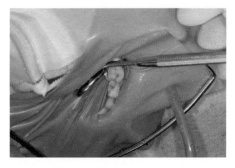

Fig. 8.23 A non-vital left lower primary molar.

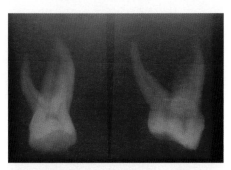

(a)

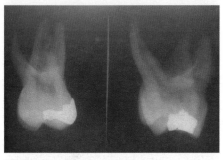

(b)

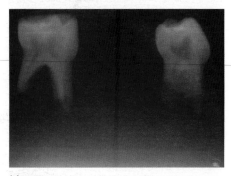

(c)

Fig. 8.24 Root canal morphology of primary molars, (a) maxillary first primary molar; (b) maxillary second primary molar; (c) mandibular primary molars. Reproduced with the kind permission of Prof. H. S. Chawla, PGIMER, India.

Access pulp chamber as described for the pulpotomy procedure.

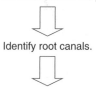

Identify root canals.

Debride root canals gently with hedstrom files and copious irrigation with normal saline or 0.5% solution of sodium hypochlorite. With the help of a good preoperative radiograph, care should be taken to keep files 2–3 mm short of apex to avoid damage to developing tooth germ.

Prepare the canals to no more than file size 30.

Dry root canals with paper points.

Select a spiral root canal filler that is two-sizes smaller than the last file used in the root canal (to avoid it being caught in the root canal), thereby minimizing the risk of it fracturing in the root canal.

Mix zinc oxide eugenol as a slurry and with the help of spiral paste fillers spin this into the root canals. Alternatively, the paste can be carried into the root canals with gutta percha points.

Fill the pulp chamber with cement.

⬇

Restore the crown, usually with a stainless-steel crown.

Fig. 8.25 The Pulpectomy Technique.

Indications for pulpectomy

- Irreversible pulpitis involving both the coronal and radicular pulp.
- Non-vital primary molars or incisors that need to be maintained in the arch.
- Abscessed primary molars.
- Primary molars with radiographic evidence of furcation pathology.

The steps for performing a pulpectomy are shown in the flow diagram. (Figure 8.25).

Figure 8.27 shows a diagrammatic representation of the technique In some cases where there is acute infection or persistent discharge from the root canals, it may be necessary to defer the root canal obturation to a *second visit*. In such cases a medicated cotton pledget, barely moistened with formocresol is sealed in the pulp chamber with either glass ionomer cement or IRM. (For those who are concerned about the safety of formocresol, Ledermix would be a suitable alternative.) In the second visit the pledget is removed and the pulpectomy procedure completed.

Follow-up and review

Though the pulpectomy technique carries a good prognosis, the outcome is not as good as a vital pulpotomy. Clinical follow-up augmented by one periapical radiograph

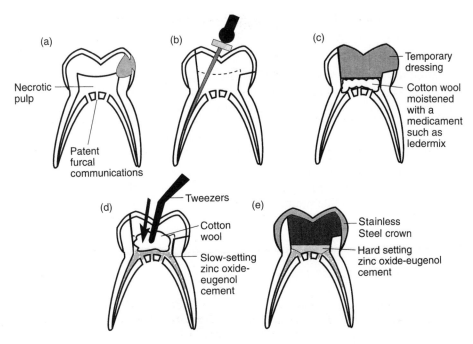

Fig. 8.26 Non-vital pulp therapy—primary tooth. (a) A carious, but restorable, non-vital primary molar. (b) Caries is eliminated and access made to the pulp. Gentle canal debridement is undertaken with small files and irrigation. (c) Disinfection of the canal system. A pledget of cotton wool barely moistened with ledermix is sealed into the pulp chamber for 7–10 days. (d) The tooth is reopened at a second visit, and, after irrigation and drying, a soft mixture of slow-setting zinc oxide–eugenol cement is gently packed into the canals with the cotton-wool pledget. (e) The pulp chamber is packed with accelerated zinc oxide–eugenol cement before definitive restoration of the tooth.

on a yearly basis is required (Fig. 8.27(a)–(b)). The following clinical and radiographic parameters can be taken as indications of success:

Clinical

- alleviation of acute symptoms;
- tooth free from pain and mobility.

Radiographic

- improvement or no further deterioration of bone condition in the furcation area.

Root canal treatment of primary incisors

The technique described above can also be used to treat non-vital or abscessed primary incisors. Increasingly, parents are reluctant to have their child's upper anterior teeth extracted. In a modern society, where a child's self-esteem is important, it is the duty of the dentists to maintain aesthetics wherever possible. Many primary incisors with abscesses that are extracted can be retained with the help of a pulpectomy technique, and the root canal morphology is such that this can easily be performed (Fig. 8.28), the only limiting factor being the child's co-operation. Indications for a pulpectomy in primary incisors include carious or traumatized primary incisors with pulp exposures or acute or chronic abscesses. Figure 8.29 shows an example of primary central incisors treated with pulpectomy.

> **Key Points**
> - A pulpectomy should be considered wherever it is essential to preserve a primary tooth that cannot be treated with other means, such as a pulpotomy.
> - Both primary molars and incisors can be treated with a pulpectomy technique.

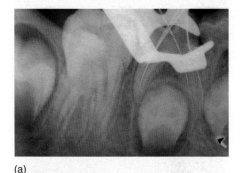

(a)

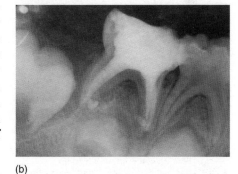

(b)

Fig. 8.27 (a) Periapical radiograph showing files placed in the root canals of left lower second primary molar. (b) Root canals have been filled with pure zinc oxide eugenol. Reproduced with the kind permission of Prof. H. S. Chawla, PGIMER, India.

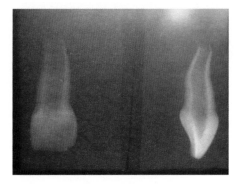

Fig. 8.28 Radiograph showing the typical morphology of the root canal in upper primary incisors.

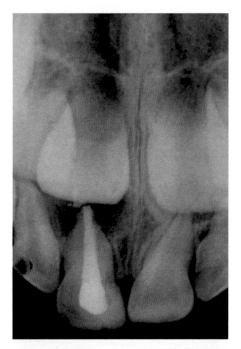

Fig. 8.29 Root canal filling in an upper primary central incisor.

8.9 TREATMENT OF A CHILD WITH HIGH CARIES RATE

It is absolutely true that restoration of children's teeth without adequate prevention is like replacing windows in a burning house. When presented with a child with a high caries rate, establishing a good preventive regime should be the first and foremost item in the treatment plan. However, it would be a folly to think that prevention alone will maintain the child in a pain free state. Restorative treatment or extraction of decayed teeth that are not suitable for restoration should be planned alongside securing good prevention. Therefore, when dealing with a high caries risk child, a comprehensive visit by visit treatment plan that deals with the preventive and restorative care of the child should be established.

Table 8.4 Prevention of rampant caries in children and adolescents

Primary dentition	*0–6 years*
Dietary advice	Dietary counselling with parents on good nursing techniques
Fluoride therapy	Toothpaste (1000+ ppm F) Drops/tablets if in area without water fluoridation Topical varnish application every 3 months
Plaque control	Oral hygiene instructions to parents Toothbrushing with parental supervision
Early visit to dentist at about 12 months of age with 3–6 month recall	
Mixed dentition	*6–12 years*
Dietary advice	Dietary counselling with parents and patients
Fluoride therapy	Toothpaste (1000+ ppm F) Tablets if in area without water fluoridation Mouthrinse (0.05% daily) Topical gel/varnish application every 3 months
Plaque control	Oral hygiene instructions to patient Toothbrushing without parental supervision Disclosing tablets
Fissure sealants	
3–6 month recalls	
Permanent dentition	*12 years+*
Dietary advice	Dietary counselling with parents and patients
Fluoride therapy	Toothpaste (1450+ ppm F) Mouthrinse (0.05% daily) Topical gel/varnish application every 3 months
Plaque control	Oral hygiene instructions to patient Toothbrushing Disclosing tablets Interdental cleaning with floss or wood sticks
Fissure sealants	
3–6 month recalls	

The type of treatment instituted for patients with rampant caries depends on the patients' and parents' motivation towards dental treatment, the extent of decay, and the age and co-operation of the child. Initial treatment, including temporary restorations, diet assessment, oral hygiene instruction, and home and professional fluoride treatments, should be performed before any comprehensive restorative programme commences. However, in patients presenting with acute and severe signs and symptoms of gross caries, pain, abscess, sinus, or facial swelling, immediate treatment is indicated. This may involve extractions and even a general anaesthetic in a young child. It is wiser to extract all the teeth with a dubious prognosis under one general anaesthetic rather than have an acclimatization programme interrupted by a painful episode in the future.

Table 8.4 summarizes the preventive regimens that should be employed for rampant caries in different age groups.

Once rampant caries is under control, then comprehensive restorative treatment can be undertaken. This should aim to retain the primary dentition with the methods described in this chapter and in Chapter 7, and deliver the child pain free into adolescence and adulthood.

8.10 SUMMARY

1. A full preventive programme must be instituted before any definitive restorations in a child with a high caries rate.
2. Repetitive treatment should be avoided and with careful treatment planning and choice of restorative materials long-lasting restorations can be carried out in children.
3. The stainless-steel metal crown is the most durable restoration in the primary dentition for large cavities and endodontically treated teeth.
4. Resin-modified glass ionomers and polyacid-modified composite resins may have an increased role in the future in the restoration of primary teeth.
5. Rubber dam should be placed, if at all possible, prior to the restoration of all teeth.
6. Careful evaluation of the state of pulp inflammation should be carried out before the placement of proximal restorations in primary teeth. Wherever the pulp is deemed to be involved, pulp therapy should be carried out prior to the coronal restoration.
7. Formocresol is likely to be replaced with newer, safer medicaments such as Ferric Sulphate.

8.11 ACKNOWLEDGEMENTS

Some parts of this text have been reproduced from Dental Update, with the kind permission of George Warman Publications.

8.12 FURTHER READING

Curzon, M. E. J. and Roberts, J. S. (1996). *Kennedy's paediatric operative dentistry* (4th edn). Wright, London. (*A comprehensive text on the technical aspects of operative dentistry for children.*)

Dental Practice Board (1997). *Setting standards in dental care for children.* Dental Practice Board, Eastbourne. (*An attempt to give guidance to dentists in General Dental Practice.*)

Duggal, M. S., Curzon, M. E. J., Fayle, Toumba, K. J., and Robertson, A. J. (2002). *Restorative techniques in paediatric dentistry* (2nd edn). Taylor & Francis, London (*A superb colour atlas and pictorial guide.*)

Duggal, M. S., Gautum, S. K., and Nicol, R. (2003). Paediatric dentistry in the new millennium: 4. Cost effective restorative techniques for primary molars. *Dental Update*, **30**, 410–15.

Faculty of Dental Surgery Clinical Effectiveness Committee (1999). *UK national clinical guidelines in paediatric dentistry. 1. Stainless steel pre-formed crowns for primary molars; 2. Management of the stained fissure in the first permanent molar.* Dental Practice Board for England and Wales, Eastbourne. (*Invaluable clinical guidelines and aide-memories.*)

Faculty of General Dental Practitioners (1998). *Selection criteria for dental radiography.* FGDP (UK), London. (*An excellent guide as to when to take radiographs for the diagnosis of caries in children.*)

Kidd, E. A. M., Smith, B. G. N. and Watson, T. (2003). *Pickard's manual of operative dentistry* (8th edn). Oxford University Press, Oxford. (*An ideal reference manual for the restoration of permanent teeth.*)

Paterson, R. C., Watts, A., Saunders, W. P., and Pitts, N. B. (1991). *Modern concepts in the diagnosis and treatment of fissure cries.* Quintessence, London. (*A very practical and clear approach to the problem.*)

Reid, J. S., Challis, P. D., and Patterson, C. J. W. (1991). *Rubber dam in clinical practice.* Quintessence, London. (*This guide will prove to you that you can easily use rubber dam.*)

8.13 REFERENCES

Duggal, M. S., Nooh, A., and High, A. (2002). Response of the primary pulp to inflammation: a review of the Leeds studies and challenges for the future. *European Journal of Paediatric Dentistry*, **3**, 111–14.

Harris, C. A. (1839). *The dental art.* Armstrong and Berry, Baltimore, MD.

Marks, L. A. M., Weerheijm, K. L., and van Amerongen, W. E. (1999). Dyract versus Tylin class II restorations in primary molars: 36 months evaluation. *Caries Research*, **33**, 387–92.

Pitts, N. B. and Longbottom, C. (1995). Preventative care advised (PCA)/operative care advised (OCA)-categorising caries by the management option. *Community Dentistry and Oral Epidemiology*, **23**, 55–9.

Welbury, R. R., Shaw, A. J., Murray, J. J., Gordon, P. H., and McCabe, J. F. (2000). Clinical evaluation of paired compomer and glass ionomer restorations in primary molars: final results after 42 months. *British Dental Journal*, **189**, 93–7.

9

Operative treatment of dental caries
in the young permanent dentition

9 Operative treatment of dental caries in the young permanent dentition

J. A. Smallridge and B. Williams

9.1 INTRODUCTION

Caries is still a considerable problem in children and adolescents. In the recent report from the 2002/2003 BASCD Survey which looked at dental disease levels in 77,693 14-year-old children in England and Wales, Pitts *et al.* (2004) found that on average half of the children examined had dentinal decay, with a mean of three permanent teeth decayed into dentine.

The first permanent teeth erupt into the mouth at approximately 6 years of age, but may appear as early as the age of 4. The eruption of the anterior teeth usually causes great excitement, as it is associated with 'the fluttering of tooth fairy wings'. However, the eruption of the first permanent molars largely goes unnoticed until there is a problem. The mean eruption time for first permanent molars has been determined as, 6.1 years in girls and 6.3 years in boys, but there is a tremendous variation in both the time of eruption and the time it takes for the tooth to emerge into the mouth. It takes 12–18 months for a first or second molar to erupt fully. The first permanent molars are teeth that commonly exhibit disrupted enamel; the reported incidence of defects range from 3.6–25%. The occlusal surfaces of these molar teeth account for about 90% of caries in children.

Restoration of the young permanent dentition is part of a continuum and cannot be regarded in isolation. The restoration is only one small part of the child's treatment and is the 'surgery' to remove the carious infected area of the tooth and replace it with a suitable restorative material. It does nothing to cure the disease and must form part of a much wider treatment modality, which includes identification of the risk factors contributing to the disease followed by introduction of specific prevention counter measures.

Efforts must be applied to all of these areas to attempt to provide the optimum conditions for future tooth survival. These risk factors and preventive measures are addressed in other chapters, such that the authors can confine themselves to appraisal of methods of treatment of caries in the young permanent dentition. They cannot hope to completely cover every aspect of operative treatment in one chapter; there are other texts that should be read to give a fuller account of the available techniques (see sections 9.15 and 9.16). However, the authors intend to give an outline of some of the options available.

9.2 ASSESSMENT OF CARIES RISK

Caries risk must influence decisions on when to treat, when to monitor, which material to use, etc.; the authors will review it briefly, despite the fact that it has been discussed in Chapter 3. The idea of a caries risk assessment for each child patient is to ensure that the chosen diagnostic tests, preventive treatment, and any provided restorations, are geared specifically to the need of that patient.

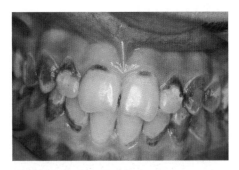

Fig. 9.1   An example of caries in a 12-year-old
girl, who sucked polos non-stop, '6 packets per day'.

Factors requiring consideration are:

(1)   present caries activity;

(2)   past caries activity;

(3)   parent /sibling caries activity;

(4)   sugar consumption;

(5)   oral hygiene;

(6)   fluoride exposure;

(7)   teeth morphology;

(8)   *Streptococcus* mutans levels;

(9)   saliva characteristics, flow rate, and consistency.

Factors (1)–(7) will become clear when a full history and examination are carried
out; while (8) and (9) will only come into play if there is rampant caries, which the
dentist cannot explain from the history (Fig. 9.1).

9.3 TREATMENT DECISIONS

The clinician must always give consideration to whether it is better either to treat a
carious lesion or remineralize it.

9.3.1 Important points in relation to treatment

1.   Gaining access to the caries inevitably means destruction of sound tooth tissue.
     The operator must keep this to a minimum, consistent with complete caries
     eradication.

2.   Once the operator places an initial restoration, he or she cannot 'undo' it and
     that tooth will inevitably require further restoration in its lifetime.

3.   Every time an operator places a restoration, he or she destroys more of the
     original tooth structure, thereby weakening the tooth.

4.   Even though the occlusion in a young person changes as growth occurs
     and teeth erupt, it is important to realize, that when the operator places
     restorations, he or she must replicate the original occlusal contacts in the
     tooth. Although, it may be tempting to keep the restoration totally out of the
     occlusion, teeth will move back into the occlusion, which will thereafter
     be slightly different and the cumulative effect of a lot of little changes can
     severely disrupt the occlusion in the long term.

5.   When treating an approximal lesion on one tooth with an adjacent neighbour,
     the operator will almost certainly damage the latter. The important surface layer
     of the neighbouring tooth, which contains the highest level of fluoride is the
     most resistant, so damage inflicted increases the chances of the adjacent surface
     of the neighbouring tooth becoming carious. It also creates an area of rough-
     ness on that surface, which in turn will accumulate more plaque, thereby
     increasing the risk of further decalcification.

6.   When placing an interproximal restoration it is inevitable that there is some
     damage to the periodontal tissues. There is the transient damage caused by
     placement of the matrix band and wedge, and there is also an enduring effect
     caused by the presence of the restoration margin. The very presence of the
     new restoration results in a contour change of the interstitial space. However
     smooth the operator attempts to make it, the altered state will increase plaque
     accumulation.

Key Point

Every time a restoration is placed, more of the original tooth structure will be destroyed, thereby weakening the tooth.

9.3.2 Important points in relation to remineralization

1. Early smooth surface lesions are reversible in the right conditions.
2. There is little evidence to suggest that remineralization occurs in lesions already into dentine.
3. The rate of caries progression is usually slow but can be rapid in some individuals, particularly younger children. In general, the older the child is at diagnosis of a carious lesion the slower the progress of the lesion, assuming constancy of other risk factors.
4. The remineralized tissue of early caries is less susceptible to further caries.
5. Small restorations are generally more successful than large, so a balance has to be struck, allowing preventive procedures adequate time to function, against the risk of lesion enlargement.

The progression rate of approximal caries can vary from tooth to tooth within the same mouth. It is thought that if the circumstances for remineralization are favourable, clinicians should use the modality, as opposed to a restoration that has a finite but limited lifespan (Figs 9.2 and 9.3).

Remineralization sources available are:

- fluoride rinse,
- fluoride varnish,
- chlorhexidine thymol varnish,
- oral hygiene measures,
- adjacent glass ionomer restorations.

Determination of the most effective method to retard the progression of approximal caries requires not only identification of the most effective remineralizing agent but also the frequency with which to employ it.

Key Point

The remineralized tissue of early caries is less susceptible to further caries.

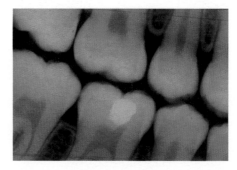

Fig. 9.2 A bitewing radiograph of a 13-year-old boy showing early caries upper right first permanent premolar and molar, and both lower molars.

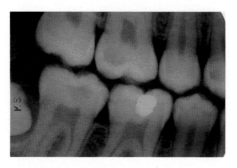

Fig. 9.3 The same boy, 18 months later, showing rapid progress of caries in the upper first premolar, molar, and the lower second molar, with little or no change in the lower second premolar and first molar.

Existing studies indicate that fluoride varnishes, solutions, and toothpastes all provide a significant effect on the progression of approximal caries in permanent molars when assessed radiographically. However, most of these studies were of limited duration (3 years). It would be interesting to know what happened after the completion of the studies and poses the following questions:

- Would the lesions have developed to the restorative stage?
- What is an acceptable frequency to monitor the lesions radiographically if this is the only acceptable way of determining progress?
- Is the cost of remineralization therapy less than restorative treatment, particularly if it entails multiple attendances of the patient?

Progress of caries through the enamel seems to be fairly slow but once the dentine is reached it accelerates. So as a rule of thumb, restore approximal surfaces once the lesion reaches the enamel/dentine interface.

9.4 DIAGNOSIS

While most dentists would agree that approximal caries is best diagnosed from bitewing radiographs, detection of occlusal caries is much more difficult. Where there is no overt or open cavity, diagnosing the status of a discoloured or stained fissure can be incredibly difficult if not impossible on occasions. Many methods have been proposed, both alone and in combination. These include:

- visual methods (dry tooth);
- probe/explorer;
- bitewing radiographs;
- electronic;
- fibre optic transillumination;
- laser diagnosis.

When two or three methods are used in combination, there is greater accuracy and higher rates of detection of caries. The most widely used combination is visual inspection under a good light, to examine a dry tooth for stains, opacities, etc., along with a good quality bitewing radiograph. Drying the tooth to be examined is essential as early lesions will only become visible, where the demineralization is minimal, when there is a dry surface. Different recommendations are made for the timing of bitewing radiographs and these are discussed in Chapter 3. Bitewing radiographs will show dentinal caries in teeth that are designated as clinically sound but there will also be teeth visually designated as carious in which there are no radiological signs of caries, hence the need for more than one method of diagnosis.

In making a diagnosis of caries, the operator has to decide, not only that there is a lesion present but also:

- Whether or not demineralization is present.
- The depth of the lesion.
- The rate of progression of the lesion.
- Whether it is an arrested or active lesion.

It would be nice to have a method of quantifying these factors. Measurements of electrical conductance and laser fluorescence have the potential to chart lesion progression/retardation as they provide a quantitative record, which if repeated over several appointments will demonstrate whether the lesion is active or arresting. They can be repeated safely more frequently than radiographs. However, it should be remembered that the electrical conductance and laser fluorescence methods would incorrectly interpret hypomineralization as caries and that similarly the laser-based instrument will routinely interpret staining to be caries.

Key Point

Diagnosis of early caries is important to be able to plan the whole treatment package.

9.5 FISSURE SEALING

Fissure sealants cannot be discussed in isolation from caries diagnosis or treatment of pit and fissure caries. The authors discuss use of these materials both preventively and therapeutically.

Toothbrush bristles cannot access the pit and fissure system because the dimensions of the fissures are too small. As a result micro-organisms remain undisturbed within the fissure system. The tooth is most susceptible to plaque stagnation during eruption, that is, a period of between 12 and 18 months. During this time, children need extra parental help in maintaining their oral hygiene. Lesion formation takes place in the plaque stagnation area at the entrance to the fissure and commences with subsurface demineralization. Demineralized enamel is more porous than sound enamel. The more demineralized and porous the affected enamel, the more it shows up both clinically and on radiographs.

> **Key Point**
>
> To detect the earliest white spots the tooth must be dried to render them more obvious.

Once the initial lesion has developed, caries may spread laterally such that a small surface lesion may hide a much greater area of destruction below the surface (Figs 9.4 and 9.5).

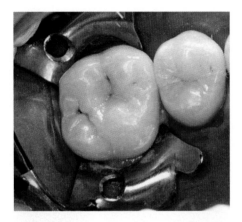

Fig. 9.4 Hidden caries—although the occlusal surface looks mostly intact it hides extensive caries.

Remineralization of occlusal lesions is much more difficult to achieve. Fissure sealing, 6 monthly 2.26% fluoride varnish application with oral hygiene instruction, and a weekly 0.2% sodium fluoride rinse, have all been found to help stabilize the disease and retard the progress of occlusal caries, but the fissure sealing group exhibited the best effectiveness. Many studies have shown that generally as the caries rates decline, the proportion of caries that affects pits and fissures of molar teeth increases, and also that the caries appears to be concentrated in a smaller cohort of children—most of the decay occurs in 25% of the child population. This predilection has meant that correct use of fissure sealants should have a maximal effect.

There is no dispute that when correctly applied and monitored, fissure sealants are highly effective at preventing dental caries in pits and fissures, but interpretation of the correct application and monitoring requires scrutiny.

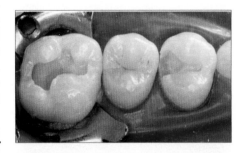

Fig. 9.5 Caries has been removed. The size of the cavity emphasizes the extent of the lesion.

> **Key Point**
>
> Fissure sealants reduce caries incidence but must be carefully monitored and maintained.

9.5.1 Who will benefit?

Not every fissure will become carious if it is not sealed. Therefore, each tooth for each child must be assessed on its own merits. The clinician must assess the risk factors for that tooth developing pit or fissure caries. As a general guide to who will benefit, review the British Society for Paediatric Dentistry Policy Document (Nunn *et al.*, 2000).

The main beneficiaries are:

1. Children and young people with medical, intellectual, physical, and sensory impairments, such that their general health would be jeopardized by either the development of oral disease or the need for dental treatment. In such children all susceptible sites in both the primary and permanent dentitions should receive consideration.

2. All susceptible sites on permanent teeth should be sealed in children and young people with caries in their primary teeth (dmfs = 2 or more).

3. Where occlusal caries affects one permanent molar, the operator should seal the occlusal surfaces of all the other molars.

4. If the anatomy of the tooth is such that surfaces are deeply fissured, then these should be sealed.

5. Where potential risk factors, such as dietary factors or oral hygiene factors, indicate a high risk of caries, then all sites at risk should be sealed.

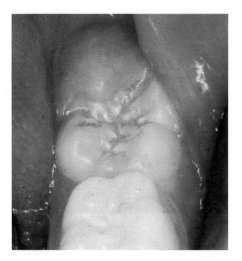

Fig. 9.6 This tooth which is too early to seal with resin, should be painted with fluoride varnish or if the caries risk is very high should be sealed with glass ionomer until further eruption has taken place.

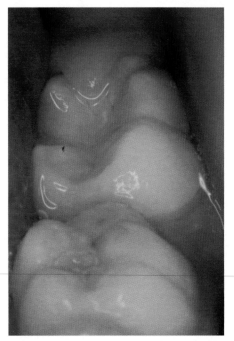

Fig. 9.7 This molar is just at the correct stage to apply fissure sealant. The very small operculum of gingival tissue can be held away from the tooth gently with a flat plastic.

6. Where there is a doubt about the caries status of a fissure or it is known to have caries confined to the enamel, fissure sealants may be used therapeutically. After application, it is essential to monitor the surface both clinically and radiologically.

Sealant use must be based on personal, tooth, and surface risk, and the clinician must assess these risks since it might change at any time in the life of the patient. So whereas it was traditionally stated that dentists should complete sealant application up to a year or two after eruption, he or she should assess the potential risk factors regularly, and place the sealant, when indicated irrespective of age. Failure rates are higher when sealants are placed on newly erupted teeth and in mouths with higher previous caries experience. Monitoring the integrity of sealant is vital in those circumstances and any deficiencies in a sealant should be corrected (Figs 9.6 and 9.7).

9.5.2 Clinical technique

Pretreatment prior to sealant application

Tooth preparation with pumice and a rotary brush results in a good clinical retention rate. Dry brushing achieves similar results. Air polishing, using a 'Prophy-Jet', an early air abrasion system that uses sodium bicarbonate particles as the abrasive medium, provides good bond strength and sealant penetration but has not received general acceptance, probably, because most dental surgeries do not possess this equipment.

Some researchers have advocated the use of 'Enameloplasty', a more aggressive intervention into the tooth, that is, mechanical enlargement of the fissures with a bur or with air abrasion, to improve sealant penetration and reduce micro-leakage. Although some studies have confirmed these claims, the authors feel that this is an unnecessary extra procedure to subject the child to, and do not recommend it.

Etching

All the methods of cleaning the tooth, discussed above, should be accompanied with etching of the enamel surface. Etching for just 20 s with a range of concentrations of acid but most often, 35–37.5% phosphoric acid is the tried and tested method. Its one drawback is the susceptibility of the etched surface to saliva or moisture contamination, which reduces the bond strength. Salivary contamination results in significantly reduced bond strengths unless removed by thorough washing. Re-etching of the surface is usually necessary if salivary contamination has occurred.

Bonding agents

Bonding agents used as an additional layer under a resin sealant yield bond strengths significantly greater than the bond strength obtained when using sealant alone. Initial results of clinical trials also show increased retention of the sealant when an intermediate bond is used. New bonding techniques are proving to be less technique sensitive, with respect to moisture control than erstwhile procedures.

The use of a bonding agent under a sealant on wet contaminated surfaces yields bond strengths equivalent to the bond strength obtained when sealant is bonded directly to clean etched enamel without contamination. Most of the data on the subject of using a bonding agent as part of the sealant procedure supports its use. Use of a bonding agent would tend to increase the time and cost of the sealant application but in cases where maintaining a dry surface is difficult or where there are areas of hypomineralization on the surface, it would have many advantages.

Logically, combination of these technologies to achieve better penetration with less steps in the application sequence would be beneficial and there is some evidence already in the use of self-etching primer–adhesive systems. As yet, there has only been a 2-year follow-up but the early results are promising in relation to retention. Other studies have shown that there are concerns about micro-leakage compared with conventional acid etching. The big bonus of the self-etching primer–adhesive system is the speed with which the operator can apply it. In the application procedure for the Prompt-L-Pop system, the operator brushes the self-etching adhesive on to the surface; air thins it, and follows this by immediate placement of the sealant and polymerization. In the study, the average time operators took for the procedure was 1.8 min compared with 3.1 min for conventional technique. Such time saving is very useful in young fidgety children. At present, therefore, there are conflicting views on these systems but with technology moving ever onwards it does seem likely that in the future it should be possible to achieve good etching and bonding with a simpler application method.

Most clinicians will employ a resin-based sealant, because they have a good track record. Many clinical trials have demonstrated the effectiveness of resin sealants and there are several long-term studies, which show the benefits. Fifteen years after a single application, resin sealants have shown 28% complete retention of sealants and 35% partial retention on first permanent molars. Where researchers re-applied sealant to those surfaces that had deficient sealant as determined by yearly exams, 65% complete retention was obtained and only 13% of the surfaces had caries or restorations after 20 years.

Retreatment

Sealants placed in the first permanent molars in children of ages 6, 7, and 8 and in second permanent molars in children of ages 11 and 12 required more re-application than those placed in older teeth. If the clinician places fissure sealant in newly erupted teeth it is more likely to fail, but should still be placed as early as possible, because the teeth are more vulnerable to caries at this time.

Modifying the resin to incorporate fluoride is a logical rationale. However, fluoride release occurs only for a very short time and at a very low level. Many studies over 2–3-year periods have reported good retention but with a similar caries incidence to conventional sealant. Since the addition of fluoride to sealant resin does not have any detrimental effect it could certainly be used, but until the chemistry can be adapted to readily unlock the fluoride, the anti-cariogenicity cannot be attributed to the fluoride.

Greater release of fluoride can be achieved using glass ionomer (poly-alkenoate). Such cements have high levels of fluoride available for release but they suffer from the drawback of poor retention. Even with the very poor retention rates, sealing with glass ionomer does seem to infer some caries protective effect. This may be due to both the fluoride released by the glass ionomer and residual material retained in the bottom of the fissure, invisible to the naked eye.

Hence, glass ionomers, used as sealants can be classed as a fissure sealant but more realistically as a fluoride depot material. They can be usefully employed to seal partially erupted molars in high risk children since eruption of the molars takes 12–18 months and during this time they are often very difficult to clean. Once the teeth are sufficiently erupted the operator may place a resin sealant. They are also useful in children where there are difficulties with the level of co-operation, as the technique does not depend on absolute moisture control.

Logically, improvement in glass ionomer technology has occurred and both resin-modified glass ionomers (RMGI) and compomers have been used as sealants. As yet, studies of these materials used as fissure sealants while available, show no improvement over resin-based sealants and so there is nothing to recommend them in preference to resins.

Filled or unfilled resins?

Retention is better for unfilled resins probably because it penetrates into the fissures more completely. It also does not need occlusal adjustment as it abrades very rapidly.

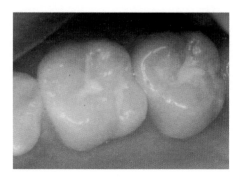

Fig. 9.8 White fissure sealants can easily be check at recall, they are also visible to show the patient and parent to help them understand the procedure.

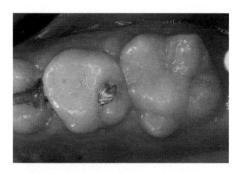

Fig. 9.9 Clear fissure sealant is less easy to see though its presence can be checked, if an area is giving cause for concern, by etching.

If a filled resin is not adjusted there is a perceptible occlusal change, possible discomfort, and wear of the opposing antagonist tooth.

Coloured or clear material?

Opaque sealants have the advantage of high visibility at recall. It has been found that identification error for opaque resin was only 1% while for clear resin the corresponding figure was 23% with the most common error being false identification of the presence of clear resin on an untreated tooth. The disadvantage of opaque sealant is that the dentist cannot examine the fissure visually at future recalls (Figs 9.8 and 9.9). The choice of an opaque versus a clear sealant is usually one of personal choice.

Safety issues

There has only been one report of an allergy to the resin used for pit and fissure sealing and concern has been raised about the oestrogenicity of resin-based composites. The proposed culprit, bis-phenol A (BPA), is not a direct ingredient of fissure sealants, but is a chemical that appears in the final product when the raw materials fail to fully react. The amount released orally is undetectable in the systemic circulation and concerns about potential oestrogenicity are probably unfounded.

Sealant bulk in relation to application

It is important to remember that the sealant must be kept to a minimum, consistent with the coverage of the complete fissure system including buccal and lingual pits. Overfilling can lead to reduction in retention and increased micro-leakage.

Sealant monitoring

Once the sealant has been placed the operator must monitor it at recall appointments and repair or replenish as necessary. Teeth lose is between 5% and 10% of sealant volume per year. Partial loss of resin sealant allows ingress of bacteria into the fissure system. This leaves that surface equally at risk from caries compared to an unsealed surface.

Cost-effectiveness

Cost-effectiveness will depend on the caries rate for the children in the population. Where there is a higher caries rate, generalized sealing will protect more surfaces that would have become carious in the future. However, if the caries rate is very high, then the risk of developing interproximal lesions is also higher and may lead to a two surface restoration even when the fissure sealed surfaces remain caries free. In low caries areas, the cost-effectiveness of sealant application *en masse* is questionable and the dentist should assess each child's individual risk factors. In contrast to this general concept, one study has shown that it is 1.6 times as costly to restore the carious lesions in the first permanent molars in an unsealed group of 5–10-year-old children living in a fluoridated area than it is to prevent them with a single application of pit and fissure sealant. This study also revealed a greater number of lesions if sealant was not utilized.

Sealing over caries

Once caries has been diagnosed it is important to determine its extent. If there is clear unequivocal evidence that the lesion does not extend beyond the enamel, then the surface may be sealed and monitored both clinically and radiologically. If the lesion extends into the dentine, the dentist would normally place either a preventive resin restoration (PRR), or if in an area of occlusal load, a conventional restoration.

However, several authors have shown that dentinal carious lesions do not progress under intact sealants. Nevertheless, if the sealant were to fail immediately or shortly after application, then the lesion would have 4–6 months to progress before the next review. We do not advocate sealing over caries except in very exceptional circumstances, that is, very nervous children who cannot cope with even minimal intervention dentistry.

9.6 RUBBER DAM

Although often perceived as difficult to apply on children, the use of rubber dam creates a better working environment for both the dentist and the child. Once the technique is mastered it can be applied both quickly and with minimal discomfort. The advantages of the rubber dam are:

1. It protects the soft tissues (tongue, cheeks, and gingivae) from damage from instruments or medicaments.
2. It reduces the risk of swallowing and inhalation of instruments, and particles and debris.
3. It makes the salivary aerosol produced by high speed rotary instruments easier to control thereby reducing the risk of infection to the dental staff.
4. If used with inhalation sedation it will reduce the amount of mouth breathing thereby allowing less nitrous oxide to be used and thus reducing the gas level in the general environment of the dental surgery.
5. It often makes the child feel isolated from the treatment, thus helping the child to feel more relaxed and able to cope.
6. It provides the best possible dry field; for materials where moisture control is essential its use is imperative (Fig. 9.10).

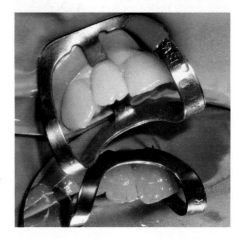

Fig. 9.10 Rubber dam in place protecting gingivae and eliminating moisture.

Other texts give full details of the various application techniques of the rubber dam. It must be remembered that good analgesia is very important, as placement of rubber dam particularly when a clamp is used is painful. An infiltration backed up by intra-papillary injections is usually needed.

9.7 ANTERIOR CARIES

Caries of permanent anterior teeth in childhood and adolescence, is not that common and usually occurs either where there is defect in the formation of the teeth, which leads to plaque accumulation, or in children with rampant caries, where the sugar intake is so high that the dentition is overwhelmed. The best material for restoring anterior teeth is composite resin. The use of this material in the treatment of patients affected by either trauma or as a solution for cosmetic problems is described in Chapters 10 and 12.

In patients suffering 'normal' caries, with interproximal cavities, composite restoration is the material of choice. In patients with rampant caries it may be preferable to use glass ionomer to restore the lesions as an interim measure while the risk factors are addressed.

9.8 OCCLUSAL CARIES

Where the dentist has established a diagnosis that a stained fissure is a carious lesion into dentine, restorative treatment is indicated. If the lesion is limited to areas of the tooth not bearing occlusal loads then a PRR is appropriate (Smallridge *et al.*, 2000).

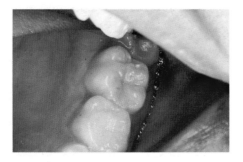

Fig. 9.11 Unrestored carious first molar. Caries identified in mesial fossa on radiograph.

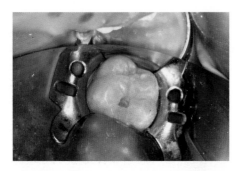

Fig. 9.12 Cavity preparation commenced after local analgesia and application of rubber dam. Access and outline form should only be of a size that enables removal of caries.

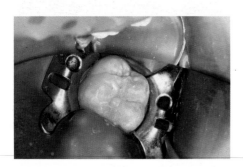

Fig. 9.13 Tooth restored with glass ionomer.

If the lesion is more extensive, then the clinician should consider a composite or an amalgam restoration.

9.8.1 The preventive resin restoration

Clinical technique

1. Administer local analgesia, after application of topical anaesthetic paste at the injection site.
2. Place rubber dam.
3. Explore the suspect area of the fissure system with a high speed small bur, removing only enough enamel to gain access to the caries. The access must by wide enough to ensure that the operator can remove caries from the peripheral tissue. If the radiographs show dentinal caries, even if the enamel seems intact, access must progress into dentine. Undermined enamel can be left *in situ* as the bis-GMA resin restoration virtually restores the original strength of the tooth.
4. Line the cavity with calcium hydroxide. There is some debate as to whether it is necessary to line these cavities. Some studies report no pulpal problems in teeth where the operator has directly etched and bonded the dentine.
5. Etch. Precise details are dependent on the chosen 'restorative' system for steps (5)–(8) and the manufacturers instructions must be followed.
6. Wash.
7. Dry.
8. Bond.
9. Place the chosen composite in the cavity. In smaller cavities glass ionomer cement is an alternative.
10. Seal all the remaining fissure system with fissure sealant.
11. Check the occlusion.
12. Review the integrity of the sealant at the routine recall appointments. If the visual appearance is inconclusive, re-etch the surface to identify sealant retention.

The technique is shown in Figs 9.11–9.20.

Where the diagnostic methods are inconclusive, the clinician should explore the fissure to validate caries free status or eradicate occult caries. Depending on the extent of any lesion, restoration by fissure sealing or composite completes the procedure.

9.8.2 Occlusal restorations in young permanent teeth

If caries affects most of the occlusal fissure system, the clinician should place a classical class I restoration. The choice of material for this restoration is dependent on the

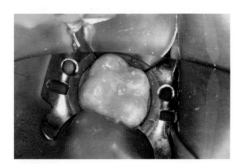

Fig. 9.14 Restoration covered with fissure sealant.

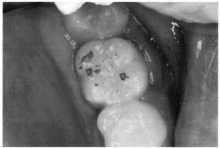

Fig. 9.15 Rubber dam removed and occlusion checked.

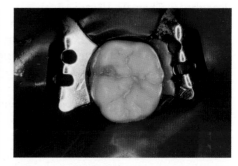

Fig. 9.16 The same principles can apply with a slightly larger lesion.

operator and appropriately informed parent. The plethora of available tooth coloured materials together with the continuing development and introduction of new materials makes choice both extensive and difficult.

Silver amalgam

Silver amalgam is the standard material against which the success of alternative materials is often judged (Rugg-Gunn *et al.*, 2000). Amalgam has a known track record. Dentists have used it for restoring teeth for more than 150 years. When looking at the literature it must be remembered that amalgam technology has evolved over a very long period and those amalgam alloys available today are probably very different in composition to those used even as recently as 15 years ago. Various studies have compared amalgam with composite resin. One such study found no significant differences between them, when the materials were used in small occlusal situations.

Amalgam has many useful properties:

1. It is easy to handle.
2. Has good durability.
3. Has relatively low cost.
4. It exhibits reducing micro-leakage with time (high copper amalgams can take up to 2 years for a marginal seal to be produced, double the time for low copper amalgams, but high copper amalgams are not as susceptible to corrosion phenomena and resulting porosity and therefore retain their strength.)
5. It is less technique sensitive compared with other restorative materials.

It is still important to control moisture as excess moisture causes delayed expansion particularly in zinc-containing alloys, and for this reason rubber dam should always be used if possible.

Despite these good properties, amalgam has two main disadvantages (1) it is not aesthetic and (2) it contains mercury, a known poison. Little can be done to combat the poor aesthetics. Remembering to polish amalgams does improve characteristics, including appearance and leads to a significant reduction in their replacement.

Clinicians concerned about the toxicity of silver amalgam seek re-assurance on the continuing use of the alloy. There are four main areas of concern:

(1) Inhalation of mercury vapour or amalgam dust;
(2) The ingestion of amalgam;
(3) Allergy to mercury;
(4) Environmental considerations.

Inhalation of amalgam dust is most likely to occur during removal of a previous restoration. This effect is transient and the effects minimized, if the operator uses rubber dam and high speed aspiration. It is not in dispute that mercury is released from amalgam restorations, during placement, polishing, chewing, and removal, but the amounts are very small and come nowhere near the amounts ingested from other daily sources, for example, air, water, and diet. True allergy to amalgam is rare. There have been only 50 cases reported in 100 years. Many countries are trying to reduce all industrial uses of mercury for environmental reasons and better mercury hygiene in dental practice is one of the areas targeted.

In small occlusal restorations the only difference needed in the tooth preparation between composite and amalgam is that when an amalgam is to be placed, undermined enamel must be removed. In both cases a resin sealant material should be placed over the margins of the restoration and the remaining fissure system.

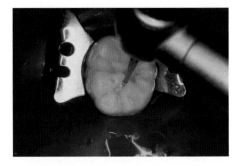
Fig. 9.17 Undermined enamel can be left as long as the operator can reach all the caries.

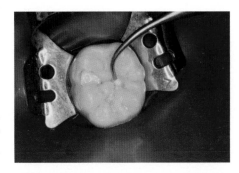
Fig. 9.18 Place a calcium hydroxide lining in the deep parts of the cavity.

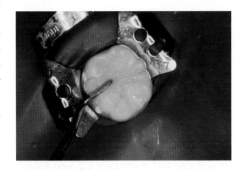
Fig. 9.19 After etching and bonding, place composite resin incrementally.

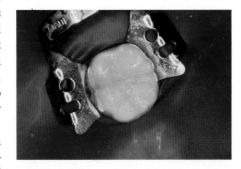
Fig. 9.20 Finish the restoration with fissure sealing.

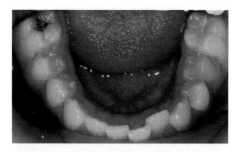

Fig. 9.21 After restoration with amalgam, place fissure sealant to cover the amalgam and seal the fissure system.

Researchers report very high success rates when amalgam is used in this manner (Fig. 9.21).

Composite resins

Many dentists advocate the use of composite as a restorative in the treatment of children. Since their introduction in the 1970s, there have been many modifications. Abrasive wear of many composite systems is comparable to that of silver amalgam in the region of 10–20 μm/year, and colour stability is now excellent compared with earlier materials.

After placement and occlusal adjustment of the restorative material, the operator should place a layer of sealant on the finished surface to fill any micro-cracks within the surface of the resin, followed by curing the resin to ensure maximal polymerization.

> **Key Point**
>
> Composite resin restorations are extremely technique sensitive. They should only be placed when isolation is guaranteed.

Before making decisions concerning the most appropriate restorative material in the treatment of children, the clinician should consider:

1. *Moisture exclusion.* Is it realistic for this patient?
2. *Patient compliance.* Will the patient sit still through the restoration?
3. *The size of the cavity.* Lesion extent determines operative duration.
4. *Patient compliance after the procedure.* Will he or she return for monitoring and review?

As long as the clinician allows due consideration in relation to these provisos concerning use of the material, it will be appropriate to employ it restoratively, since its inherent properties make it an excellent choice in the treatment of children for occlusal cavities. As long as the responses to questions 1, 2, and 4 are affirmative and the restoration is relatively small, the composite can be used with confidence.

The advent of dentine bonding systems has enabled clinicians to achieve bonding of materials, to the dentine as well as to the enamel, thereby improving the strength of the restoration. Dentine bonding is very technique sensitive. Adherence to manufacturer instructions is axiomatic at all times. Initially the technique consisted of etching and rinsing followed by application of primer containing a solvent resin monomer to wet and penetrate the collagen meshwork. Finally the operator applied a bonding agent, which penetrates into the primed dentine.

One-bottle systems in which the primer and the bonding agent are combined within one solution are now on the market. When combined, they require a moist surface to facilitate etching and bonding. With such agents there is some evidence to suggest that patients may suffer a high incidence of postoperative sensitivity.

There are also a few systems in the market, where the manufacturer has combined etch, prime, and bond solutions into a single solution. There is little independent research as yet to support these systems in relation to long-term performance, but initial results appear to indicate that there is very low postoperative sensitivity. The potential time-saving advantage would, of course, be welcome if researchers prove in the future that these systems provide high bond strength between the polymerized material and the dentine.

Key Point

New techniques and materials will always emerge in the market, but it is essential for the practitioner to be sceptical until researchers report clinical trials of adequate design and duration. Extrovert exponents of a particular technique or material frequently sway us into purchasing a material prematurely, but to our cost later.

Glass ionomer cements

This group of materials tend to be more brittle than composites, but have the advantage of adherence to both enamel and dentine without etching. The coefficient of expansion of glass ionomer is very close to that of dentine and once set, these materials remain dimensionally stable in the mouth despite constantly changing moisture and temperature levels. Their biggest advantage over composites is that they are able to release fluoride over an extended period of time. Their lack of strength limits their use in the permanent dentition but they can be used in PRRs where there is no occlusal load and as an interim restoration while caries is brought under control (Figs 9.22 and 9.23). They are also the authors' choice of material for cementing stainless-steel crowns.

Resin-modified glass ionomer

Reinforcement of glass ionomer with resin has been used to produce a fast setting cement but these materials require etching prior to placement. On modifying the materials, fracture toughness/resistance and abrasion resistance improve, and they still retain biocompatibility, fluoride ion hydrodynamics, favourable thermal expansion and contraction characteristics, and most important of all, they retain physico-chemical bonding to tooth structure.

Compomer (polyacid-modified resin-based composite)

These materials are a combination of composite and ionomer. They have better aesthetics than glass ionomer as a single material and have the advantage of some fluoride release, but there is still a need to etch during the restorative procedure. However, it would appear that they suffer from the disadvantages of loss of retention together with gap formation between the material and tooth substance. Despite these generally accepted limitations there is one recent report of a 92.3% success rate using compomer in stress bearing restorations in permanent posterior teeth. Further studies will clarify the issue.

9.9 APPROXIMAL CARIES

In children caries occurs more often occlusally than approximally, but as they progress to adulthood, the relative level of approximal caries increases. The authors advocate managing occlusal caries immediately by sealing or PRRs. They also support remineralization techniques as an early intervention approach in approximal caries, where the lesion has not reached the dentine. Whichever way the clinician chooses to restore approximal caries, it will always entail loss of some sound tooth tissue. In approximal restorations, sufficient tooth preparation just to gain access to the carious dentine is necessary. Shape the outline form only to include the carious dentine and to remove demineralized enamel. Finish the cavo surface margins to remove unsupported enamel.

Amalgam works well in these situations but clinicians are equally using composite resins more frequently in approximal restorations of young permanent teeth. Although there are some studies reporting good success rates, the overall consensus

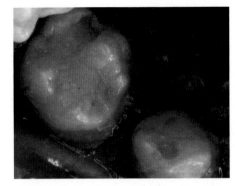

Fig. 9.22 A deficient glass ionomer restoration seen after a year.

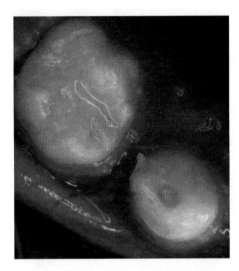

Fig. 9.23 The operator simply adds more glass ionomer to the deficient restoration.

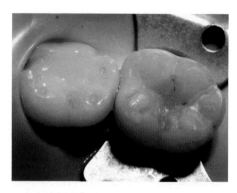

Fig. 9.24 Mesial caries in a lower first molar. The lesion is not readily apparent.

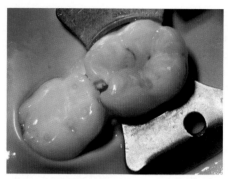

Fig. 9.25 The lesion is opened. This view shows the extent of the caries more clearly. The operator does not need to extend for prevention.

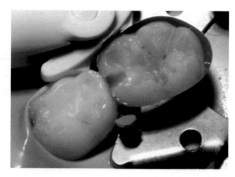

Fig. 9.26 The caries has been removed, a band placed with wedge, and the cavity lined.

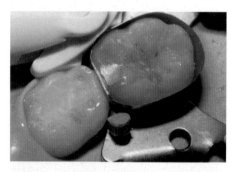

Fig. 9.27 The operator has packed amalgam into the mesial slot.

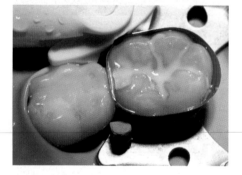

Fig. 9.28 The operator has sealed the remainder of the fissure system.

seems to be that tooth coloured restorations are prone to earlier failure than amalgam restorations. Operators should inform parents of this proviso when discussing the choice of restorative material. (See Figs 9.24–9.28.)

9.10 EXTENSIVE/DEEP CARIES

Unfortunately, a situation sometimes arises where the caries is already extensive prior to the initial consultation, and the clinician needs to consider preservation versus extraction issues.

Rampant caries does occur in the permanent dentition as well as the primary dentition and once again treatment planning has to consider the person as a whole—indeed with children, sometimes the whole family—not just the teeth involved in one particular individual. This involves decision-making on

- The advisability of restoration versus planned extraction.
- How to restore if that is the favoured modality.
- How to prevent onset of further lesions, that is, reduce the risk factors by examining diet, oral hygiene, fissure sealing, fluoride treatment, and a rigid recall regime.

9.10.1 Extraction considerations

If there is extensive caries affecting the first permanent molars it may be expedient to consider extraction rather than restoration. It is however, important to check for the presence and development of the second premolars before prescribing extraction of the first permanent molars since lack of the premolars necessitates all possible measures to attempt to retain the first permanent molars. The decision on extraction is dependent on the age of the child, the stage of development of the dentition, and the occlusion. This is discussed in detail in Chapter 14.

Whereas there may be different treatment options with regard to carious first permanent molars, the clinician should usually attempt to retain incisors and/or canines, with extensive caries whenever possible.

9.10.2 Conservative treatment options

Various techniques have a part to play in conservation of teeth with deep caries.

- Indirect pulp capping.
- Direct pulp capping

- Pulpotomy
- Pulpectomy

When the tooth erupts its roots are incompletely formed and approximately 20–40% shorter than the mature root. It may take up to 5 years after eruption for the root to complete its formation and develop an apical constriction.

> **Key Point**
> Whenever it is thought that caries removal might result in a pulpal exposure, efforts should be made to preserve pulp vitality in order to enable normal root maturation to occur.

Indirect pulp capping

If it is thought that exposure is likely to occur with full caries removal then sometimes it is expedient to leave caries in the deepest part of the lesion. Place a radio-opaque, biocompatible base over the remaining carious dentine to stimulate healing and repair. It is important to completely remove caries from all the lateral walls of the cavity before placement of a restoration since failure to do so will result in spread of secondary caries and the need for future intervention.(See Figs 9.29–9.33.)

Traditionally operators have used calcium hydroxide for indirect pulp capping because it has a good success rate. Alternatives suggested include adhesive resins, and glass ionomer cements, but as yet there are no published studies looking at these techniques in permanent teeth. Whichever material is utilized, the crucial factor is to isolate the pulp well from the oral environment. Re-investigation of these teeth after about 6 months when the pulp has had an opportunity to lay down reparative dentine used to be recommended. However studies have found that the residual carious dentine mostly re-mineralizes and hardens and caries progression does not occur in the absence of micro-leakage. Returning to the operative site, to complete caries removal increases the risk of pulp exposure, therefore the authors consider it wiser to perform the indirect pulp capping and definitive restoration in one appointment.

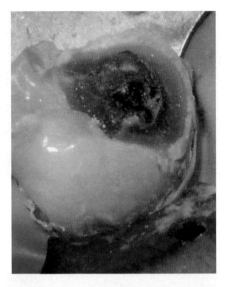

Fig. 9.29 A very large carious lesion with a definite risk of pulp exposure.

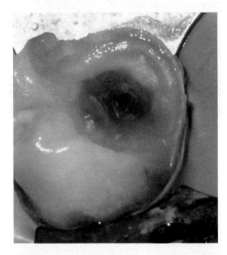

Fig. 9.30 Remove caries from the amelo-dentinal junction.

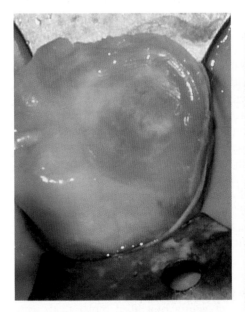

Fig. 9.31 Remove further caries from all areas except where the operator considers such removal will expose the pulp.

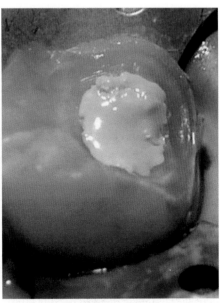

Fig. 9.32 Place a calcium hydroxide dressing.

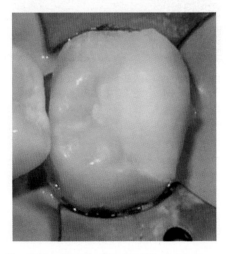

Fig. 9.33 Cover the dressing with glass ionomer prior to preparation for a stainless steel crown.

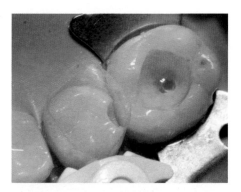

Fig. 9.34 Where a pulp exposure occurs, in an immature permanent molar, cut out the superficial pulp tissue (about 1 mm) with a high-speed diamond bur. Bleeding should cease easily.

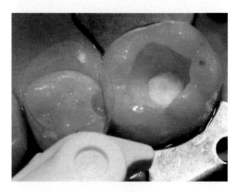

Fig. 9.35 Pressure with saline soaked cotton wool pledglet consolidates the position. It is important to stress that the haemorrhage must cease before placing the lining.

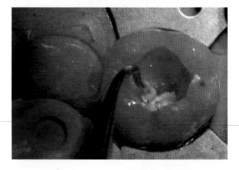

Fig. 9.36 Place a calcium hydroxide lining.

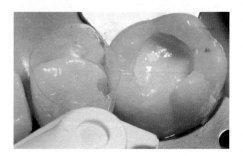

Fig. 9.37 Place a glass ionomer base over the calcium hydroxide.

The direct pulp cap

When a small exposure is encountered during cavity preparation the operator can place a direct pulp cap. The concept once again is to preserve the vitality of the pulp. Calcium hydroxide has traditionally been used as the direct capping agent. Total etching and sealing with a dentine-bonding agent has been tried but this resulted in increased non-vitality, so it is now contraindicated. As in traumatic exposures, pulp capping has given disappointing results compared with the technique of partial pulpotomy, so should only be used if a pulpotomy cannot be performed.

For all techniques in which the pulp is preserved it is important to assess the situation correctly before embarking on the treatment:

- There should be no history of spontaneous pain.
- There should be no swelling, mobility, discomfort to percussion.
- A normal periodontal appearance should be present radiographically.
- Pulp tissue should appear normal and vital.
- Cessation of bleeding from the pulp exposure site should occur with isotonic irrigation within 2 min.

Pulpotomy

Pulpotomies are successful in young teeth due to their increased pulpal circulation and ability to repair. The procedure consists of applying rubber dam after local analgesia and then clearing all lateral margins around the exposure and the pulpal floor of any caries. The superficial layer of the exposed pulp and the surrounding dentine are excised to a depth of 2 mm using a high speed diamond bur. The technique is the same as the Cvek pulpotomy described in Chapter 12 for pulp exposure in traumatized teeth. Only tissue judged to be inflamed should be removed. Whether sufficient tissue has been removed is ascertained by gently irrigating the remaining pulp surface with isotonic saline until bleeding stops. If bleeding does not cease easily, it is probable that the tissue is still inflamed and a further millimetre of pulp tissue is removed. Similarly if there is no bleeding at all then further pulp tissue should be removed until bleeding is found. After haemostasis has been obtained a soluble paste of calcium hydroxide is applied to the wound surface. It is important that there is no blood clot between the wound surface and the dressing as this will prevent repair and reduce the chances of success. Recently, MTA (mineral trioxide aggregate) has been proposed for pulp capping and pulpotomy dressings, but most of the published studies so far on this topic have been performed on animals. Hence at present calcium hydroxide, the tried and tested remedy should still be used. In order to aid repair, the clinician should apply dry sterile pellets of cotton wool carefully with modest pressure to adapt the calcium hydroxide medicament to the prepared cavity and remove excess water from the paste.

As in pulp capping it is essential that the operator fills the cavity with a material that provides a good hermetic seal. The latter can be the final restoration as there is no need to re-enter the wound site. Although the presence of a dentinal bridge radiographically represents a success, its absence does not indicate failure. After a year, success is represented by a tooth where there are no signs of clinical or radiographic pathology and where the root has developed apically and thickened laterally. The pulpotomy technique has much to recommend it, *viz.* a good success rate and continued root development. It is therefore considered the treatment of choice when there has been a pulp exposure in an immature permanent tooth.(See Figs 9.34–9.38.)

Pulpectomy

Root canal therapy following pulpectomy has a poor success rate in young permanent molars. In a recent study only 36% of young root filled molar teeth were considered a success. Hence, pulpectomy should be reserved only for cases exhibiting symptoms where the pulp is irreversibly damaged.

9.11 HYPOMINERALIZED, HYPOMATURE, OR HYPOPLASTIC FIRST PERMANENT MOLARS

As caries has declined generally, it has become more apparent that there is another problem that commonly affects first permanent molars and incisors. Very recently this condition has been called 'molar-incisor hypomineralization' (MIH). This term covers a range of developmental anomalies from small white, yellow, or brown patches to extensive loss of tissue from almost the whole enamel surface. It is characterized by a very rapid breakdown of the enamel, which can be extremely sensitive. The breakdown may even occur in a few months while the tooth is still erupting. The difficulties of cleaning a partially erupted tooth are then compounded by the sensitivity. This produces an area where plaque builds up and which leads to rapid carious attack. As is always the case with first permanent molars, exfoliation of primary molars does not precede their eruption, so children and parents are often unaware of their presence and thus they do not seek treatment until the teeth start to cause problems.

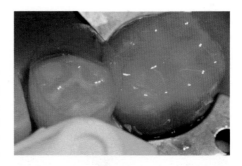

Fig. 9.38 Restore with etched, bonded, composite resin to provide a hermetic seal. There is no need to re-investigate the site, so consider the restoration as definitive.

Molar-incisor hypomineralization has been defined as 'hypomineralization of systemic origin of one to four permanent molars frequently associated with affected incisors'. The expression of the phenomenon can vary in severity between patients but also within a mouth, so in one quadrant there may only be a small hypomineralized area, while in others almost total destruction of the occlusal surface.(See Figs 9.39 and 9.40.)

Usually the incisors do not suffer the same breakdown of the surface and sensitivity as the molars. However, they do frequently cause a cosmetic defect. This can be treated as the child becomes conscious of it, either by coverage with composite (veneer) or partial removal of the defect and coverage with composite (localized composite restoration). Details of these treatment techniques will be covered in Chapter 10.

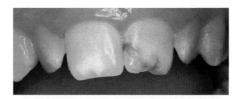

Fig. 9.39 MIH effects on the incisors; a mild white patch on one tooth can occur in the same mouth as more severe brown discolouration with some surface breakdown.

The first problem to remedy in molars is the sensitivity. Various desensitizing agents theoretically and anecdotally do help, but no clinical trials specifically related to MIH have been reported. They include:

- Repeated application of 5% sodium fluoride varnish (Duraphat).
- Commercially available 'sensitive tooth toothpastes'.
- Daily use of 0.4% stannous fluoride gels.

Fissure sealants can be useful where the affected areas are small and the enamel is intact. The use of bonding agents as described above under the resin sealant should help with bonding if the margin of the sealant is left on an area of hypomineralized enamel. The application of the bonding agents alone, once polymerized may reduce the sensitivity in the affected teeth *per se*. It is important to remember to monitor fissure sealants in these teeth very carefully as there is a high chance of marginal breakdown. If there is surface breakdown the tooth will require some form of restoration. The first decision to make is whether the clinician needs to maintain the tooth throughout life or if it is more pragmatic to consider extraction (Chapter 14). If the decision is that the first molars will be extracted as part of a long-term orthodontic plan, it is probable that they will still need temporisation because of the high level of sensitivity. These teeth are very difficult to anaesthetize, often staying sensitive when the operator has given normal levels of analgesic agent. If a child complains during treatment of a hypomineralized molar tooth, credibility should be given to their grievance. If a child experiences pain or discomfort during treatment, they will become increasingly anxious in successive treatments. This has been shown to be true for 9-year-old children, where dental fear, anxiety, and behaviour management were far more common in those children with severely hypomineralized first permanent molars when compared with unaffected controls.

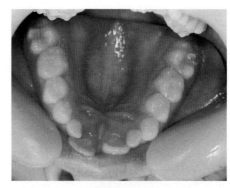

Fig. 9.40 MIH affecting the first permanent molars; some breakdown of the hypomineralised enamel is already occurring.

Inevitably, a balance has to be made between using simpler methods, such as dressing with a glass ionomer cement that may well need replenishment often on

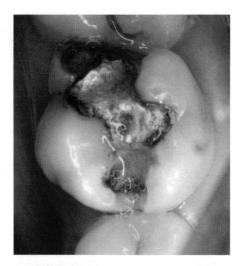

Fig. 9.41 Caries and further breakdown around an amalgam in a hypomineralised molar.

several occasions before the optimum time for extraction, and deciding early within the treatment to provide a full coverage restoration, for example. a stainless-steel crown which should last without requiring replacement prior to extraction time. All adjuncts to help the analgesia, such as inhalation sedation should be used, if indicated. It is also useful to use rubber dam for all the usual reasons plus the protection afforded by exclusion of spray from the other three un-anaesthetized molars, which probably will also be very sensitive.

If the intention is to maintain the molar in the long term, then the choice of restorative techniques expands. If the area of breakdown of the hypomineralized enamel is relatively confined then the operator should use conventional restorative techniques. It is however difficult to determine where the margins of a preparation should be left as sometimes seemingly normal enamel (to visual examination) undergoes breakdown.

Amalgam is of limited use, because, further breakdown often occurs at the margins, and it is non-adhesive so does not restore the strength of the tooth. Composite resins, on the other hand, when used with an appropriate bonding agent in well, demarcated lesions, should have a good success rate. Deciding where to leave the margin in these teeth presents difficulty. Fayle (2003) described his approach of investigating abnormal looking enamel at the margins of the defect with a slow rotating steel bur extending into these areas until good resistance is detected. This approach is at present not backed up by clinical studies but is a technique adopted by many dentists and could help avoid unnecessary sacrifice of sound tissue. (See Fig. 9.41.)

Most hypomineralized molars with surface breakdown involving one cusp or more will need a restoration with greater coverage. Either stainless-steel crowns or cast adhesive copings provide the most satisfactory options.

9.11.1 Preformed metal crowns (stainless–steel crowns)

The advantages of these are:

1. Single visit for placement.
2. Relatively quick and simple procedure.
3. Usually reduce sensitivity totally, because they cover the whole tooth.
4. Inexpensive compared with cast restorations.
5. Good retention rate.

The disadvantages are:

1. Require more tooth preparation than cast preparations.
2. Once a tooth has been prepared for a stainless-steel crown, it will need a full coverage restoration eventually. It has been suggested that placing orthodontic separators 1 or 2 weeks prior to preparation reduces the amount of tissue requiring removal. However, some reduction is usually necessary.
3. Gingival margins are sub-gingival.

Operative technique

1. Obtain adequate anaesthesia.
2. Isolate the tooth to be crowned.
3. Select the crown size.
4. Remove any carious dentine and enamel.
5. Replace tooth bulk with glass ionomer.
6. Reduce the occlusion minimally.
7. Reduce the mesial and distal surfaces, slicing with a fine tapered bur. Depending on the natural anatomy of the tooth it may be necessary to create a peripheral chamfer on the buccal and lingual surfaces.

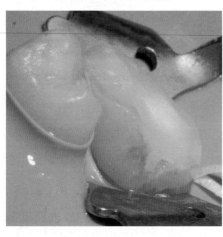

Fig. 9.42 Stainless-steel crown preparation. The occlusal surface is reduced minimally just enough to allow room to place the crown without disrupting the occlusion.

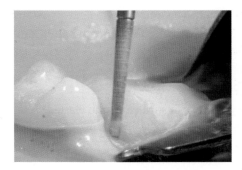

Fig. 9.43 Stainless-steel crown preparation. Obtain mesial and distal reduction with a fine tapered diamond bur with minimal buccal and palatal reduction that is just sufficient to allow the operator to place the crown. It is tempting not to effect any distal reduction if there is no erupted second permanent molar but remember it is important not to change the proportions of the tooth or create an overhang that will impede second molar eruption.

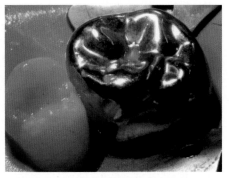

Fig. 9.44 Stainless-steel crown is tried in and fit determined. This crown will now need to be contoured and smoothed around the margins so that they fit evenly 1 mm below gingival level around the whole periphery. It is important that the crown has a good contact point mesially. Contour the tooth with the correct pliers.

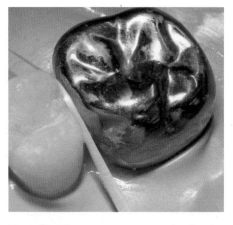

Fig. 9.45 Glass ionomer cement is placed in the crown, and overfilled to prevent voids forming under the crown. Excess cement is removed with cotton wool rolls and hand instruments, and the interstitial area cleared with dental floss.

8. Try the selected crown; adjust the shape cervically, such that the margins extend ~1 mm below the gingival crest evenly around the whole of the perimeter of the crown. Sharp Bee Bee scissors usually achieve this most easily, followed by crimping pliers to contour the edge to give spring and grip. Permanent molar preformed metal crowns need this because they are not shaped accurately cervically. This is because there is such a variation in crown length of the first permanent molars.

9. After the contouring, smooth and polish the crown to ensure that it does not attract excessive amounts of plaque.

10. After test fitting of the crown remove the rubber dam to check the occlusion then re-apply for cementation.

11. Cement the crown usually with a glass ionomer based cement.

12. Remove excess cement carefully with an explorer and knotted floss. Finally recheck the occlusion. (See Figs 9.42–9.46.)

9.11.2 Cast adhesive copings

This type of restoration offers two main advantages over preformed metal crowns:

- avoids unnecessary approximal reduction;
- enables margins to remain supragingival.

However three disadvantages are:

- still needs local analgesia;
- takes two visits to complete;
- technique is more expensive.

(See Fig 9.47.)

Operative technique (Harley and Ibbetson, 1993)

Visit 1.

1. Local analgesia.
2. Rubber dam.

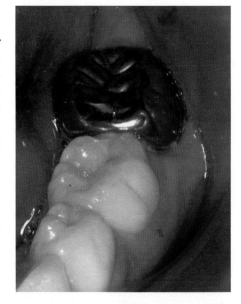

Fig. 9.46 A stainless-steel crown that was placed 1 year previously

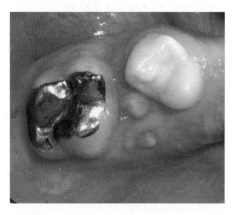

Fig. 9.47 An etched coping covering the occlusal surface of a hypoplastic molar.

3. Preparation to remove any carious or softened enamel.
4. Gingival retraction with cords (to prevent crevicular fluid and other moisture contaminating the preparation site and impressions).
5. Impression with rubber base material.
6. Temporization if much tooth tissue has been removed.

The casting is constructed in the laboratory, and the fit surface is sand blasted.
Visit 2.

7. Local analgesia.
8. Rubber dam.
9. Tooth is brushed with pumice, washed, and dried.
10. Casting is tried in to check marginal adaptation and fit.
11. Casting is re-sandblasted to obtain optimum conditions for bonding.
12. Tooth is etched, washed, and dried.
13. Cement is applied to fit surface of casting ensuring there are no bubbles.
14. The casting is held in position under pressure for 3 min.
15. Excess cement is removed.
16. Oxygen inhibiting material (oxyguard) is applied over the margins of the casting and maintained in position for a further 3 min.
17. The oxyguard is removed by washing; margins rechecked; and occlusion checked.

9.12 ALTERNATIVES TO CONVENTIONAL CAVITY PREPARATION

9.12.1 Air abrasion

There has recently been a resurgence of interest in air abrasion technology with several different commercial units available. With air abrasion machines, aluminium oxide particles (27 or 50 μm) are blasted against the teeth under a range of pressures (30–160 psi) with variable particle flow rates.

One very obvious concern is the safety aspect due to the presence of quantities of free aluminium oxide in the surgery environment. In theory aluminium oxide is considered harmless. It is found in a wide variety of products from toothpastes to polishing wheels. The size of the particles is considered too big to enter the distal airways or alveoli of the lungs. What dust does enter the lungs should be easily removed by ciliary action. However, anyone who has used one of these units will know that control of the dust is an ongoing challenge; rubber dam and very good suction help, but it still seems to spread.

Air abrasion produces a cavity preparation with both rounded cavo-surface margins and internal line angles. The surface it creates is irregular with many fine voids and defects. Initially it was considered that this surface might provide enough retention without etching but studies show this as erroneous.
Some of the clear advantages proposed for air abrasion are:

- Elimination of vibration, less noise, and decreased pressure.
- Reduction in pain during cavity preparation; 85% of patients do not require local analgesia.
- Less damaging pulpal effects than with conventional hand-piece usage, when used at higher pressures of 160 psi and with smaller particle size of 27 μm.
- Less fracture and crazing of enamel and dentine during cavity preparation.
- Root canal access through porcelain crowns without fracturing porcelain.

Air abrasion has been proposed for:

- Cleaning and removing stains and incipient caries from pits and fissures prior to sealant and PRRs.
- Small class I, III, IV, and V cavity preparations and selected class II preparations.
- Repair and removal of composites, glass ionomers, and porcelain restorations.
- Cleaning and preparation of castings, orthodontic bands, and brackets prior to cementation.

What it cannot do is remove leathery dentinal caries or prepare extensive cavities requiring classical retentive form.

To use it successfully, the clinician must learn a new technique as the tip does not touch the tooth and therefore there is no tactile feedback. The tip width and the tip to tooth distance seem to have most influence on the cavity width and depth. Increasing the distance produces larger shallower cuts. Increasing the tip diameter produces larger deeper cuts. Therefore, the most precise removal of tooth tissue is achieved with a small inner diameter tip (0.38 mm), held 2 mm from the tooth surface. If cutting a class II cavity, it is essential to protect the adjacent tooth. Care must also be taken around the soft tissues to prevent surgical emphysema. Glass/mirror surfaces may be damaged by the dust.

In the preparation of PRRs, this technique gives as good a result as conventional methods. It was thought that cavities would be smaller with air abrasion but this has not been realized practically.

In conclusion, air abrasion may be useful in preparation of small cavities with reduced patient discomfort, when combined with acid etching to obtain a good bond with adhesive materials, and when correctly and carefully used. However, the dust is a practical problem.

9.12.2 Ozone therapy

Dental treatments are constantly evolving. One such innovation, ozone therapy (healozone) has hit the media headlines, spiking much public interest. The technology is available and costly devices for delivery of ozone for dental purposes exist, but as yet the superiority of this modality over conventional treatment has not been proven with properly conducted clinical trials.

The theory of the action of ozone is that it kills micro-organisms, by oxidizing their cell walls to rupture their cytoplasmic membranes, that is, it is bactericidal. In laboratories it has been shown that ozone can substantially reduce the numbers of micro-organisms within carious dentine on short exposures of 10–20 s. However, the clinical significance of this has not been established. It has been postulated that the use of ozone together with a remineralizing regime of fluoride paste and rinse, oral hygiene instruction, and dietary advice would be beneficial and that it would arrest primary root caries to a greater extent than remineralizing regime alone. It has also been suggested that ozone treatment can stabilize pit and fissure caries preventing further deterioration. However, the authors will stay with more traditional methods of caries control until proper controlled trials of reasonable duration (>4 years) have been reported.

9.12.3 Lasers

The public perception of lasers in dentistry is that they can do remarkable things painlessly, so obviously this appeals to a greater number of people. However, the number of dentists offering lasers as an option in their practices is still small. The cost of equipment is obviously a significant factor, but as with all new technologies it is important that each dentist considers the proven clinical outcomes, that is, what the recorded literature states regarding the safety, efficacy, and effectiveness.

With lasers this is further complicated by the fact that there are many different types of lasers, with different uses and new types and applications being produced constantly.

Laser types and uses

• Carbon dioxide lasers	Soft tissue incision/ablation Gingival troughing Aesthetic contouring of gingivae Treatment of oral ulcers Fraenectomy and gingivectomy De-epithelization of gingival tissue during periodontal regenerative procedures
• Nd : YAG	Similar to above plus removal of incipient caries but because of the depth of penetration there is a greater risk of collateral damage than with dioxide lasers.
• Er : YAG	Caries removal Cavity preparation in both enamel and dentine Preparation of root canals
• Argon laser	Resin curing Tooth bleaching Treatment of ulcers Aesthetic gingival contouring Fraenectomy and gingivectomy

Lasers produce light energy within a narrow frequency range. They are named after the active element within them, which determines the wavelength of the light emitted. So some of the commoner lasers have the following characteristics

- Neodymium : yttrium-aluminium-garnet (Nd : YAG) wavelength $= 1.064 \mu m$
- Carbon dioxide lasers wavelength $= 10.6 \mu m$
- Erbium : YAG $= 2.94 \mu m$
- Argon $= 457–502$ nm
- Gallium-Arsenide (diode) $= 904$ nm
- Holmium : YAG $= 2.1 \mu m$

The wavelength of light is the primary determinant of the degree to which the target material absorbs light. The deeper the laser energy penetrates, the more it scatters and distributes throughout the tissue, for example, carbon dioxide laser penetrates 0.01–0.03 mm into the tissue while Nd : YAG laser penetrates 2–5 mm. The light from dental lasers is absorbed and converted to heat, while the thermal effects caused depend on the tissue composition and the time the beam is focused on the target tissue. The increase in temperature may cause the tissue to change in structure and composition, for example, denaturation, vapourization, carbonization, and melting followed by recrystallization. The argon laser has a major advantage over the other lasers in that the wavelength at which it operates is absorbed by haemoglobin and therefore provides excellent haemostasis.

Let us look first at safety. In order for a procedure to be deemed safe, collateral damage must be within acceptable limits, that is, the risk–benefit ratio must be small with the benefit to the patient being significant; for example, laser-induced tissue trauma to the surgical site can add several more days to the healing process and cause dramatically abnormal appearances for up to 10–14 days postoperatively. Balanced against this, postoperative pain is usually minimal.

Using an Er : YAG laser for cavity preparation and caries removal

Proposed advantages:

- Laser use results in clean sharp margins in enamel and dentine.
- The pulp is protected and safe as the depth of energy penetration is negligible. (There is one study that shows deeper damage to nerve terminals and fibres visible under electron microscope examination though its clinical significance is unknown.)
- Patients report little or no pain with the use of Er : YAG laser in cavity preparation.
- Time taken for cavity preparation is short.

Disadvantages:

- Cost.
- The need to learn a new technique in which there is no proprioceptive feedback since the laser tip does not impinge dental tissue.

Laser caries detection/laser fluorescence

This is a low-power laser application, which does not raise safety concerns. The system is commercially available and known as 'Diagnodent'(KaVo). Many workers have studied it and reported the laser fluorescence system overscores lesions while the conventional visual method underscores them. The problem with the laser fluorescence instrument is that it cannot differentiate between caries and hypomineralisation. Furthermore, staining is interpreted as caries and the presence of plaque deleteriously affects performance. Therefore, it should only be used as an adjunct to clinical examination and diagnosis.

Argon laser irradiation as a preventive treatment

At certain settings Nd : YAG laser irradiation of sound enamel has been reported to increase surface micro-hardness. Some researchers report that argon laser irradiation produces a surface with enhanced caries resistance. Several authors have studied these by creating plaque retentive areas on teeth destined to be removed for orthodontic reasons and recorded the effect that different pre-treatments had prior to 6 weeks of plaque accumulation. Pre-treatment with an argon laser led to less lesion formation and improved further if combined with topical fluoride application. The results seem very impressive but need replication in the long term, in the form of controlled clinical trials, to determine the significance in a population as a whole instead of specific artificially created caries prone areas. If proven they may yield a simple non-invasive and pain free technique for reducing caries susceptibility of enamel.

Resin curing

Argon lasers are able to polymerize composite resins in a shorter time than conventional light sources. The use of this type of laser has the additional advantage of increasing the ability of tooth structure to resist cariogenic challenges and may also increase resistance of the enamel surrounding the polymerized resin. One study also found that laser polymerization lowered the proportion of non-polymerized monomer and slightly improved the physical properties of the resin in comparison to visible-light methods of curing. It is important to remember that resins cured with lasers do not necessarily have superior physical properties and it is particularly important to check that the initiators within the resin are activated at the specific wavelength of the laser. Again there is a paucity of clinical studies to support these concepts.

Laser bleaching

Both carbon dioxide and argon lasers have been suggested as a method of tooth whitening. There have been no controlled clinical studies and there are concerns regarding the pulpal safety in connection with carbon dioxide lasers, so the use of this type of laser is not recommended. In one study an argon ion laser produced less temperature rise when used to increase the activity of a bleaching gel compared with conventional quartz tungsten; hence, plasma arc lights may be acceptable.

Enamel etching

It has been suggested that laser irradiation may eliminate the need for etching, but as yet there is not scientific literature to back this claim.

In summary, some of the preliminary reports on the use of lasers give much room for optimism. They not only suggest that it might be possible to use lasers to help prevent decay, but it may also be possible to perform certain surgeries and prepare cavities with little pain for the patient. However, greater clinical trial validation of these claims is needed before lasers can be considered superior to conventional methods, so that failure to utilize the former will be considered as a disservice to the patients. As yet the equipment cost and the need for different laser types for various types of treatment make their use prohibitive for most UK dentists.

9.13 RAMPANT CARIES

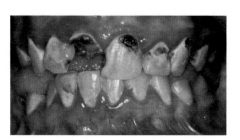

Fig. 9.48 Rampant caries in a 13-year-old girl. She only attended because the incisor had fractured. Her whole attitude to dentistry needs to change in order to treat her successfully.

It is important to consider the many factors that determine the treatment of a child with a high caries rate (Fig. 9.48). If the child presents with an acute problem of pain or swelling, then immediate treatment is indicated to relieve the child of the pain. After that, it is important that the clinician considers the attitude of the child and his or her parents together with motivation towards dental treatment, the co-operation of the child, the age, and the extent of decay.

It may be possible to place temporary restorations while preventive strategies are commenced. These will include:

1. Dietary analysis and appropriate advice to the child and the parent.
2. Plaque control, oral hygiene instruction depending on age to the child or the parent, the techniques of toothbrushing, and disclosure.
3. Fluoride
   –tooth paste
   –mouth rinse;
   –varnish application every 6 months.
4. Fissure sealants
5. Regular recall.

Once the caries is under control, definitive restorative treatment can commence.

9.14 SUMMARY

1. A full preventive programme, to attempt to treat the cause of the caries, must accompany any restorative treatment.
2. Utilize rubber dam if at all possible prior to the restoration of all teeth.
3. Early treatment of occlusal surface caries saves tooth tissue but with early approximal lesions use remineralization wherever the lesion has not reached the dentine.

4. Consideration should be given to pulp preservation in deep lesions in immature permanent teeth.

5. Hypomineralized first molars deteriorate rapidly, can be extremely sensitive and require early treatment

6. New materials and technologies constantly appear for evaluation. Treat with caution until long-term clinical trial results verify the claims of the initial researchers.

9.15 FURTHER READING

Kidd, E. A. M., Smith, B. G. N., and Watson, T. F. (2003). *Pickard's manual of operative dentistry*, (8th edn). Oxford Medical Publications, Oxford University Press, Oxford. (*A very full and informative guide to restoration of permanent teeth.*)

Reid J. S., Challis, P. D., and Patterson, C. J. W. (1991). *Rubber dam in clinical practice.* Quintessence, London. (*This provides a guide to the simple use of rubber dam.*)

9.16 REFERENCES

Fayle, S. A. (2003). Molar Incisor Hypomineralisation: restorative management. *European Journal of Paediatric Dentistry*, **4**(3), 121–6.

Harley, K. E. and Ibbetson, R. J. (1993). Dental anomalies: are adhesive castings the solution? *British Dental Journal*, **174**, 15–22.

Nunn, J. H., Murray, J. J., and Smallridge, J. (2000). British Society of Paediatric Dentistry: a policy document on fissure sealants in paediatric dentistry. *International Journal Paediatric Dentistry*, **10**(2), 174–7.

Pitts, N. B., Boyles, J., Nugent, Z. J., Thomas, N., Pine, C. M. (2004). The dental caries experience of 14-year-old children in England and Wales. Surveys co-ordinated by the British Association for the Study of Community Dentistry in 2002/2003. *Community Dental Health*, **21**(1), 45–57.

Rugg-Gunn, A. J., Welbury, R. R., and Toumba, J. (2000). BSPD Policy Document: A policy document on the use of amalgam in paediatric dentistry. *International. Journal of Paediatric Dentistry*, **11**, 233–8.

Smallridge, J. Faculty of Dental Surgery, and Royal College of Surgeons (2000). UK national clinical guidelines in paediatric dentistry. Management of the stained fissure in the first permanent molar. *International Journal of Paediatric Dentistry*, **10**(1), 79–83.

Advanced restorative dentistry

10 Advanced restorative dentistry

N. M. Kilpatrick and R. R. Welbury

10.1 INTRODUCTION

The aim of this chapter is to cover the management of more complicated clinical problems associated with children and adolescents; tooth discolouration, inherited enamel and dentine defects, hypodontia and tooth surface loss. There is considerable overlap in the application of the various restorative techniques; therefore the chapter is divided into two parts: the first outlines the clinical steps involved in the various procedures, while the second covers the more general principles of management of the particular dental problems.

10.2 ADVANCED RESTORATIVE TECHNIQUES

It is not the remit of this chapter to cover advanced restorative dentistry in detail, but many of the techniques used in children are the same as those for adults (Tables 10.1 and 10.2).

With the aid of some clinical examples, seven of the restorative procedures will be described in simple stages. Omitted from this list are the stages involved in the provision of full crown restorations and bridgework, which are the specific remit of a restorative dentistry textbook. However, the provision of porcelain veneers, more commonly associated with adult patients, will be mentioned briefly.

10.2.1 The hydrochloric acid–pumice microabrasion technique

This is a controlled method of removing surface enamel in order to improve discolorations that are limited to the outer enamel layer. It is achieved by a combination of abrasion and erosion—the term 'abrosion' is sometimes used. In the clinical technique that will be described no more than 100 μm of enamel are removed. Once completed the procedure should not be repeated again in the future. Too much enamel removal is potentially damaging to the pulp and cosmetically the underlying dentine colour will become more evident.

Indications

(1) fluorosis;
(2) idiopathic speckling;
(3) postorthodontic treatment demineralization;
(4) prior to veneer placement for well-demarcated stains;
(5) white/brown surface staining, e.g. secondary to primary predecessor infection or trauma (Turner teeth).

Table 10.1 Advanced restorative techniques

Hydrochloric acid—pumice microabrasion technique
Non-vital bleaching
Vital bleaching—chairside and nightguard
Localized composite resin restorations
Composite veneers—direct and indirect
Porcelain veneers
Adhesive metal castings
Full crowns
Bridgework—adhesive and fixed

Table 10.2 Ideal features of restorative treatments

Resolve sensitivity
Restore function
Aesthetic
Have proven durability
Cause insignificant loss of tooth structure
Preserve dental hard tissues
Enhance periodontal health
Simple, quick and tolerable to the patient

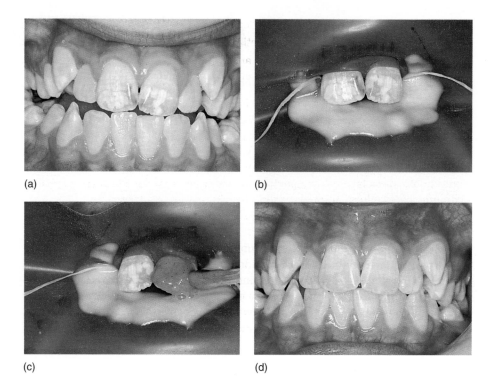

Fig. 10.1 (a) Characteristic appearance of fluorotic discoloration. (b) Rubber dam isolation with bicarbonate of soda in position. (c) Application of hydrochloric acid—pumice slurry with a wooden stick. (d) Appearance at 2 years' post-treatment.

Armamentarium

(1) bicarbonate of soda/water;
(2) Copalite varnish or vaseline;
(3) fluoridated toothpaste;
(4) non-acidulated fluoride (0–2 years: drops);
(5) pumice;
(6) rubber dam;
(7) rubber prophylaxis cup;
(8) Soflex discs (3M);
(9) 18% hydrochloric acid.

Technique

1. Perform preoperative vitality tests, take radiographs and photographs (Fig. 10.1(a)).
2. Clean the teeth with pumice and water, wash, and dry.
3. Isolate the teeth to be treated with rubber dam, and paint Copalite varnish around the necks of the dam or vaseline under the dam.
4. Place a mixture of sodium bicarbonate and water on the dam behind the teeth, as protection in case of spillage (Fig. 10.1(b)).
5. Mix 18% hydrochloric acid with pumice into a slurry and apply a small amount to the labial surface on either a rubber cup rotating slowly for 5 s or a wooden stick rubbed over the surface for 5 s (Fig. 10.1(c)), before washing for 5 s directly into an aspirator tip. Repeat until the stain has reduced, up to a maximum of 10×5-s applications per tooth. Any improvement that is going to occur will have done so by this time.
6. Apply the fluoride drops to the teeth for 3 min.
7. Remove the rubber dam.

8. Polish the teeth with the finest Soflex discs.
9. Polish the teeth with fluoridated toothpaste for 1 min.
10. Review in 1 month for vitality tests and clinical photographs (Fig. 10.1(d)).
11. Review biannually checking pulpal status.

Critical analysis of the effectiveness of the technique should not be made immediately, but delayed for at least 1 month as the appearance of the teeth will continue to improve over this time. Experience has shown that brown mottling is removed more easily than white, but even where white mottling is incompletely removed it nevertheless becomes less perceptible. This phenomenon has been attributed to the relatively prismless layer of compacted surface enamel produced by the 'abrosion' technique, which alters the optical properties of the tooth surface.

Long-term studies of the technique have found no association with pulpal damage, increased caries susceptibility, or significant prolonged thermal sensitivity. Patient compliance and satisfaction is good and any dissatisfaction is usually due to inadequate preoperative explanation. The technique is easy to perform for the operator and patient, and is not time consuming. Removal of any mottled area is permanent and achieved with an insignificant loss of surface enamel. Failure to improve the appearance by the HCl–pumice microabrasion technique has no harmful effects and may make it easier to mask some lesions with veneers.

10.2.2 Non-vital bleaching

This technique describes the bleaching of teeth that have become discoloured by the diffusion into the dentinal tubules of haemoglobin breakdown products from necrotic pulp tissue.

Indications

(1) discoloured non-vital teeth;
(2) well-condensed gutta percha root filling;
(3) no clinical or radiological signs of periapical disease.

Contraindications

(1) heavily restored teeth;
(2) staining due to amalgam.

Armamentarium

(1) rubber dam;
(2) zinc phosphate or IRM cement;
(3) 37% phosphoric acid;
(4) bleaching agent, for example, hydrogen peroxide, carbamide peroxide, or sodium perborate;
(5) cotton wool;
(6) glass ionomer cement;
(7) white gutta percha temporary restorative;
(8) composite resin;
(9) non-setting calcium hydroxide.

Technique

1. Take preoperative periapical radiographs; these are essential to check for an adequate root filling (Fig. 10.2(a)).

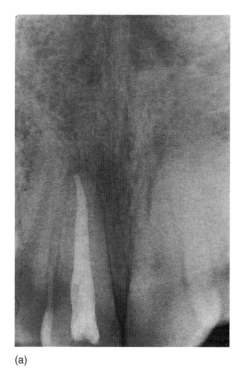
(a)

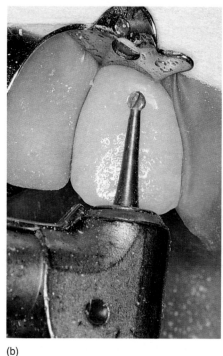
(b)

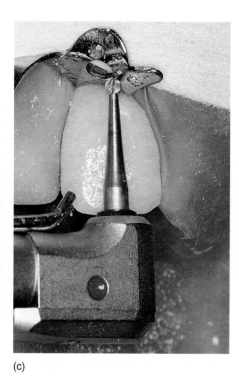
(c)

Fig. 10.2 (a) Radiograph of upper right central incisor with a well-condensed root filling. (b) Standard bur in a contra-angled head may not reach the dentogingival junction. (c) Correct depth achieved using a standard bur in a miniature head.

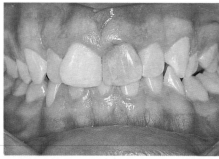
(a)

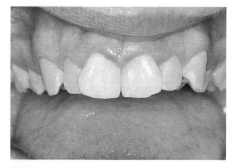
(b)

Fig. 10.3 (a) and (b) Intensely darkened, non-vital, upper left central incisor treated by four changes of bleach.

2. Clean the teeth with pumice and make a note of the shade of the discoloured tooth.

3. Place rubber dam, isolating the single tooth. Ensure adequate eye and clothing protection for the patient, operator, and dental nurse.

4. Remove palatal restoration and pulp chamber restoration.

5. Remove root filling to the level of the dentogingival junction—you may need to use adult burs in a mini-head (Fig. 10.2(b) and (c)).

6. Place 1 mm of cement over the gutta percha.

7. Freshen dentine with a round bur. Do not remove excessively.

8. Etch the pulp chamber with 37% phosphoric acid for 30–60 s, wash, and dry—this will facilitate the ingress of the hydrogen peroxide.

9. Place the bleaching agent, either alone or on a cotton wool pledget into the pulp chamber. Place into the tooth, either alone with a flat plastic instrument or on a cotton-wool pledget.

10. Place a dry piece of cotton wool over the mixture.

11. Seal the cavity with glass ionomer cement.

12. Repeat the process at weekly intervals until the tooth is slightly overbleached.

13. Place non-setting calcium hydroxide into the pulp chamber for 2 weeks. Seal with glass ionomer cement.

14. Finally, restore the tooth with white gutta percha (to facilitate reopening the pulp chamber again, if necessary, at a later date) and composite resin.

Figures 10.3(a) and (b) show an example of a highly successful result. If the colour of a tooth has not significantly improved after three changes of bleach then it is unlikely to do so, and further bleaching should be abandoned. The maximum number of bleach applications is usually accepted as 10. Failure of a tooth to bleach could be due to either inadequate removal of filling materials from the pulp chamber or to 'time expired' bleaching agent. Both these factors should be checked before abandoning a procedure.

Slight overbleaching is desirable, but the patient should be instructed to attend the surgery before the next appointment if marked overbleaching has occurred.

Non-vital bleaching has a reputation of causing brittleness of the tooth. This is probably the result of previous injudicious removal of dentine (which only needs to be 'freshened' with a round bur), rather than a direct effect of the bleaching procedure itself.

This method of bleaching has been associated with the later occurrence of external cervical resorption. The exact mechanism of this association is unclear, but it is thought that the hydrogen peroxide diffuses through the dentinal tubules to set up an inflammatory reaction in the periodontal ligament around the cervical region of the tooth. In a small number of teeth there is a gap between the end of the enamel and the beginning of the cementum, and in these cases the above explanation is tenable. The purpose of the 1-mm layer of cement is to cover the openings of the dentinal tubules at the level where there may be a communication to the periodontal ligament. In the same way, non-setting calcium hydroxide is placed in the pulp chamber for 2 weeks prior to final restoration in order to eradicate any inflammation in the periodontal ligament that may have been initiated.

Clinical studies have demonstrated that regression can be expected with this technique. The longest study after 8 years gave a 21% failure rate. However, if white gutta percha has been placed within the pulp chamber then it is readily removed and the tooth easily rebleached.

The advantages of the technique are many: easy for operator and patient; conservation of tooth tissue and maintenance of the original crown morphology; no irritation to gingival tissues; no problems with changing gingival level in young patients compared to veneers or crowns; no technical assistance required.

10.2.3 The inside/outside bleaching technique

Recently, an alternative approach to the management of the discoloured endodontically treated tooth has been described. Known as the inside/outside bleaching technique, it is essentially a combination of the walking and vital bleaching techniques. Tooth preparation is the same as described for the walking bleach technique (section 10.2.2) with particular attention being paid to removal of the gutta percha below the cemento-enamel junction followed by the placement of a barrier (usually a glass ionomer cement or zinc oxide eugenol cement) to seal the root canal from the oral cavity. A custom made tray (see Fig. 10.5 (b)) is constructed as a vehicle for the bleaching gel. However, rather than creating space labially as in the vital bleaching technique a small reservoir is created palatal to the affected tooth only. The gel, 10% carbamide peroxide, is placed by the patient into both the access cavity of the non-vital tooth and the tray. The tray is then worn full time for up to 4 days, the gel being replaced every 2–4 h. Once an aesthetically acceptable result is achieved the access cavity is refilled appropriately. Long-term results are not yet available for this approach with relapse being as likely as any of the other bleaching techniques.

10.2.4 Vital bleaching—chairside

This technique involves the external application of hydrogen peroxide to the surface of the tooth followed by its activation with a heat source. The technique has achieved considerable success in the United States, but it is a lengthy and time-consuming procedure that requires a high degree of patient compliance and motivation.

Indications

(1) very mild tetracycline staining without obvious banding;
(2) mild fluorosis;
(3) yellowing due to ageing;
(4) single teeth with sclerosed pulp chambers and canals.

Armamentarium

(1) rubber dam with clamps and floss ligatures;
(2) Orabase gel;
(3) topical anaesthetic;
(4) gauze;
(5) 37% phosphoric acid;
(6) heating light with rheostat;
(7) 30-volume hydrogen peroxide;
(8) polishing stones;
(9) fluoride drops (0–2 years: drops).

Technique

1. Take preoperative periapical radiographs and perform vitality tests. Replace any leaking restorations.
2. Clean the teeth with pumice and water to remove extrinsic staining. Take preoperative photographs with a tooth from a 'Vita' shade guide registering the shade, adjacent to the patient's teeth.
3. Apply topical anaesthetic to gingival margins.
4. Coat the buccal and palatal gingivae with Orabase gel as extra protection from the bleaching solution.
5. Isolate each tooth to be bleached using individual ligatures. The end teeth should be clamped (usually from second premolar to second premolar).
6. Cover the metal rubber dam clamps with damp strips of gauze to prevent them from getting hot under the influence of the heat source.
7. Etch the labial and a third of the palatal surfaces of the teeth with the phosphoric acid for 60 s, wash, and dry. Thoroughly soak a strip of gauze in the 35% hydrogen peroxide and cover the teeth to be bleached.
8. Position the heat lamp 13–15 inches (33–38 cm) from the patient's teeth. Set the rheostat to a mid-temperature range and increase it until the patient can just feel the warmth in their teeth, and then reduce it slightly until no sensation is felt.
9. Keep the gauze damp by reapplying the hydrogen peroxide every 3–5 min using a cotton bud. Make sure the bottle is closed between applications as the hydrogen peroxide deactivates on exposure to air.
10. After 30 min remove the rubber dam, clean off the Orabase gel, and polish the teeth using the shofu stones. Apply the fluoride drops for 2–3 min.
11. Note that postoperative sensitivity may occur and should be relieved with paracetamol.
12. Assess the change—it may be necessary to repeat the process 3–10 times per arch. Treat one arch at a time. Keep the patient under review as rebleaching may be required after 1 or more years.
13. Take postoperative photographs with the original 'Vita' shade tooth included.

This technique is very time consuming and retreatment may be necessary so the patient must be highly motivated. The technique can be used in the treatment of discolouration caused by pulp chamber sclerosis (Fig. 10.4(a)–(c)). These cases require isolation of the single tooth.

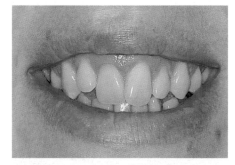

(a)

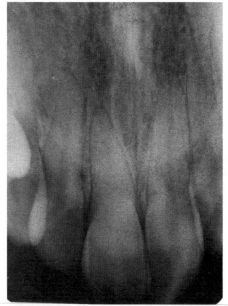

(b)

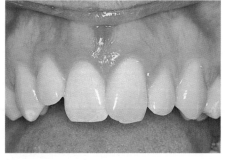

(c)

Fig. 10.4   (a) and (b) A discoloured, upper right central incisor with radiograph confirming sclerosis of the pulp chamber and root canal. (c) Appearance of upper right central incisor after four chairside bleaching treatments.

10.2.5 Vital bleaching—nightguard

This technique involves the daily placement of carbamide peroxide gel into a custom-fitted tray of either the upper or the lower arch. As the name suggests, it is carried out by the patient at home and is initially done on a daily basis.

Indications

(1) mild fluorosis;

(2) moderate fluorosis as an adjunct to hydrochloric acid–pumice microabrasion;

(3) yellowing of ageing.

Armamentarium

(1) upper impression and working model;

(2) soft mouthguard—avoiding the gingivae;

(3) 10% carbamide peroxide gel.

Technique

1. Take an alginate impression of the arch to be treated and cast a working model in stone.

2. Relieve the labial surfaces of the teeth by about 0.5 mm and make a soft, pull-down, vacuum- formed splint as a mouthguard (Fig. 10.5(a)). The splint should be no more than 2 mm in thickness and should not cover the gingivae. It is only a vehicle for the bleaching gel and not intended to protect the gingivae.

3. Instruct the patient on how to floss their teeth thoroughly. Perform a full mouth prophylaxis and instruct them how to apply the gel into the mouth-guard (Fig. 10.5(b)).

4. Note that the length of time the guard should be worn depends on the product used.

5. Review about 2 weeks later to check that the patient is not experiencing any sensitivity, and then at 6 weeks, by which time 80% of any colour change should have occurred.

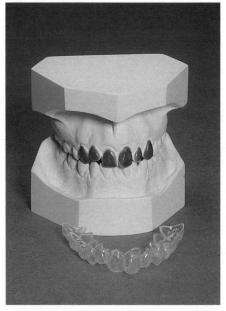

(a)

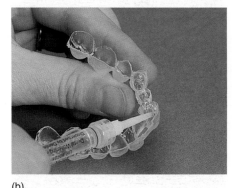

(b)

Fig. 10.5 (a) Model of upper arch with wax relief for construction of a night guard. (b) Mouthguard being loaded with carbamide peroxide gel.

Carbamide peroxide gel (10%) breaks down in the mouth into 3% hydrogen peroxide and 7% urea. Both urea and hydrogen peroxide have low molecular weights, which allow them to diffuse rapidly through enamel and dentine and thus explains the transient pulpal sensitivity occasionally experienced with home bleaching systems.

Pulpal histology with regard to these materials has not been assessed, but no clinical significance has been attributed to the changes seen with 35% hydrogen peroxide over 75 years of usage, except where teeth have been overheated or traumatized. By extrapolation, 3% hydrogen peroxide in the home systems should therefore be safe.

Although most carbamide peroxide materials contain trace amounts of phosphoric and citric acids as stabilizers and preservatives, no indication of etching or a significant change in the surface morphology of enamel has been demonstrated by scanning electron microscopy analysis. There was early concern that bleaching solutions with a low pH would cause demineralization of enamel when the pH fell below the 'critical' pH of 5.2–5.8. However, no evidence of this process has been noted to date in any clinical trials or laboratory tests, and this may be due to the urea (and subsequently the ammonia) and carbon dioxide released on degradation of the carbamide peroxide elevating the pH.

There is an initial decrease in bond strengths of enamel to composite resins immediately after home bleaching but this returns to normal within 7 days. This effect has been attributed to the residual oxygen in the bleached tooth surface which inhibits polymerization of the composite resin. The home bleaching systems do not affect the colour of restorative materials. Any perceived effect is probably due to superficial cleansing.

Minor ulceration or irritation may occur during the initial treatment. It is important to check that the mouthguard does not extend on to the gingivae and that the edges of the guard are smooth. If ulceration persists a decreased exposure time may be necessary. If there is still a problem then allergy is a possibility.

There are no biological concerns regarding the short-term use of carbamide peroxide. It has a similar cytotoxicity on mouse fibroblasts as zinc phosphate cement and Crest toothpaste, and has been used for a number of years in the United States to reduce plaque and promote wound healing. However, there are no long-term studies on its safety; laboratory studies have shown that carbamide peroxide has a mutagenic potential on vascular endothelium and there may be harmful effects on the periodontium, together with delayed wound healing.

Published clinical studies of 1–2 years' duration have shown that the yellowing of ageing responds best to treatment. Although this would appear to take home bleaching out of the remit of paediatric dentistry, it may still have a part to play in the preliminary lightening of tetracycline-stained teeth prior to veneer placement, and also in cases of mild fluorosis. Irrespective of the clinical application, evidence suggests that annual retreatment may be necessary to maintain any effective lightening. This further highlights the importance of more research into the long-term effects of this treatment on the teeth, the mucosa, and the periodontium.

The exact mechanism of bleaching in any of the three methods described is unknown. Theories of oxidation, photo-oxidation, and ion exchange have been suggested. Conversely, the cause of rediscolouration is also unknown. This may be a combination of chemical reduction of the oxidation products previously formed, marginal leakage of restorations allowing ingress of bacterial and chemical byproducts, and salivary or tissue fluid contamination via permeable tooth structure.

10.2.6 Localized composite resin restorations

This restorative technique uses recent advances in dental materials science to replace defective enamel with a restoration that bonds to and blends with enamel.

Indications

1. Well-demarcated white, yellow, or brown hypomineralised enamel.

Armamentarium

(1)   rubber dam/contoured matrix strips (Vivadent);

(2)   round and fissure diamond burs;

(3)   enamel/dentine bonding kit;

(4)   new generation, highly polishable, hybrid composite resin;

(5)   Soflex discs (3M) and interproximal polishing strips.

Technique

1.   Take preoperative photographs and select the shade (Fig. 10.6(a)).
2.   Apply rubber dam or contoured matrix strips.
3.   Remove demarcated lesion with a round diamond bur down to the amelodentinal junction (ADJ).
4.   Chamfer the enamel margins with a diamond fissure bur to increase the surface area available for retention.
5.   Etch the enamel margins—wash and dry.
6.   Apply the dentine primer to dentine and dry.

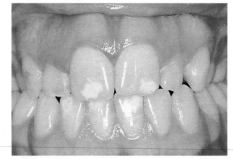

(a)

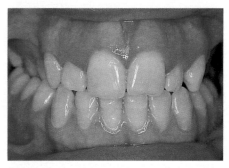

(b)

Fig. 10.6   (a) and (b) Well-demarcated white opacities on the upper central incisors treated by localized composite restorations.

7. Apply the enamel- and dentine-bonding agent and light-cure.

8. Apply the chosen shade of composite using a brush lubricated with the bonding agent to smooth and shape, and light-cure for the recommended time.

9. Remove the matrix strip/rubber dam.

10. Polish with graded Soflex discs (3M), finishing burs, and interproximal strips if required. Add characterization to the surface of the composite.

11. Take postoperative photographs (Fig. 10.6(b)).

The localized restoration is quick and easy to complete. Despite the removal of defective enamel down to the ADJ there is often no significant sensitivity and therefore no need for local anaesthesia. If the hypoplastic enamel has become carious and this extends into dentine then a liner of glass ionomer cement (correct shade) prior to placement of the composite resin will be necessary. Local anaesthesia will probably be required in these cases. Advances in bonding and resin technology make these restorations simple and obviate the need for a full labial veneer. Disadvantages are marginal staining, accurate colour match, and reduced composite translucency when lined by a glass ionomer cement.

10.2.7 Composite resin veneers

Although the porcelain jacket crown (PJC) may be the most satisfactory long-term restoration for a severely hypoplastic or discoloured tooth, it is not an appropriate solution for children for two reasons: (1) the large size of the young pulp horns and chamber; and (2) the immature gingival contour.

Composite veneers may be direct (placed at initial appointment) or indirect (placed at a subsequent appointment having been fabricated in the laboratory). The conservative veneering methods may not just offer a temporary solution, but a satisfactory long-term alternative to the PJC. Most composite veneers placed in children and adolescents are of the 'direct' type, as the durability of the indirect composite veneers is as yet unknown.

Before proceeding with any veneering technique, the decision must be made whether to reduce the thickness of labial enamel before placing the veneer. Certain factors should be considered:

1. Increased labiopalatal bulk makes it harder to maintain good oral hygiene. This may be courting disaster in the adolescent with a dubious oral hygiene technique.

2. Composite resin has a better bond strength to enamel when the surface layer of 200–300 mm is removed.

3. If a tooth is very discoloured some sort of reduction will be desirable, as a thicker layer of composite will be required to mask the intense stain.

4. If a tooth is already instanding or rotated, its appearance can be enhanced by a thicker labial veneer.

New generation, highly polishable, hybrid composite resins can replace relatively large amounts of missing tooth tissue as well as being used in thin sections as a veneer. Combinations of shades can be used to simulate natural colour gradations and hues.

Indications

(1) discolouration;

(2) enamel defects;

(3) diastemata;

(4) malpositioned teeth;

(5) large restorations.

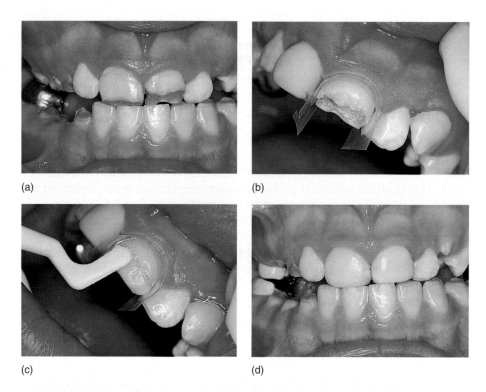

Fig. 10.7   (a) A young patient with amelogenesis imperfecta. (b) Contoured matrix strip in position. (c) Incremental placement of dentine shade composite. (d) Postoperative view showing final composite veneers.

Contraindications

(1)   insufficient available enamel for bonding;
(2)   oral habits, e.g. woodwind musicians.

Armamentarium

(1)   rubber dam/contoured matrix strips (Vivadent);
(2)   preparation and finishing burs;
(3)   new generation, highly polishable, hybrid composite resin;
(4)   Soflex discs (3M) and interproximal polishing strips.

Technique

1.   Use a tapered diamond bur to reduce labial enamel by 0.3–0.5 mm. Identify the finish line at the gingival margin and also mesially and distally just labial to the contact points.
2.   Clean the tooth with a slurry of pumice in water. Wash and dry and select the shade (Fig. 10.7(a)).
3.   Isolate the tooth either with rubber dam or a contoured matrix strip. Hold this in place by applying unfilled resin to its gingival side against the gingiva and curing for 10 s (Fig. 10.7(b)).
4.   Etch the enamel for 60 s, wash, and dry.
5.   Where dentine is exposed apply dentine primer.
6.   Apply a thin layer of bonding resin to the labial surface with a brush and cure for 15 s. It may be necessary to use an opaquer at this stage if the discolouration is intense.
7.   Apply composite resin of the desired shade to the labial surface and roughly shape it into all areas with a plastic instrument, then use a brush lubricated with unfilled resin to 'paddle' and smooth it into the desired shape. Cure 60 s

gingivally, 60 s mesioincisally, 60 s distoincisally, and 60 s from the palatal aspect if incisal coverage has been used. Different shades of composite can be combined to achieve good matches with adjacent teeth and a transition from a relatively dark gingival area to a lighter more translucent incisal region (Fig. 10.7(c)).

8. Flick away the unfilled resin holding the contour strip and remove the strip.

9. Finish the margins with diamond finishing burs and interproximal strips and the labial surface with graded sandpaper discs. Characterization should be added to improve light reflection properties (Fig. 10.7(d)).

The exact design of the composite veneer will be dependent upon each clinical case, but will usually be one of four types: intraenamel or window preparation; incisal bevel; overlapped incisal edge; or feathered incisal edge (Fig. 10.8).

Tooth preparation will not normally expose dentine, but this will be unavoidable in some cases of localized hypoplasia or with caries. Sound dentine may need to be covered by glass ionomer cement prior to placement of the composite veneer.

Figure 10.9(a) and (b) show an example of successful composite veneers that have been in place for 5 years. Studies have shown that composite veneers are durable enough to last through adolescence until a more aesthetic porcelain veneer can be placed. This is normally only considered at about the age of 18–20 years

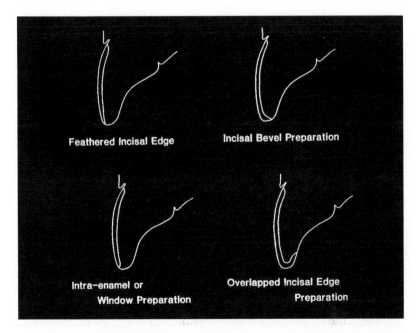

Fig. 10.8 Types of veneer preparation.

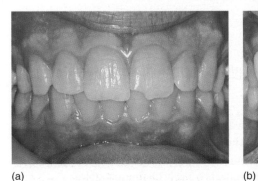

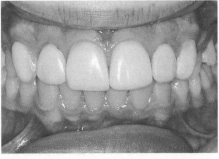

(a)   (b)

Fig. 10.9 (a) Teenaged girl with dark, tetracycline discoloration and an enamel fracture. (b) 5 years' postplacement of composite veneers.

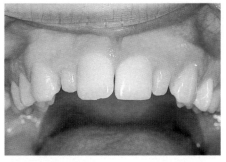

(a)

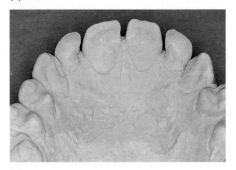

(b)

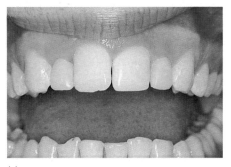

(c)

Fig. 10.10 (a) Peg-shaped lateral incisors in a 15-year old. (b) Laboratory model showing three-quarter wrap-around, porcelain veneers on the upper laterals. (c) Final restorations on the upper laterals 2 years' postcementation.

when the gingival margin has achieved an adult level and the standard of oral hygiene and dental motivation are acceptable.

10.2.8 Porcelain veneers

Porcelain has several advantages over composite as a veneering material: its appearance is superior; it has a better resistance to abrasion; and it is well tolerated by the gingival tissues. However, it is vital that the porcelain fits exactly and that the film thickness of the luting cement is kept to a minimum. These luting cements are only moderately filled composite resins and they absorb water, hydrolyse, and stain. This coupled with the apical migration of the gingival margin in young patients can result in an unacceptable aesthetic appearance in a relatively short time.

Instruction in standard porcelain veneer preparation is covered in restorative dentistry textbooks. If there are occasions when they are used at an earlier age then the same principles apply. However, a non-standard application that is being used more frequently at a younger age is the restoration of the peg lateral incisor (Fig. 10.10(a)). This utilizes a no-preparation technique and the technician is asked to produce a three-quarter wrap-around veneer finished to a knife edge at the gingival margin (Fig. 10.10(b)). An elastomeric impression is taken after gingival retraction to obtain the maximum length of crown, and cementation should be under rubber dam (Fig. 10.10(c)).

10.2.9 Adhesive metal castings

The development of acid-etched, retained cast restorations has allowed the fabrication of cast occlusal onlays for posterior teeth and palatal veneers for incisors and canines. These restorations are manufactured with minimal or no tooth preparation and are ideal for cases where there is a risk of tooth tissue loss.

Indications

(1)   amelogenesis imperfecta;

(2)   dentinogenesis imperfecta;

(3)   dental erosion, attrition, or abrasion;

(4)   enamel hypoplasia.

Armamentarium

(1)   gingival retraction cord;

(2)   elastomeric impression material;

(3)   facebow system;

(4)   semi-adjustable articulator;

(5)   rubber dam;

(6)   Panavia Ex (Kuraray).

Technique

1.   Obtain study models (these are essential) and photographs if possible.

2.   Perform a full mouth prophylaxis.

3.   Ensure good moisture isolation.

4.   Place retraction cord into the gingival crevices of the teeth to be treated and remove immediately prior to taking the impression.

5.   Take an impression using an elastomeric impression material—a putty/wash system is the best and check the margins are easily distinguishable.

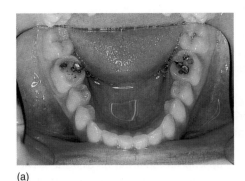

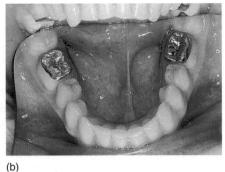

(a)   (b)

Fig. 10.11 (a) Marked occlusal enamel loss of lower first permanent molars. (b) Cast occlusal onlays *in situ* after replacement of amalgam restorations with composite resin.

6. Take a facebow transfer and interocclusal record in the retruded axis position.
7. Mount the casts on a semi-adjustable articulator.
8. Construct cast onlays, a maximum of 1.5 mm thick occlusally in either nickel/chrome or gold.
9. Grit-blast the fitting surfaces of the occlusal onlays.
10. Return to the mouth and check the fit of the onlays.
11. Polish the teeth with pumice and isolate under rubber dam where possible.
12. Cement onlays using Panavia Ex.
13. Check occlusion.
14. Review in 1 week for problems, and regularly thereafter.

Figure 10.11(a) and (b) show gold onlays cemented on to the lower first permanent molars of a 16-year-old boy with erosive tooth surface loss. Such cast restorations may be provided for both posterior and anterior teeth with very little or no tooth preparation. Nevertheless, some children may find this treatment challenging as it demands high levels of patient co-operation. Local anaesthesia may be needed as the hypoplastic teeth are often sensitive to the etching and washing procedure and the placement of gingival retraction cord can be uncomfortable. Furthermore, moisture control can be difficult and, while preferable, rubber dam is not always feasible.

When used to protect the palatal aspect of upper anterior teeth there may be an aesthetic problem as the metal may 'shine through' the translucent incisal tip of young teeth. The durability of this form of restoration has now been confirmed by 10-year evaluation studies.

10.2.10 Indirect composite resin onlays

An alternative to cast metal onlays are indirect composite onlays. In addition to the obvious aesthetic advantages these restorations can be modified relatively easily. This is particularly useful for conditions such as erosion where the disease process may well be ongoing and therefore the tooth and/or restoration may require repair or additions. Studies suggest that these restorations are durable in the anterior region, however, in response to patient demand indirect composite onlays are increasingly being used in the posterior region (Fig. 10.12 (a)–(c)), where their durability is currently unclear. The disadvantage of these restorations is that they need to be thicker than their cast counterparts, are bulkier and can cause greater increases in vertical dimension. However, in young patients, providing the occlusion remains balanced and there is no periodontal pathology, then increases in vertical dimension appear well tolerated.

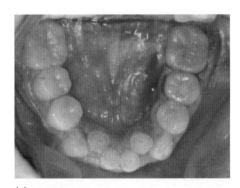

(a)

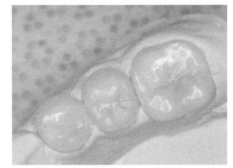

(b)

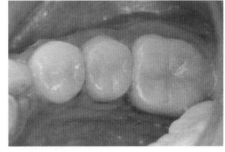

(c)

Fig. 10.12 Direct Composite Onlays made for lower posterior quadrants.

10.3 TOOTH DISCOLOURATION

The colour of a child's teeth can be of great importance. Peer-group pressure can be very strong and teasing about the size, position, and colour of the teeth can be very harmful to a child or adolescent.

The causes of discoloured teeth may be classified in a number of ways: congenital/ acquired; enamel/dentine; extrinsic/intrinsic; systemic/local. The most useful method of classification for the clinical management of discolouration is one that identifies the main site of discolouration (Table 10.3). Once the aetiology of the discolouration had been identified the most appropriate method of treatment can be chosen. Ideal and permanent results may not be realistic in the young patient; however, significant improvements are achievable which do not compromise the teeth in the long term.

The approach to treatment for all forms of discolouration should be cautious, with the emphasis on minimal tooth preparation. For example, in a case of fluorosis the microabrasion technique may produce some improvement but the patient/parent may still be dissatisfied. Composite veneers can then be placed, although if the child requires subsequent fixed appliance treatment these may be damaged and require replacement before placing porcelain veneers as the definitive restoration in the late teenage years.

Discolouration originating in the dentine is often difficult to treat. The single, non-vital dark incisor presents particular problems. In the young patient, the apex

Table 10.3   The aetiology of tooth discolouration

Extrinsic staining	
Beverages/food	
Smoking	
Poor oral hygiene (chromogenic bacteria): green/orange stain	
Drugs	
Iron supplements: black stain	
Minocycline: black stain	
Chlorhexidine: brown/black stain	
Intrinsic discolouration	
Enamel	
Local causes	caries
	idiopathic
	injury/infection of primary precessor
	internal resorption
Systemic causes	amelogenesis imperfecta
	drugs, e.g. tetracyclines
	fluorosis
	idiopathic
	systemic illness during tooth formation
Dentine	
Local causes	caries
	internal resorption
	metallic restorative materials
	necrotic pulp tissue
	root-canal filling materials
Systemic causes	bilirubin (haemolytic disease of newborn)
	congenital porphyria
	dentinogenesis imperfecta
	drugs, e.g. tetracyclines

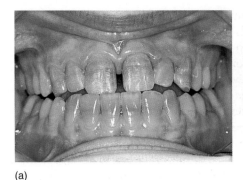

(a)

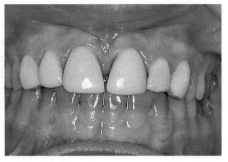

(b)

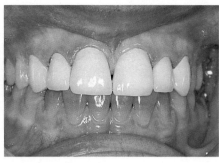

(c)

Fig. 10.13 (a) Severe tetracycline discolouration in a 14 year old. (b) Composite veneers placed under opaqueing agents to mask the discoloration. (c) Porcelain jacket crowns were provided at 20 years of age.

may be immature, root canal therapy incomplete, and non-vital bleaching therefore precluded. A composite veneer can improve the aesthetics but may fail to adequately disguise the discolouration even with the use of opaqueing agents. Ultimately, a jacket crown may be the best option in the older patient. Similarly, moderate-to-severe tetracycline discolouration, which fortunately is less common today, is very difficult to treat in the young patient. Long-term full crowns or porcelain veneers often provide definitive treatment, but composite veneers can be acceptable in the adolescent without completely masking the underlying discolouration (Fig. 10.13(a)–(c)). Indirect composite veneers, placed with minimal tooth preparation, may be useful in the management of this problem but this technique has yet to be evaluated.

> **Key Points**
> - Microabrasion should be the first line of treatment in all cases of enamel opacities.
> - Composite should be used in preference to porcelain in children.

Finally, it is very important to bear in mind the expectations of the patient and, often more importantly, the parent. An unrealistically high expectation of brilliant white 'film star' teeth will result in postoperative disappointment. For instance, in fluorosis cases it is the excessively white, mottled areas which will be removed by the microabrasion technique resulting in a uniform colour that is the same as the original background colour, but some patients will feel their treated teeth are 'too yellow'. Adequate preoperative explanation, preferably with photographic examples, may help to minimize this problem. Nevertheless, there will remain a group of dissatisfied patients and for medico-legal reasons careful documentation of all cases of cosmetic treatment should be kept.

10.4 TOOTH SURFACE LOSS

Dentists have been aware of the problem of tooth wear or non-carious loss of tooth tissue for a long time. However, it is only more recently that it has been increasingly associated with our younger population. There are three processes that make up the phenomenon of tooth wear:

(1) *attrition*—wear of the tooth as a result of tooth-to-tooth contact;

(2) *erosion*—irreversible loss of tooth substance brought about by a chemical process that does not involve bacterial action;

(3) *abrasion*—physical wear of tooth substance produced by something other than tooth-to-tooth contact.

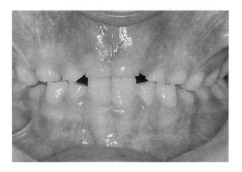

Fig. 10.14 Primary incisors showing physiological wear.

Table 10.4 Clinical signs of tooth wear (Smith and Knight 1984)

Pulp exposure
Loss of vitality attributable to tooth wear
Exposure of secondary dentine
Exposure of dentine on buccal or lingual surfaces
Cupped occlusal or incisal surfaces
Wear in one arch more than the other
Restorations projecting above the surface of the tooth
Wear producing sensitivity
Reduction in length of incisal teeth so that the length is out of proportion to the width

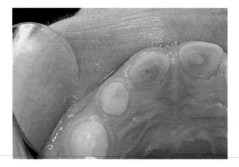

Fig. 10.15 Primary incisors showing pathological wear and pulp exposure.

Table 10.5 Examples of foods and drinks with erosive potential

Citrus fruits, for example, lemons, oranges, grapefruits
Tart apples
Vinegar and pickles
Yoghurt
Fruit juices
Carbonated drinks, including low calorie varieties, sparkling mineral water, and 'sports' drinks
Vitamin C tablets

In children, abrasion is relatively uncommon. The most frequent cause of abrasion is overzealous toothbrushing, which tends to develop with increasing age. Attrition during mastication is common, particularly in the primary dentition where almost all upper incisors show some signs of attrition by the time they exfoliate (Fig. 10.14). However, over the past decade the contribution of erosion to the overall process of tooth wear in the younger population has been highlighted. While erosion may be the predominant process, attrition and abrasion may be compounding factors, for example, toothbrush abrasion may be increased if brushing is carried out immediately after the consumption of erosive foodstuffs or drinks. It is often difficult to identify a single causative agent in a case of tooth wear so the general term 'tooth surface loss' may be more appropriate.

10.4.1 Prevalence

The problem with trying to assess the prevalence of tooth wear is that a degree of tooth tissue loss is a part of the normal physiological process of ageing; however, when it is likely to prejudice the survival of the teeth it can be said to be pathological. Smith and Knight in 1984 described a Tooth Wear Index (TWI), which included certain features that they felt were diagnostic of pathological tooth wear. These features are shown in Table 10.4.

There is very little published evidence on the prevalence or severity of tooth wear in children. In 1993 the National Child Dental Health Survey included an assessment of the prevalence of erosion of both primary and permanent incisor teeth for the first time. The survey reported that 52% of 5-year-old children had erosion of the palatal surfaces of their primary incisors, with 24% showing progression into the pulp (Fig. 10.15). The prevalence of erosion of the palatal surfaces of permanent incisors was also alarmingly high—27% of 15 year olds; however, only 2% showed progression into the pulp. What is unclear at the present time is whether the problem of tooth surface loss is actually increasing or whether these figures reflect an increased awareness.

10.4.2 Aetiology

In young patients there are three main causes of tooth surface loss:

(1) dietary;

(2) gastric regurgitation; and

(3) parafunctional activity.

In addition to these three factors certain environmental factors have been linked to tooth wear. However, with the exception of frequent use of chlorinated swimming pools, most environmental and occupational hazards do not apply to children.

Dietary causes of tooth surface loss

The most common cause of erosive tooth surface loss is an excessive intake of acidic food or drink. Table 10.5 shows the types of foodstuffs implicated in erosive tooth surface loss in young patients.

Acidic drinks, in particular, are available to all age groups of children. Pure 'baby' fruit juices are marketed for consumption by infants and these have been shown to have pH values below the critical pH for the dissolution of enamel (pH = 5.5). Many of these drinks are given to infants in a feeding bottle, and the combination of the highly acidic nature of the drink and the prolonged exposure of the teeth to the acidic substrate may result in excessive tooth surface loss as well as dental caries. While a wide range of foods and drinks are implicated in the aetiology of tooth surface loss, soft drinks make up the bulk of the problem. Soft drink consumption has increased dramatically over the past 40 years to a staggering 151 litres per capita of the population in the United Kingdom in 1991, with adolescents accounting for up to 65% of these purchases. Pure fruit juices do contribute to this figure, but, increasingly, carbonated drinks make up a large part of the younger population's intake and are now widely available in vending machines located in schools, sports centres, and other public areas. Both normal and so-called 'diet' carbonated drinks have very low pH values and are associated with tooth surface loss. While there is no direct relationship between the pH of a substrate and the degree of tooth surface loss, pH does give a useful indication as to the potential to cause damage. Other factors such as titratable acidity, the influence on plaque pH, and the buffering capacity of saliva will all influence the erosive potential of a given substrate. In addition, it has been shown that erosive tooth surface loss tends to be more severe if the volume of drink consumed is high or if the intake occurs at bedtime.

> **Key Points**
>
> The degree of erosive, tooth-surface loss may be related to:
>
> * the frequency of intake;
> * the timing of intake;
> * toothbrushing habits.

The pattern of dietary, erosive tooth surface loss depends on the manner in which the substrate is consumed. Carbonated drinks are not uncommonly held in the mouth for some time as the child 'enjoys' the sensation of the bubbles around the mouth. This habit may result in a generalized loss of surface enamel (Fig. 10.16(a) and (b)). Note the chipping of the incisal edges of the upper anterior teeth in Fig. 10.16—this is an example of attrition contributing to the overall pattern of tooth surface loss. A generalized loss of the surface enamel of posterior teeth is often evident particularly on the first permanent molars, and characteristic saucer-shaped lesions develop on the cusps of the molars. This phenomenon is known as perimolysis. More peculiar habits are not uncommon; Fig. 10.17 shows the dentition of a young cyclist who very frequently consumed a lemon drink via a straw in his bicycle's drink bottle. Figure 10.18 is an example of a young adult who, for many years, daily consumed 2 lbs (almost 1 kg) of raw Bramley cooking apples. The extent of tooth surface loss has left his amalgam restorations 'proud'.

Gastric regurgitation and tooth surface loss

The acidity of the stomach contents is below pH 1.0 and therefore any regurgitation or vomiting is potentially damaging to the teeth. As many as 50% of adults with signs of tooth surface loss have a history of gastric reflux. The aetiology of gastric regurgitation may be divided into two categories: (1) those with upper gastrointestinal disorders; and (2) those with eating disorders.

In young patients, long-term regurgitation is associated with a variety of underlying problems (Table 10.6).

In addition, there are a group of patients who suffer from gastro-oesophageal reflux disease (GORD). This may be either symptomatic—in which case the individual knows what provokes the reflux—or, more insidiously, asymptomatic GORD, where the patient is unaware of the problem and continues to ingest reflux-provoking foods.

Unexplained, erosive tooth surface loss is one of the principal signs of an eating disorder. There are three such disorders to be aware of: anorexia nervosa; bulimia nervosa; and, more rarely, rumination (this is a condition of unknown aetiology in which food is voluntarily regurgitated into the oral cavity and either expelled or swallowed again).

Anorexia nervosa is a sociocultural disease mainly affecting middle-class, intelligent, females between 12 and 30 years of age. Like bulimia nervosa it is a secretive disease with sufferers denying illness and refusing therapy. People with anorexia exhibit considerable weight loss (up to 25% of their body weight in severe cases), have a fear of growing fat, and a distorted view of their body shape. While those with bulimia suffer

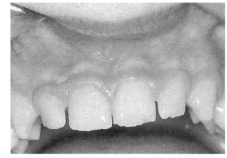

(a)

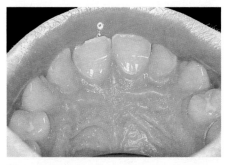

(b)

Fig. 10.16 (a) and (b) Teeth of a teenager who consumed considerable amounts of carbonated drinks. Note chipping of incisal edges and characteristic palatal tooth surface loss.

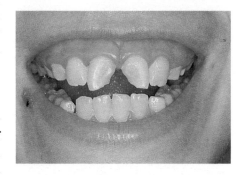

Fig. 10.17 A 12 year old with an unusual pattern of tooth surface loss.

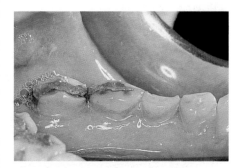

Fig. 10.18 Marked tooth surface loss may eventually leave an amalgam restoration 'proud'.

Table 10.6 Conditions in children associated with chronic regurgitation

Gastro-oesophageal reflux
Oesophageal strictures
Chronic respiratory disease
Disease of the liver/pancreas/biliary tree
Overfeeding
Feeding problems/failure to thrive
  conditions
Children with mental handicap
Reye's syndrome
Rumination

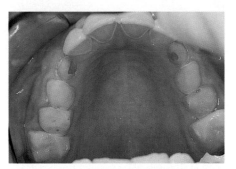

(a)

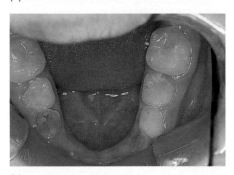

(b)

Fig. 10.19 (a) and (b) Upper and lower arch of a 10-year-old boy with chronic gastro-oesophageal reflux.

characteristic binges on 'junk foodstuffs' and follow this with self-induced vomiting, overzealous exercise, and the use of laxatives to prevent weight gain—they may subsequently develop GORD, which causes typical signs of heartburn and oesophagitis.

The pattern of erosive tooth loss seen in all patients who suffer from chronic gastric regurgitation is similar, with marked erosion of the palatal surface of upper incisors and premolars. There is a surprising lack of tooth sensitivity. Over time, the buccal and occlusal surfaces of the lower molars and premolars also become affected (Fig. 10.19(a) and (b)).

As a result of the asymptomatic nature of some of the gastrointestinal disorders and the secretive nature of the eating disorders, dentists may well be the first professionals to see the signs of gastric regurgitation. The presence of erosive tooth surface loss may be the only sign of an underlying disorder, and such a finding should be taken seriously and handled carefully in communication with medical colleagues.

Parafunctional activity

Localized, tooth surface loss frequently occurs in patients who exhibit abnormal parafunctional habits. The excessive grinding that is a feature of this problem is not always apparent to the patient; however, apart from the marked tooth tissue loss, other signs of bruxism may be evident including hypertrophy of the muscles of mastication, cheek biting, and tongue faceting. An example of erosion and parafunction having a disastrous effect on the dentition may be seen (and heard) in children who have cerebral palsy. These children often have chronic gastric regurgitation and also severe bruxism resulting in excessive tooth surface loss.

10.4.3 Management

Immediate

The most important aspect of the management of tooth surface loss is early diagnosis. While it is important to treat any dental sensitivity resulting from the tooth surface loss it is essential to establish the aetiology and, where possible, to eliminate the cause. This may not always be possible—the existence of an underlying eating disorder cannot be resolved quickly or simply. Indeed, as with all forms of behaviour modification, the elimination of dietary causes of erosion will often be difficult, particularly in young adolescents who are no longer under parental control and who often find it hard to adjust to alternative life-styles and dietary habits. Ideally, the cause of the tooth surface loss should be eliminated before restorative treatment is started. In order to achieve this, all patients and parents should be given dietary counselling which should be personal, practical, and positive. It is important not to simply advise against all carbonated drinks but to offer positive alternatives, and to suggest that such drinks may be taken as a treat occasionally and that intake should be limited to meal times. Table 10.7 gives some

Table 10.7 Practical prevention of erosion

Inform patients of the types of foods and drinks that have the greatest erosive potential
  (see Table 10.5)
Consume still/non-carbonated drinks as an alternative
Limit the intake of acidic foods/drinks to meal times
Advocate consumption of a neutral food immediately after a meal, e.g. cheese
Advise use of neutral fluoride mouthwash or gel for daily use to try and minimize the
  effect of the acids
Encourage use of bicarbonate of soda mouthrinse in cases of recurrent gastric reflux
Where attrition is marked, neutral fluoride gel placed into an occlusal guard during
  the night or during episodes of vomiting may be helpful

practical suggestions that may be made to patients depending on the aetiology of the problem.

In young patients dental sensitivity may be a problem. Erosive tooth loss may be rapid and with the large pulp chambers pulpal inflammation is common and secondary dentine does not have time to form. The use of glass ionomer cements or resin-based composites as temporary coverage may resolve the sensitivity and also act as a diagnostic aid.

Definitive treatment

In many cases, if the tooth surface loss is diagnosed early, preventive counselling may be sufficient. It is a good idea to make study casts of all patients with signs of tooth surface loss and to give these to the patient to keep. The rate of progression of the wear can then be monitored. However, in more advanced cases, where there are sensitivity or cosmetic problems, active intervention is required. Table 10.8 shows the relative merits of the options available.

Key Points

Main treatment objectives for tooth-surface loss:

- resolve sensitivity;
- restore missing tooth surface;
- prevent further tooth tissue loss;
- maintain a balanced occlusion.

Table 10.8 Treatment techniques for tooth surface loss

Technique	Advantages	Disadvantages
Cast metal (nickel/chrome or gold)	Fabricated in thin section—require only 0.5 mm space Very accurate fit possible Very durable Suitable for posterior restorations in parafunction. Does not abrade opposing dentition	May be cosmetically unacceptable due to 'shine through' of metallic grey Cannot be simply repaired or added to intraorally
Composite Direct	Adequately durable for labial veneers only Least expensive May be used as a diagnostic tool	Technically difficult for palatal veneers Limited control over occlusal and interproximal contour Inadequate as a posterior restoration
Indirect	Can be added to and repaired relatively simply intraorally Aesthetically superior to cast metal Control over occlusal contour and vertical dimension	Requires more space—minimum of 1.0 mm Unproven durability
Porcelain	Best aesthetics Good abrasion resistance Well tolerated by gingival tissues	Potentially abrasive to opposing dentition Inferior marginal fit Very brittle—has to be used in bulk section Hard to repair

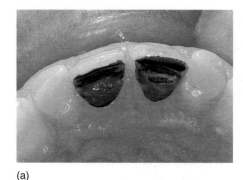
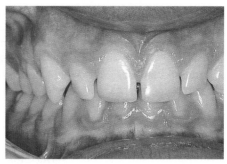

(a)   (b)

Fig. 10.20   (a) and (b) Cast palatal veneers on upper central incisors. Note the 'shine through' despite placement of labial composite veneers.

In some cases there will be only localized tooth wear and an incomplete overbite, leaving enough space to place the restorations. Figure 10.20(a) and (b) show the same patient as shown earlier in Fig. 10.16(a) and (b) who consumed considerable quantities of carbonated drinks in association with sporting activities. This habit caused considerable palatal wear of his upper incisors with characteristic chipping of the incisal edges. Cast adhesive veneers were placed on the palatal aspect of the upper incisors to protect from further wear, and direct resin-based composite labial veneers were used to restore the aesthetics. Note in this case the slight grey 'shine through' effect on the incisal tips due to the cast restorations.

In many other cases compensatory growth, which will help to maintain the occlusal vertical dimension, or the presence of a significant malocclusion, may result in inadequate space for the necessary restorations. Figure 10.21(a) shows a case of a 12-year-old boy who has a class II, division II malocclusion and who consumed three cans of carbonated drinks everyday. The combination of the erosive drink and the attrition brought about by the close tooth-to-tooth contact has resulted in a loss of palatal tooth tissue from the upper central incisors. There is insufficient space palatally to place any form of restoration, but a simple removable orthodontic appliance with a flat anterior bite plane can be used to reduce the overbite (Fig. 10.21(b)). In children this occurs relatively quickly (within 6 weeks) principally by compensatory overeruption of the posterior segments. Once sufficient space has been created cast metal palatal veneers can be placed.

Alternatively, if there has been marked wear of the posterior teeth, as shown in Fig. 10.22(a), it will be necessary to restore the occlusal surfaces and protect them from further wear prior to placing anterior restorations. Cast adhesive occlusal onlays are recommended in these cases (Fig. 10.22(b)). Young patients will accommodate the increase in vertical dimension easily, providing a balanced occlusal contact is achieved. The use of a facebow record facilitates this. The main advantage of using cast metal onlays is the minimal thickness of material needed and its resistance to abrasive wear. Indirect composite veneers are a recent addition to our armamentarium and they offer considerable advantages, particularly in cases where the aetiology is unclear or the patient cannot stop the habit/problem. These restorations facilitate future additions and repairs (using direct composite) if the erosion continues or restarts. However, if there is an element of attrition or signs of parafunction composite onlays will not be adequately durable in the posterior segments, so cast restorations are recommended.

Long-term review

All patients with tooth surface loss should be reviewed regularly for three reasons:

(1)   to monitor future tooth surface loss;
(2)   to maintain the existing restorations; and
(3)   to provide support for the patient.

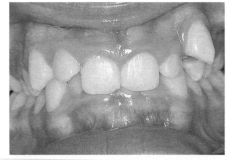

(a)

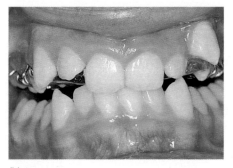

(b)

Fig. 10.21   (a) Skeletal pattern II with deep overbite compounding palatal erosion in a 12-year-old boy. (b) An upper removable appliance in position to reduce the overbite.

Patients with eating disorders in particular are prone to periods of relapse and the dentist is in an ideal position to diagnose these periods. The dentist can develop a special and trusting relationship with the young patient over the longer term, which is based not simply on seeing the patient when they are 'ill' and therefore to admonish them, but also when they are well to support and encourage them. Likewise in patients with dietary erosion, continual reinforcement of good dietary habits is needed throughout the child's life and into adulthood. People change their diet as they get older—one example is the young adolescent who manages to stop drinking Coca Cola but starts drinking lager to excess instead and the erosion continues!

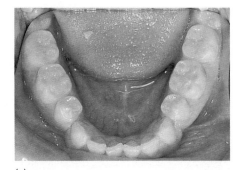

(a)

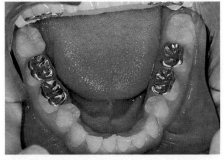

(b)

10.5 INHERITED ANOMALIES OF ENAMEL AND DENTINE

Chapter 13 covers the whole range of dental anomalies; however, the treatment of amelogenesis imperfecta and dentinogenesis imperfecta poses specific challenges to the dentist. In view of the wide variety of presentations and degree to which each individual case is affected, it is difficult to make generalizations. Early diagnosis of these conditions is important to their long-term prognosis; parents need to be educated as to the implications of the condition; monitoring of the amount of tooth wear can start, and, where necessary, teeth can be protected. There are four main clinical problems associated with inherited enamel and dentine defects:

Fig. 10.22 (a) A 16-year-old boy with marked tooth surface loss of lower permanent molars. Note the perimolysis of the first molars. (b) Postcementation of gold onlays on the permanent molars.

(1) poor aesthetics;

(2) chipping and attrition of the enamel;

(3) exposure and attrition of the dentine causing sensitivity; and

(4) poor oral hygiene, gingivitis, and caries.

While it is impossible to draw up a definitive treatment plan for all cases, it is possible to define the principles of treatment planning for this group of patients. It is important to realize that not all children with amelogenesis imperfecta or dentino- genesis imperfecta are affected equally. Many will not have marked tooth wear or symptoms, and will not require advanced intervention. Table 10.9 describes the principles of treatment in terms of the age of the child/adolescent and with regard to the three aspects of care: prevention, restoration, and aesthetics.

Table 10.9 Principles of treatment for amelogenesis and dentinogenesis imperfecta

	Prevention	Restoration	Aesthetics
Primary dentition (0–5 years)	Diet advice Fluoride supplements Oral hygiene instruction	Glass ionomer cement (GIC) Stainless-steel crowns (SSCs) (particularly on E's)	Minimal intervention GICs
Mixed dentition (6–16 years)	Diet advice Fluoride supplements Oral hygiene instruction ±chlorhexidine	SSCs on primary molars Adhesive castings on first permanent molars Localized composite/GIC	Direct ⎱ ⎰ Composite veneers Indirect ⎰
Permanent dentition (16+ years)	Oral hygiene instruction Topical fluoride	Adhesive castings on premolars Full mouth rehabilitation	Porcelain veneers Full crowns Over dentures Complete dentures

Prevention

Prevention is an essential part of the management of children with enamel and dentine anomalies. Oral hygiene in these children is often poor, due in part to the rough enamel surface which promotes plaque retention and to the sensitivity of the tooth to brushing. As a result there may be marked gingival inflammation and bleeding. The combination of gingival swelling and enamel hypoplasia can result in areas of food stagnation and a generally low level of oral health. Oral hygiene instruction must be given sympathetically, with plenty of encouragement, and should be continually reinforced. In some cases it may be necessary to carry out some restorative/cosmetic treatment before good oral hygiene measures can be practised. For example, the placement of anterior composite veneers may reduce dentine sensitivity and improve the enamel surface so that the patient can brush their teeth more effectively. Conventional caries prevention with diet advice, fluoride supplements, and topical fluoride applications is mandatory. In this group of children it is particularly important to preserve tooth tissue and not allow caries to compromise further the dental hard tissues.

Restoration

Restorative treatment varies considerably depending on the age of the child and extent of the problem. The basic principle of treatment is that of minimal intervention. If there is sensitivity or signs of enamel chipping, techniques to cover and protect the teeth should be considered. In the very young child it is often impossible to carry out extensive operative treatment, but the placement of glass ionomer cement over areas of enamel hypoplasia is simple and effective. In older/more co-operative children stainless-steel (or nickel/chrome) preformed crowns should be placed on the second primary molars to minimize further wear due to tooth on tooth contact (Chapter 8). It is advisable (and usually possible) to place such restorations with minimum tooth preparation because of the pre-existing tooth tissue loss.

Young children with dentinogenesis imperfecta often pose the greatest problems. The teeth undergo such excessive wear that they become worn down to gingival level and are unrestorable. Teeth affected by dentinogenesis imperfecta are also prone to spontaneous abscesses due to the progressive obliteration of the pulp chambers. In these cases pulp therapy is unsuccessful and extraction of the affected teeth is necessary.

As the permanent dentition develops close monitoring of the rate of tooth wear will guide the decision about what intervention is needed. Cast occlusal onlays on the first permanent molars not only protect the underlying tooth structure but also maintain function and control symptoms. The resulting increase in the vertical dimension is associated with a decrease in the vertical overlap of the incisors. Within a few weeks full occlusion is usually re-established, the whole procedure being well tolerated by young patients. As the premolars erupt similar castings may be placed if wear is marked (Fig. 10.23(a)–(c)). Alternatively, localized composite or glass ionomer cement restorations may be placed over areas of hypoplasia.

The emphasis should remain on minimal tooth preparation until the child gains adulthood. At this point, if clinically indicated, full mouth rehabilitation may be considered and should have a good prognosis in view of the conservative approach

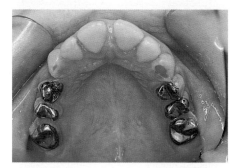

(a)

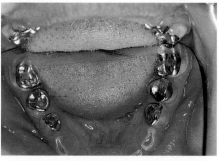

(b)

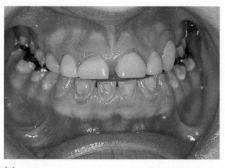

(c)

Fig. 10.23 Upper and lower arches of a 14-year-old girl with dentinogenesis imperfecta showing cast onlays on the second permanent molars and the premolars, and labial and palatal composite veneers on the upper incisors.

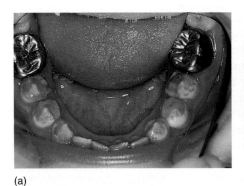

(a)

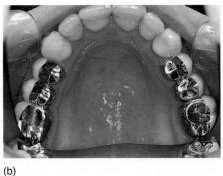

(b)

Fig. 10.24 (a) A 14-year-old boy with severe amelogenesis imperfecta. Stainless-steel crowns were placed on the first permanent molars at 9 years of age (lower arch). (b) At 20 years of age a full mouth rehabilitation was completed (upper arch).

that has been adopted throughout the early years (Fig. 10.24(a) and (b)). Patients with dentinogenesis imperfecta should be treated with caution. The characteristic form of the teeth in this condition is unfavourable for crowning; the teeth being supported by short, thin roots. The permanent dentition, like the primary dentition, is prone to spontaneous abscesses and the prognosis for endodontic treatment is very poor. The long-term plan for these patients is often some form of removable prosthesis, either an overdenture placed over the worn permanent teeth or a more conventional complete denture. The role of implants in these patients has yet to be defined fully.

Aesthetics

Aesthetics is not usually a problem in the primary dentition. Where the child is sufficiently co-operative the use of glass ionomer cements to restore and improve the appearance of primary incisors can be useful in gaining the respect and support from the patient and parent. In a few exceptional cases the loss of primary teeth may cause upset, but can be compensated for by constructing dentures. In cases of dentinogenesis imperfecta where the teeth are very worn but remain asymptomatic, overdentures can be constructed to which young children adapt remarkably well. These will need to be remade regularly as the child grows.

As the permanent incisors erupt they must be protected from chipping of the enamel. The placement of composite veneers not only improves the appearance but also promotes better gingival health and protects the teeth from further wear. In a few cases the quality of the enamel is so poor that the bond between composite and tooth will be unsuccessful. It should be noted that in these cases porcelain veneers are also likely to be unsuccessful and full coronal restorations are the only option.

Early consultation with an orthodontist is advisable in order to keep the orthodontic requirements simple. Treatment for these patients is possible and in many cases proceeds without problems. The use of removable appliances, where appropriate, and orthodontic bands rather than brackets will minimize the risk of damage to the abnormal enamel. The problem is twofold: there may be frequent bond failure during active treatment or the enamel may be further damaged during debonding. Some orthodontists prefer to use bands even for anterior teeth, while others will use glass ionomer cement as the bonding agent in preference to more conventional resin-based agents. In other instances cosmetic restorative techniques (veneers and crowns) may be more appropriate than orthodontic treatment.

10.6 HYPODONTIA

Individuals with missing teeth may present at any age requesting replacement of their missing teeth for both aesthetic and functional reasons. A detailed discussion on the management of hypodontia is beyond the remit of this text, however, there are a few principles that can be considered. During infancy and early school years there is rarely a need for any active intervention. An exception may be infants with Ectodermal Dysplasia who can have multiple teeth missing. In such cases the provision of removable partial or even complete dentures can be highly successful. However, as children move through the mixed and permanent dentition phases, aesthetics become increasingly important. Replacing one or two teeth may be relatively straightforward using either removable partial dentures or adhesively retained bridges (Fig. 10.25 (a)–(e)). However, those individuals with multiple missing teeth often have associated skeletal and dentoalveolar discrepancies which demand a multidisciplinary approach (Fig. 10.26(a)–(c)). The core to such a clinical team includes a paediatric dentist, orthodontist, and prosthodontist. In addition a periodontist and a maxillofacial surgeon may be required for implants, bone grafting, and/or orthognathic surgery in later years. Finally, access to a geneticist with expertise in orofacial

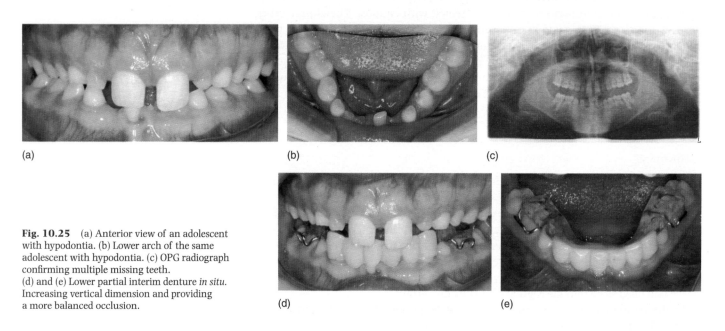

(a)   (b)   (c)

(d)   (e)

Fig. 10.25 (a) Anterior view of an adolescent with hypodontia. (b) Lower arch of the same adolescent with hypodontia. (c) OPG radiograph confirming multiple missing teeth. (d) and (e) Lower partial interim denture *in situ*. Increasing vertical dimension and providing a more balanced occlusion.

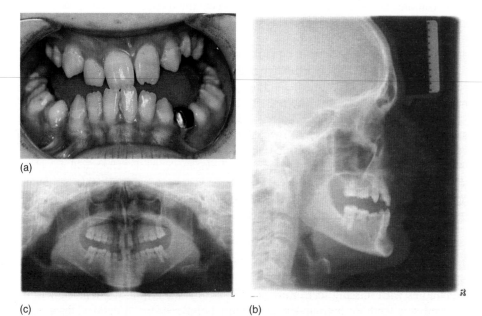

(a)

(c)   (b)

Fig. 10.26 (a) Anterior clinical view of a 15-year-old male with a significant skeletal discrepancy, posterior open bites, and multiple missing teeth. (b) and (c) Radiographs of the same 15-year-old male.

anomalies can be beneficial as adolescents begin to contemplate the implications of their dental anomaly on family planning.

Children with multiple missing teeth and their families should be referred early to a multidisciplinary team for discussion and preliminary planning. Consideration needs to be given to the number and position of the missing dental units, the age of the child, their level of and attitude towards oral health, and importantly the wishes and expectations of the individual and their family. The aim of orthodontic treatment is to consolidate the spacing and place the existing teeth in the optimum position to support the definitive restorations. However consideration also needs to be given to any underlying skeletal discrepancy or dentoalveolar deficiency that may require a more surgical approach. Interim restorative solutions, such as removable dentures, composite veneer, or partial veneer restorations, can be placed during the mixed dentition phase but will require maintenance throughout adolescence. Proactive preventive strategies need to be supported in order to achieve optimum dental and periodontal health. This is essential for the long-term success of definitive prosthodontic solutions which may include removable dentures, porcelain veneers or crowns, fixed conventional or adhesively retained bridges, and osseointegrated implants.

Key Points

- Children with multiple missing teeth should be:
  —referred early to a multidisciplinary clinical team;
  —exposed to proactive prevention to optimize their periodontal health.
- Treatment options may include:
  —interim measures, for example, partial dentures or composite veneers in childhood and adolescence;
  —definitive restorations, for example, crowns, bridges, veneers, and dental implants
  —surgical interventions, for example, orthognathic surgery and bone grafting

---

10.7 SUMMARY

1. The management of children with advanced restorative problems should be viewed as a long-term commitment.
2. Advanced restorative problems in children should be treated as conservatively as possible.
3. Identification of the aetiology of tooth discolouration is essential for selecting the most appropriate treatment technique.
4. Microabrasion should be the first treatment option in all cases of enamel surface discolouration.
5. Porcelain veneers should be delayed until a mature gingival contour is attained.
6. Nearly 30% of all 15 year olds have experience of erosive tooth surface loss.
7. The cause of tooth surface loss should be determined and eliminated before active treatment is started.
8. Maintenance of occlusal face height is essential in patients with amelogenesis or dentinogenesis imperfecta.

10.8 FURTHER READING

Bishop, K., Briggs, P., and Kelleher, M. (1994). The aetiology and management of localized anterior tooth wear in the young adult. *Dental Update*, **21**, 153–60. (*A good review with a lot of references and clinical examples.*)

Dahl, J. E., and Pallesen, U. (2003). Tooth bleaching: a criticial review of the biological aspects. *Critical Reviews in Oral Biology and Medicine*, **14**, 292–304. (*A well-referenced review on the efficacy of tooth bleaching.*)

Harley, K. E. and Ibbetson, R. J. (1993). Dental anomalies—are adhesive castings the solution? *British Dental Journal*, **174**, 15–22. (*A well-written study covering the clinical technique and the follow-up of 12 children with amelogenesis or dentinogenesis imperfecta.*)

Kilpatrick, N. M. and Welbury, R. R. (1993). Hydrochloric acid–pumice microabrasion technique for the removal of enamel pigmentation. *Dental Update*, **20**, 105–7. (*A clinical study assessing the effectiveness of the microabrasion technique.*)

King, P. A. (1999). Tooth surface loss: adhesive techniques. *British Dental Journal*, **186**, 321–6. (*A good description of current techniques.*)

Nunn, J. H., Carter, N. E., Gillgrass, T. J., Hobson, R. S., Jepson, N. J., Meechan, J. G., and Nohl, F. S. (2003). The interdisciplinary management of hypodontia: parts 1–5. *British Dental Journal*, **194**, 245–251, 299–304, 361–6, 423–7, 479–82. (*A comprehensive series of papers addressing the complexities of management of hypodontia.*)

Poyser, N. J., Kelleher, M. G., and Briggs, P. F. (2004). Managing discoloured non-vital teeth: the inside/outside bleaching technique. *Dental Update*, **31**, 204–10. (*A simple report of the technique.*)

Welbury, R. R. (1991). A clinical study of a microfilled composite resin for labial veneers. *International Journal of Paediatric Dentistry*, **1**, 9–15. (*A longitudinal clinical study evaluating composite veneers in adolescents.*)

10.9 REFERENCES

Smith, B. G. and Knight, J. K. (1984). An index for measuring the wear of teeth. *British Dental Journal*, **156**, 435–8.

O'Brien, M. (1994). *Children's dental health in the United Kingdom 1993*. HMSO, London.

11

Periodontal diseases in children

11 Periodontal diseases in children

P. A. Heasman and P. J. Waterhouse

11.1 INTRODUCTION

Periodontal diseases comprise a group of infections that affect the supporting structures of the teeth: marginal and attached gingiva; periodontal ligament; cementum; and alveolar bone.

Acute gingival diseases—primarily herpetic gingivostomatitis and necrotizing gingivitis—are ulcerative conditions that result from specific viral and bacterial infection. Chronic gingivitis, however, is a non-specific inflammatory lesion of the marginal gingiva which reflects the bacterial challenge to the host when dental plaque accumulates in the gingival crevice. The development of chronic gingivitis is enhanced when routine oral hygiene practices are impaired. Chronic gingivitis is reversible if effective plaque control measures are introduced. If left untreated the condition invariably converts to chronic periodontitis, which is characterized by resorption of the supporting connective tissue attachment and apical migration of the junctional epithelia. Slowly progressing, chronic periodontitis affects most of the adult population to a greater or lesser extent, although the early stages of the disease are detected in adolescents.

Children are also susceptible to aggressive periodontal diseases that involve the primary and permanent dentitions, respectively, and present in localized or generalized forms. These conditions, which are distinct clinical entities affecting otherwise healthy children, must be differentiated from the extensive periodontal destruction that is associated with certain systemic diseases, degenerative disorders, and congenital syndromes.

Periodontal tissues are also susceptible to changes that are not, primarily, of an infectious nature. Factitious stomatitis is characterized by self-inflicted trauma to oral soft tissues and the gingiva are invariably involved. Drug-induced gingival enlargement is becoming increasingly more prevalent with the widespread use of organ transplant procedures and the use of long-term immunosuppressant therapy. Localized enlargement may occur as a gingival complication of orthodontic treatment.

A classification of periodontal diseases in children is given in Table 11.1.

11.2 ANATOMY OF THE PERIODONTIUM IN CHILDREN

Marginal gingival tissues around the primary dentition are more highly vascular and contain fewer connective tissue fibres than tissues around the permanent teeth. The epithelia are thinner with a lesser degree of keratinization, giving an appearance of increased redness that may be interpreted as mild inflammation. Furthermore, the localized hyperaemia that accompanies eruption of the primary dentition can persist, leading to swollen and rounded interproximal papillae and a depth of gingival sulcus exceeding 3 mm.

Table 11.1　A classification of periodontal diseases in children

Gingival conditions without loss of connective tissue attachment	Periodontal conditions with loss of connective tissue attachment
Acute gingivitis 　herpetic gingivostomatitis 　necrotizing ulcerative gingivitis	*Chronic periodontitis* 　plaque induced 　complication of orthodontic treatment
Chronic gingivitis 　plaque induced 　puberty gingivitis	*Aggressive periodontitis*
Gingival enlargement 　drug-induced (generalized) *Traumatic gingivitis* *Mucogingival problems*	*Periodontitis as a manifestation of systemic disease* 　Papillon–Lefèvre syndrome 　Ehlers–Danlos syndrome 　hypophosphatasia 　Chediak–Higashi syndrome 　leucocyte adhesion deficiency syndrome 　neutropenias 　histiocytosis

During eruption of the permanent teeth the junctional epithelium migrates apically from the incisal or occlusal surface towards the cementoenamel junction (CEJ). While the epithelial attachment is above the line of maximum crown convexity, the gingival sulcus depth often exceeds 6 or 7 mm, which favours the accumulation of plaque. When the teeth are fully erupted, there continues to be an apical shift of junctional epithelium and the free gingival margins. Stability of the gingiva is achieved at about 12 years for mandibular incisors, canines, second premolars, and first molars. The tissues around the remaining teeth continue to recede slowly until about 16 years. Thus the gingival margins are frequently at different levels on adjacent teeth that are at different stages of eruption. This sometimes gives an erroneous appearance that gingival recession has occurred around those teeth that have been in the mouth longest.

A variation in sulcus depths around posterior teeth in the mixed dentition is common. For example, sulcus depths on the mesial aspects of Es and 6s are greater than those on the distal of Ds and Es, respectively. This is accountable to the discrepancy in the horizontal position of adjacent CEJs due to the difference in the occlusoapical widths of adjacent molar crowns.

The attached gingiva extends from the free gingival margin to the mucogingival line minus the sulcus depth in the absence of inflammation. Attached gingiva is necessary to maintain sulcus depth, to resist functional stresses during mastication, and to resist tensional stress by acting as a buffer between the mobile gingival margin and the loosely structured alveolar mucosa. The width of attached gingiva is less variable in the primary than in the permanent dentition. This may partly account for the scarcity of mucogingival problems in the primary dentition.

The periodontal ligament space is wider in children, partly as a consequence of thinner cementum and alveolar cortical plates. The ligament is less fibrous and more vascular. Alveolar bone has larger marrow spaces, greater vascularity, and fewer trabeculae than adult tissues, features that may enhance the rate of progression of periodontal disease when it affects the primary dentition.

The radiographic distance between the CEJ and the healthy alveolar bone crest for primary canine and molar teeth ranges from 0 to 2 mm. Individual surfaces display distances of up to 4 mm when adjacent permanent or primary teeth are erupting or exfoliating, respectively, and eruptive and maturation changes must be considered when radiographs are used to diagnose periodontal disease in children. When such changes are excluded, a CEJ–alveolar crest distance of more than 2 mm should arouse suspicion of pathological bone loss in the primary dentition.

> **Key Points**
> Anatomy:
> - junctional epithelium;
> - marginal gingiva;
> - attached gingiva;
> - alveolar bone.

11.3 ACUTE GINGIVAL CONDITIONS

The principal acute gingival conditions that affect children are primary herpetic gingivostomatitis and necrotizing ulcerative gingivitis. The latter is most frequently seen in young adults, but it also affects teenagers.

11.3.1 Primary herpetic gingivostomatitis

Herpetic gingivostomatitis is an acute infectious disease caused by the herpesvirus hominis. The primary infection is most frequently seen in children between 2 and 5 years of age, although older age groups can be affected. A degree of immunity is transferred to the newborn from circulating maternal antibodies so an infection in the first 12 months of life is rare. Almost 100% of urban adult populations are carriers of, and have neutralizing antibodies to, the virus. This acquired immunity suggests that the majority of childhood infections are subclinical.

Transmission of the virus is by droplet infection and the incubation period is about 1 week. The child develops a febrile illness with a raised temperature of 100–102 °F (37.8–38.9 °C). Headaches, malaise, oral pain, mild dysphagia, and cervical lymphadenopathy are the common symptoms that accompany the fever and precede the onset of a severe, oedematous marginal gingivitis. Characteristic, fluid-filled vesicles appear on the gingiva and other areas such as the tongue, lips, buccal, and palatal mucosa. The vesicles, which have a grey, membranous covering, rupture spontaneously after a few hours to leave extremely painful yellowish ulcers with red, inflamed margins (Fig. 11.1(a) and (b)). The clinical episode runs a course of about 14 days and the oral lesions heal without scarring. Very rare but severe complications of the infection are aseptic meningitis and encephalitis.

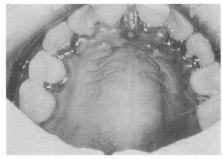
(a)

The clinical features, history, and age group of the affected children are so characteristic that diagnosis is rarely problematic. If in doubt, however, smears from recently ruptured vesicles reveal degenerating epithelial cells with intranuclear inclusions. The virus protein also tends to displace the nuclear chromatin to produce enlarged and irregular nuclei.

Herpetic gingivostomatitis does not respond well to active treatment. Bed rest and a soft diet are recommended during the febrile stage and the child should be kept well hydrated. Pyrexia is reduced using a paracetamol suspension and secondary infection of ulcers may be prevented using chlorhexidine. A mouthrinse (0.2%, two to three times a day) may be used in older children who are able to expectorate, but in younger children (under 6 years of age) a chlorhexidine spray can be used (twice daily) or the solution applied using a sponge swab. In severe cases of herpes simplex, systemic acyclovir can be prescribed as a suspension (200 mg) and swallowed, five times daily for 5 days. In children under 2 years the dose is halved. Acyclovir is active

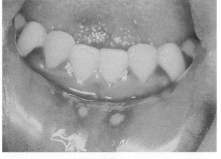
(b)

Fig. 11.1 Ulcerative stage of primary herpetic gingivostomatitis:(a) palatal gingiva; (b) lower lip mucosa.

against the herpesvirus but is unable to eradicate it completely. The drug is most effective when given at the onset of the infection.

> **Key Points**
>
> Herpetic gingivostomatitis—clinical:
> - primary/recurrent;
> - viral;
> - vesicular lesions;
> - complications rare.

> **Key Points**
>
> Herpetic gingivostomatitis—treatment:
> - symptomatic;
> - rest and soft diet;
> - paracetamol suspension;
> - acyclovir.

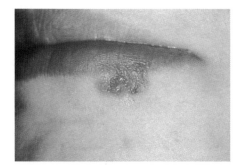

Fig. 11.2 Herpetic 'cold sore' at the vermilion border of the lower lip.

After the primary infection the herpesvirus remains dormant in epithelial cells of the host. Reactivation of the latent virus or reinfection in subjects with acquired immunity occurs in adults. Recurrent disease presents as an attenuated intraoral form of the primary infection or as herpes labialis, i.e. the common 'cold sore' on the mucocutaneous border of the lips (Fig. 11.2). Cold sores are treated by applying acyclovir cream (5%, five times daily for about 5 days).

11.3.2 Necrotizing ulcerative gingivitis

Necrotizing ulcerative gingivitis (NUG) is one of the commonest acute diseases of the gingiva. In the United States and Europe, NUG affects young adults in the 16–30 age range with reported incidence figures of 0.7–7%. In developing countries, NUG is prevalent in children as young as 1 or 2 years of age when the infection can be very aggressive leading to extensive destruction of soft and hard tissues (Fig. 11.3). Epidemic-like occurrences of NUG have been reported in groups such as army recruits and first-year college students. These outbreaks are more likely to be a consequence of the prevalence of common pre-disposing factors rather than communicability of infection between subjects.

Clinical features

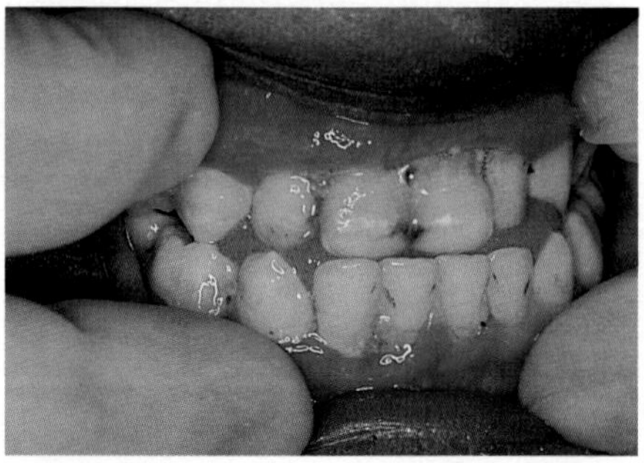

NUG is characterized by necrosis and ulceration, which first affect the interdental papillae and then spread to the labial and lingual marginal gingiva. The ulcers are 'punched out', covered by a yellowish-grey pseudomembranous slough, and extremely painful to the touch (Fig. 11.3). The acute exacerbation is often super-imposed upon a pre-existing gingivitis, and the tissues bleed profusely on gentle probing. The standard of oral hygiene is usually very poor. A distinctive halitosis is common in established cases of NUG, although fever and lymphadenopathy are less common than in herpetic gingivostomatitis.

The clinical course of NUG is such that the acute stage enters a chronic phase of remission after 5–7 days. Recurrence of the acute condition is inevitable, however, and if this acute–chronic cycle is allowed to continue then the marginal tissues lose their contour and appear rounded. Eventually, the inflammation and necrosis involve the alveolar crest and the subsequent necrotizing periodontitis leads to rapid

Fig. 11.3 A 5-year-old Ethiopian boy with necrotizing ulcerative gingivitis.

bone resorption and gingival recession. Progressive changes are also a consequence of inadequate or incomplete treatment.

Aetiology

A smear taken from an area of necrosis or the surface of an ulcer will reveal numerous dead cells, polymorphonuclear leucocytes, and a sample of the micro-organisms that are frequently associated with NUG. Fusiform bacteria and spirochaetes are both numerous and easy to detect. A fusospirochaetal complex has been strongly implicated as the causative organisms in NUG. Other Gram-negative anaerobic organisms including *Porphyromonas gingivalis, Veillonella* species, and *Selenomonas* species have been detected, which suggests that NUG could be a broad anaerobic infection.

A viral aetiology has also been suggested, primarily because of the similarity between NUG and known viral diseases. The restriction of the disease to children and young adults, for example, may infer that older subjects have undergone seroconversion (and are thus immune) as a consequence of clinical or subclinical viral infection in earlier life. The recurring episodes of the disease may also be explained by a viral hypothesis. The ability to undergo latent infection that is subject to reactivation is a characteristic of the herpesvirus. The argument for the implication of a virus in NUG is therefore valid and novel, although a specific virus has yet to be isolated from oral lesions.

Predisposing factors

Poor oral hygiene and a pre-existing gingivitis invariably reflect the patient's attitude to oral care. Many young adults with NUG are heavy smokers. The effect of smoking on the gingiva may be mediated through a local irritation or by the vasoconstrictive action of nicotine, thus reducing tissue resistance and making the host more susceptible to anaerobic infection. Smoking is obviously not a predisposing factor in young children. In underdeveloped countries, however, children are often undernourished and debilitated, which may predispose to infection. Outbreaks of NUG in groups of subjects who are under stress has implicated emotional status as an important predisposing factor. Elevated plasma levels of corticosteroids as a response to an emotional upset are thought to be a possible mechanism.

It is conceivable that all the predisposing factors have a common action to initiate or potentiate a specific change in the host such as lowering the cell-mediated response. Indeed, patients with NUG have depressed phagocytic activity and chemotactic response of their polymorphonuclear leucocytes.

> **Key Points**
> Necrotizing ulcerative gingivitis—clinical:
> * yellow-grey ulcers;
> * fusospirochaetal infection;
> * possible viral aetiology;
> * well-established predisposing factors.

Treatment

It is important at the outset that the patient is informed of the nature of NUG and the likelihood of recurrence of the condition if the treatment is not completed. Smokers should be advised to reduce the number of cigarettes smoked. A soft, multitufted brush is recommended when a medium-textured brush is too painful.

Mouthrinses may be recommended but only for short-term use (7–10 days). Rinsing with chlorhexidine (0.2% for about 1 min) reduces plaque formation, while the use of a hydrogen peroxide or sodium hydroxyperborate mouthrinse oxygenates and cleanses the necrotic tissues.

Mechanical debridement should be undertaken at the initial visit. An ultrasonic scaler with its accompanying water spray can be effective with minimal discomfort for the patient. Further, if NUG is localized to one part of the mouth, local anaesthesia of the soft tissues can allow some subgingival scaling to be undertaken.

In severe cases of NUG, a 3-day course of metronidazole (200 mg three times a day) alleviates the symptoms, but the patients must be informed that they are required to reattend for further treatment.

Occasionally, it is necessary to surgically recontour the gingival margin (gingivo-plasty) to improve tissue architecture and facilitate subgingival cleaning.

Key Points

Necrotizing ulcerative gingivitis—treatment:

- intense oral hygiene;
- remove predisposing factors;
- mechanical debridement;
- metronidazole.

11.4 CHRONIC GINGIVITIS

National Surveys (1973, 1983, and 1993) of children's dental health in the United Kingdom show that the prevalence of chronic gingivitis increases steadily between the ages of 5 and 9 years and is closely associated with the amount of plaque, debris, and calculus present (Fig. 11.4). For example, in 1993, 26% of 5-year-olds had some signs of gingivitis, and the proportion increased to 62% at the age of 9. The prevalence of gingivitis peaks at about 11 years and then decreases slightly with age to 15 years. In terms of gingivitis, there has been no improvement over the decades between surveys. Indeed, in 1993, between 11 and 14% more children of all ages between 6 and 12 years had signs of gingivitis when compared with 1983. These differences were not maintained with increasing age, however, as 52% of 15-year-olds had gingivitis in 1993 compared with 48% in 1983. Furthermore, there were no differences between 1983 and 1993, in the proportion of 15-year-olds with pockets between 3.5 and 5.5 mm (9 and 10%, respectively). These data suggest that the gingival condition of children in the United Kingdom has deteriorated over the 10 years between 1983 and 1993, whereas the periodontal status of 15-year-olds has not changed. Certainly, changes in gingival health do not mirror the dramatic improvement in the prevalence of caries over the same period. Children's mouths tended to be cleaner in 1983 than in 1973. This trend was reversed by 1993 when between 10 and 20% more children of all ages had plaque deposits. Levels of calculus were similar in both surveys.

The onset of puberty and the increase in circulating levels of sex hormones is one explanation for the increase in gingivitis seen in 11-year-olds. Oestrogen increases the cellularity of tissues and progesterone increases the permeability of the gingival vasculature. Oestradiol also provides suitable growth conditions for species of black pigmenting organisms which are associated with established gingivitis.

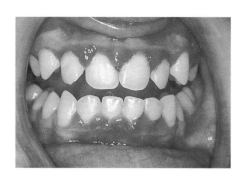

Fig. 11.4 Chronic marginal gingivitis in a 10-year-old girl.

Histopathology

The inflammatory infiltrate associated with marginal gingivitis in children is analogous to that seen in adults during the early stages of gingival inflammation. The dominant cell is the lymphocyte, although small numbers of plasma cells, macrophages, and neutrophils are in evidence. Research findings have not yet determined unequivocally whether the lymphocyte population is one of unactivated B cells or is T-cell dominated.

The relative absence of plasma cells, which are found in abundance in more established and advanced lesions in adults, confirms that gingivitis in children is quiescent and does not progress inexorably to involve the deeper periodontal tissues.

> **Key Points**
> Chronic gingivitis:
> - plaque-associated;
> - lymphocyte-dominated;
> - complex flora;
> - linked to the onset of puberty.

Microbiology

The first organisms to colonize clean tooth surfaces are the periodontally harmless, Gram-positive cocci that predominate in plaque after 4–7 days. After 2 weeks, a more complex flora of filamentous and fusiform organisms indicates a conversion to a Gram-negative infection, which, when established, comprises significant numbers of *Capnocytophaga*, *Selenomonas*, *Leptotrichia*, *Porphyromonas*, and *Spirochaete* spp. These species are cultivable from established and advanced periodontal lesions in cases of adult periodontitis. This suggests that the host response (rather than the subgingival flora) confers a degree of immunity to the development of periodontal disease in children, thus preventing spread of the contained gingivitis to deeper tissues.

Manual versus powered toothbrushes

The treatment and prevention of gingivitis are dependent on achieving and maintaining a standard of plaque control that, on an individual basis, is compatible with health. Toothbrushing is the principal method for removing dental plaque, and powered toothbrushes now provide a widely available alternative to the more conventional, manual toothbrushes for cleaning teeth.

There is considerable evidence in the literature to suggest that powered toothbrushes are beneficial for specific groups: patients with fixed orthodontic appliances—for whom there is also evidence that powered toothbrushes are effective in reducing decalcification; children and adolescents; and children with special needs. It remains questionable whether children who are already highly motivated with respect to tooth cleaning will benefit from using a powered toothbrush. It is possible that, particularly in children, any improved plaque control as a consequence of using a powered toothbrush may result from a 'novelty effect' of using a new toothbrush rather than because the powered toothbrush is more effective as a cleaning device.

A systematic review evaluating manual and powered toothbrushes with respect to oral health has made some important conclusions. Compared to manual toothbrushes, rotating/oscillating designs of powered toothbrushes reduced plaque and gingivitis by 7–17% although the clinical significance of this could not be determined. Powered brushes, therefore, are at least as effective and equally as safe as their manual counterparts with no evidence of increased incidence of soft tissue abrasions or trauma. No clinical trials have looked at the durability, reliability, and relative cost of powered and manual brushes so it is not possible to make any recommendation regarding overall toothbrush superiority.

11.5 DRUG-INDUCED GINGIVAL ENLARGEMENT

Enlargement of the gingiva is a well-recognized unwanted effect of a number of drugs. The most frequently implicated are phenytoin, cyclosporin, and nifedipine (Fig. 11.5).

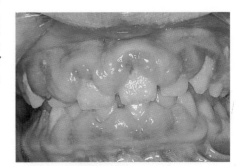

Fig. 11.5 Drug (phenytoin)-induced gingival enlargement in a 12-year-old boy.

11.5.1 Phenytoin

Phenytoin is an anticonvulsant used in the management of epilepsy. Gingival enlargement occurs in about 50% of dentate subjects who are taking the drug, and is most severe in teenagers and those who are cared for in institutions. The exact mechanism by which phenytoin induces enlargement is unclear. The gingival enlargement reflects an overproduction of collagen (rather than a decrease in degradation), and this may be brought about by the action of the drug on phenotypically distinct groups of fibroblasts that have the potential to synthesize large amounts of protein. Phenytoin-induced enlargement has been associated with a deficiency of folic acid, which may lead to impaired maturation of oral epithelia.

11.5.2 Cyclosporin

Cyclosporin is an immunosuppressant drug that is used widely in organ transplant patients to prevent graft rejection. Approximately 30% of patients taking the drug demonstrate gingival enlargement, with children being more susceptible than adults. The exact mechanism of the drug in causing enlargement is unknown. There is evidence to suggest both a stimulatory effect on fibroblast proliferation and collagen production as well as an inhibitory effect on collagen breakdown by the enzyme collagenase.

11.5.3 Nifedipine

Nifedipine is a calcium-channel blocker that is used in adults for the control of cardiovascular problems. It is also given to post-transplant patients to reduce the nephrotoxic effects of cyclosporin. The incidence of gingival enlargement in dentate subjects taking nifedipine is 10–15%. The drug blocks the calcium channels in cell membranes—intracellular calcium ions are a prerequisite for the production of collagenases by fibroblasts. The lack of these enzymes could be responsible for the accumulation of collagen in the gingiva.

Clinical features of gingival enlargement

The clinical changes of drug-induced enlargement are very similar irrespective of the drug involved. The first signs of change are seen after 3–4 months of drug administration. The interdental papillae become nodular before enlarging more diffusely to encroach upon the labial tissues. The anterior part of the mouth is most severely and frequently involved so that the patient's appearance is compromised. The tissues can become so abundant that oral functions, particularly eating and speaking, are impaired.

Enlarged gingiva is pink, firm, and stippled in subjects with a good standard of oral hygiene. When there is a pre-existing gingivitis the enlarged tissues compromise an already poor standard of plaque control. The gingiva then exhibit the classical signs of gingivitis (Fig. 11.5).

Key Points

Gingival enlargement:

- drug-induced;
- collagen accumulation;
- surgical treatment;
- superimposed gingivitis.

Management of gingival enlargement

A strict programme of oral hygiene instruction, scaling, and polishing must be implemented. Severe cases of gingival enlargement inevitably need to be surgically excised (gingivectomy) and then recontoured (gingivoplasty) to produce an architecture that allows adequate access for cleaning.

A follow-up programme is essential to ensure a high standard of plaque control and to detect any recurrence of the enlargement. As the causative drugs need to be taken on a long-term basis, recurrence is common. When a phenytoin-induced enlargement is refractory to long-term treatment, the patient's physician may be requested to modify or change the anticonvulsant therapy to drugs such as sodium valproate or carbamazepine, which do not cause gingival problems. There is no alternative medication to cyclosporin, however, and the patients inevitably require indefinite oral care.

11.6 TRAUMATIC GINGIVITIS (GINGIVITIS ARTEFACTA/FACTITIOUS GINGIVITIS)

Gingivitis artefacta has minor and major variants. The minor form results from rubbing or picking the gingiva using the fingernail, or perhaps from abrasive foods such as crisps, and the habit is usually provoked by a locus of irritation such as an area of persistent food packing or an already inflamed papilla (Fig. 11.6). The lesions resolve when the habit is corrected and the source of irritation is removed.

The injuries in gingivitis artefacta major are more severe and widespread and can involve the deeper periodontal tissues (Fig. 11.7(a)). Other areas of the mouth such as the lips and tongue may be involved and extraoral injuries may be found on the scalp, limbs, or face (factitious dermatitis) (Fig. 11.7(b)). The lesions are usually viewed with complete indifference by the patient who is unable to forward details of their time of onset or possible cause.

The treatment of these patients, other than the dressing and protection of oral wounds, does not lie with the dentist. Psychological reasons for inflicting the lesions may be complex and obscure. A psychological or psychiatric consultation, rarely welcomed either by older children or their parents, is necessary if the patient is to be prevented from ultimately inflicting serious damage upon themselves.

Key Points

Gingivitis artefacta:

- minor/major;
- self-inflicted;
- habitual;
- psychological.

11.7 MUCOGINGIVAL PROBLEMS IN CHILDREN

In adults much attention has focused on whether recession is more likely to occur locally where there is a reduced width of keratinized gingiva (KG). Conversely, of course, gingival recession inevitably leads to a narrowing of the zone of KG. It is, therefore, often difficult to determine unequivocally whether a narrow zone of KG is the cause or the effect of recession. A narrow or finite width of KG is compatible with gingival health, providing the tissues are maintained free of inflammation and chronic, traumatic insult. A wider zone of KG is considered more desirable to

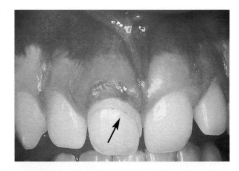

Fig. 11.6 Traumatic gingival injury inflicted by the fingernail (arrowed) that has been teased from the gingival crevice of 1|. (Reproduced with kind permission of the Editor, *British Dental Journal* and Mr P. R. Greene, General Dental Practitioner, Manchester.)

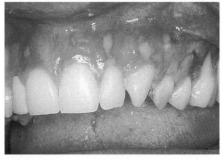

(a)

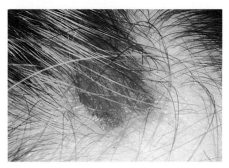

(b)

Fig. 11.7 (a) Generalized, self-inflicted ulceration of the attached gingiva and extensive loss of attachment around |6. (b) Ulcerative lesion at the hairline on the scalp. The lesions were produced by rubbing with a fingernail. (Reproduced with kind permission of the Editor, *Journal of Periodontology*.)

withstand gingival inflammation, trauma from mastication, toothbrushing, and forces from muscle pull.

Anterior teeth with narrow zones of KG are frequently encountered in children, as the width of KG varies greatly during the mixed dentition. For example, when permanent teeth erupt labially to their predecessors they frequently appear to erupt through alveolar mucosa with a complete absence of KG (Fig. 11.8). When the tooth has fully erupted an obvious width of KG is present.

The width of KG alone should not be the sole indicator of potential sites of gingival recession in children. The position of a tooth in the arch is a better guide as studies have shown that, of those permanent incisors with recession, about 80% are displaced labially. Aggravating factors such as gingivitis or mechanical irritation from excessive and incorrect toothbrushing further increase the likelihood of recession.

Gingival recession is also a common periodontal complication of orthodontic therapy when labial tipping of incisors is undertaken. When roots move labially through the supporting envelope of alveolar bone the potential for recession increases.

When gingival recession occurs in children, a conservative approach to treatment should be adopted. The maximum distance from the gingival margin to the CEJ should be recorded. Overenthusiastic toothbrushing practices are modified and a scale and polish given if necessary. The recession must then be monitored carefully until the permanent dentition is complete. Longitudinal studies of individual cases have shown that, as the supporting tissues mature, the gingival attachment tends to creep spontaneously in a coronal direction to cover at least part of the previously denuded root surface. This cautious approach is preferred to corrective surgical intervention to increase the width of KG.

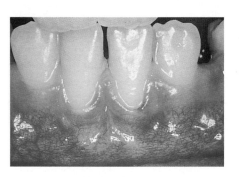

Fig. 11.8 Lower central incisors that have erupted somewhat labially to the partially erupted 2⌐2. There is only a minimal width of keratinized gingiva buccal to the 1⌐1.

> **Key Points**
>
> Gingival recession:
>
> - narrow keratinized gingiva;
> - local trauma;
> - post orthodontics;
> - conservative treatment approach.

11.8 CHRONIC PERIODONTITIS

A number of epidemiological studies (Table 11.2) have investigated the prevalence of chronic periodontitis in children. The variation in prevalence between studies is considerable and attributable to different methods of diagnosing attachment loss and the use of different cut-off levels to determine disease presence. Some workers use intraoral radiographs to measure from the CEJ to the alveolar crest, while others use a periodontal probe to determine clinically the distance from the CEJ to the base of the periodontal crevice or pocket. Radiographic studies on children with a primary or a mixed dentition indicate that loss of attachment is uncommon under the age of 9 years. A microscopic examination of the root surfaces of 200 extracted molars, however, demonstrated a mean attachment loss of 0.26 mm on two-thirds of the surfaces on 94% of teeth. Clinically, such small changes are insignificant and difficult to detect.

Cut-off levels at which disease is diagnosed in adolescents have been set at 1, 2, or 3 mm. Larger cut-off values provide more stringent criteria for the detection of attachment loss and consequently the disease appears less prevalent. An exception

Table 11.2 Key studies to determine the prevalence of periodontal disease (ALOSS) in children

Country of study (year)	Subjects	Method of diagnosis of ALOSS	Periodontal disease prevalence	Observations
UK (1974)	590 15-year-olds	Probing from CEJ ≥1 mm ≥2 mm	46% 11%	Evidence of social class gradient; lower class higher disease prevalence
UK (1975)	602 14-year-olds	Radiographs CEJ–AC > 3 mm	51.5%	Disease also diagnosed by irregular AC and widened ligament space
Norway (1984)	2409 15-year-olds	Radiographs CEJ–AC > 2 mm	11%	Maxillary first molars primarily affected
Hungary (1987)	200 extracted primary molars	Microscopic examination of root surface	Mean ALOSS 0.26 mm on two-thirds surfaces of 94% teeth	More ALOSS on maxillary (than mandibular) molars and adjacent to carious tooth surfaces
Norway (1988)	2767 14-year-olds	Radiographs CEJ–AC > 2 mm	4.5%	Previous orthodontic treatment may increase prevalence of ALOSS
UK (1990)	167 14-year-olds	Probing from CEJ ≥1 mm ≥2 mm	3% 0%	Subgingival calculus closely correlates with future ALOSS
New Zealand (1994)	317 5-year-olds	Radiographs CEJ–AC > 2 mm	2.1% Definite bone loss	Bone loss more likely with higher dmft
Sweden (1994)	8666 7–9-year-olds	Radiographs CEJ–AC > 2 mm	2–5%	Children with bone loss had more calculus and higher dfs

CEJ, cementoenamel junction; ALOSS, attachment loss; AC, alveolar crest; DMFT/S, decayed, missing, filled teeth/surfaces.

to this trend was seen in a study of 602, 14–15-year-olds in the United Kingdom; 51.5% of the subjects were diagnosed as having periodontal disease determined by a CEJ—alveolar crest distance of 3 mm. Additional radiographic features were also used, namely an irregular contour of the alveolar crest and a widened, coronal periodontal ligament space. Such observations may result from minor tooth movements following eruption of the second molars and consolidation of the occlusion, or from remodelling of bone after orthodontic treatment. It is, therefore, likely that 51.5% is a considerable overestimate of disease prevalence in this age group. If a cut-off value of 2 mm is deemed acceptable, the majority of studies put the prevalence of disease in adolescents at 1–11%. This suggests that chronic adult periodontitis initiates and progresses during the early teenage years.

Observations made with respect to periodontal disease in children include:

- When loss of attachment occurs at interproximal sites it is a consequence of pathological change and correlates closely with the presence of subgingival calculus;

- The prevalence of periodontal destruction correlates positively with DMF (decayed, missing, and filled) teeth or surfaces. This suggests either, that carious or broken down surfaces predispose to plaque accumulation, or perhaps more likely, that in the absence of oral health care, periodontal disease and caries progress independently;

- When the loss of attachment occurs on buccal or palatal surfaces, it is more often associated with trauma from an incorrect toothbrushing technique than with an inflammatory response.

Key Points

Loss of attachment:

- plaque-induced;
- trauma-induced;
- detected radiographically;
- decayed, missing, and filled (teeth) link.

11.9 RISK FACTORS FOR PERIODONTAL CONDITIONS AND DISEASES

A risk factor can be defined as a state or occurrence that increases the probability of an individual developing a disease. Risk factors for periodontal disease can be classified as local or general. Local factors, for example, an instanding lateral incisor, may serve to compromise local plaque control by hindering effective cleaning and resulting in dental plaque accumulation. On the other hand, general risk factors, such as an inherited disorder may predispose an individual to periodontal disease despite a good level of plaque control.

It is important to understand that if a child possesses a risk factor for periodontal disease, it does not necessarily follow that the child will develop the condition. Conversely, a patient may appear to have no risk factors, but the disease may develop subsequently. Bearing this in mind, risk factors (both local and general) should be considered when assessing, diagnosing, treating, and maintaining child patients with periodontal disease.

11.9.1 Local risk factors

These can be grouped simply into four areas. There may be overlap between these areas.

- Malocclusions.
- Following traumatic dental injuries.
- Plaque retentive factors.
- Ectopic eruption

Malocclusions

An instanding or rotated tooth may be difficult to clean and can cause increased plaque retention. A traumatic occlusion may result in direct damage to the periodontal support. Angle's Class II division ii malocclusions with increased and complete overbites may predispose to damage of the gingiva palatal to the upper incisor teeth. Similarly, severely retroclined upper incisor teeth may damage the labial gingiva of the lower teeth.

Following a traumatic dental injury

Luxation, intrusion and avulsion injuries all result in varying degrees of damage to the periodontal ligament and if severe, alveolar bone. This results in increased tooth mobility which is managed by providing the affected teeth with a splint.

If a traumatised tooth is left in a severely mobile state or in traumatic occlusion, the periodontal ligament fibres will not heal and further damage may ensue.

Plaque retentive factors

There is a multitude of plaque retentive factors which may serve to compromise the health of the periodontium. They may be naturally occurring (in the case of a dental anomaly) or be iatrogenic.

Examples of dental anomalies include:

* Erupted supernumerary teeth (localized malocclusion).
* Invaginated odontomes.
* Talon cusps.
* Pitted, grooved amelogenesis imperfecta (with sensitivity).
* Enamel pearls or root grooves.

Examples of iatrogenic factors include:

* Orthodontic appliances.
* Partial dentures.
* Ledges and overhangs on poorly fitting preformed metal crowns.
* Ledges and overhangs from intracoronal restorations.

11.9.2 General risk factors

General risk factors for periodontal disease may have a genetic basis, with certain inherited conditions possessing periodontal manifestations (e.g. Papillon Lefèvre Syndrome). The genetic conditions are dealt with previously in this chapter. There are also metabolic, haematological, and environmental risk factors within the general category. A full discussion of each is outwith the scope of this chapter, so the two most prevalent examples of general risk factors, diabetes mellitus and smoking will be discussed.

Diabetes mellitus

Children with Type I diabetes *with poor diabetic control* are at risk of developing periodontal disease. The link appears not to be directly with the level of plaque control but to the presence of systemic complications, such as retinal and renal problems. The overall severity of periodontal disease may increase with increasing duration of the diabetes. There are a number of factors which may contribute to a child's risk status. They may be inherited or secondary to high levels of blood glucose (hyperglycaemia).

These can be outlined as:

* Defective polymorphonuclear leucocyte function (chemotaxis, phagocytosis, and adherence);
* Disordered collagen metabolism (gingival fibroblasts produce less collagen and the polymorphonuclear leucocytes produce more of the enzyme collagenase than in non-diabetics). This results in poor wound healing;
* The hyperglycaemic state may favour certain inflammatory mediators and increase oxygen radical production by macrophages.

Tobacco smoking

Smoking is now thought to be a significant environmental risk factor for periodontal disease. Smokers have 3–6 times the level of periodontal disease when compared with non-smokers and young people are thought to be more vulnerable. Often, the signs of disease are masked because nicotine and other tobacco products cause vasoconstriction, reducing the blood supply to the gingivae and lowering the tendency to bleed.

There are a number of smoking-related mechanisms pertaining to smoking as a risk factor for periodontal disease. These include:

- Increased prevalence of some periodontal pathogens;
- Reduction in the levels of salivary IgA;
- Reduction in effective phagocytosis;
- Alterations in the numbers of certain T cell populations.

If an individual stops smoking this will allow an improved response to the management of periodontal disease, but the time taken for this 'recovery' to occur is unclear.

The underlying defect associated with general risk factors is compromised phagocytosis and or chemotaxis. The importance of polymorphonuclear leucocyte (neutrophil) function to the host response is also demonstrated in less common conditions such as the neutropaenias (see page 252).

11.10 PERIODONTAL COMPLICATIONS OF ORTHODONTIC TREATMENT

Orthodontic treatment in adolescents, particularly with fixed appliances, can predispose to a deterioration in periodontal health and a number of well-recognized complications.

11.10.1 Gingivitis

Access for interproximal toothbrushing is reduced considerably during fixed appliance therapy and the accumulation of plaque induces gingivitis (Fig. 11.9). The problem is compounded when teeth are banded rather than bonded as periodontal health is more easily maintained when the gingival sulcus is not encroached upon by metal bands.

When supragingival plaque deposits are present on teeth that are being repositioned orthodontically, the type of movement used may play an important part in the development of periodontal problems. Supragingival plaque deposits are shifted into a subgingival location by tipping movements. Conversely, bodily movements are less likely to induce a relocation of supragingival plaque.

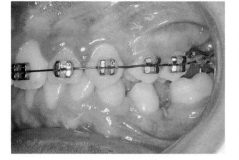

Fig. 11.9 Chronic marginal gingivitis associated with fixed appliance therapy.

11.10.2 Gingival enlargement

The anterior palatal gingiva and mucosa have a propensity for enlargement when tissues are 'rolled up' between incisors that are being retracted and the fixed anterior margin of the acrylic plate of a removable appliance (Fig. 11.10(a) and (b)). Generally, however, these changes tend to be transient and resolve when appliances are removed.

11.10.3 Attachment and bone loss

The mean, annual rate of coronal attachment loss during appliance therapy ranges from 0.05 to 0.30 mm, which compares favourably with figures for the mean annual

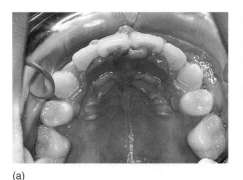

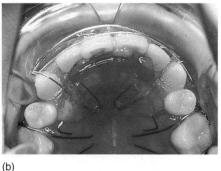

(a) (b)

Fig. 11.10 (a) Gingival enlargement on the palatal aspect of retracted maxillary incisors. (b) Appliance *in situ*. (Reproduced by kind permission of Mr N. E. Carter, Consultant in Orthodontics, Newcastle.)

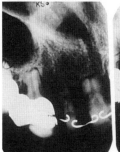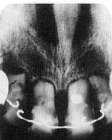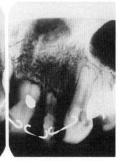

Fig. 11.11 Apical root resorption of 321|123 following orthodontic treatment. (Reproduced by kind permission of Dr I. L. Chapple, Professor of Periodontology, Birmingham, UK.)

attachment loss in untreated populations. A well-recognized complication of orthodontic tooth movement is apical root resorption, particularly when excessive forces are used (Fig. 11.11). Such changes must also be regarded as loss of attachment, albeit at an apical rather than a coronal site.

11.10.4 Gingival recession

The response of the facial periodontal tissues to labial tooth movement in anterior segments is unpredictable. Labial movement of incisors is sometimes associated with gingival recession. The risk of recession is greater when the alveolar bone plate is thin or where dehiscences or fenestrations in the bone exist.

11.10.5 Trauma

Direct local irritation of the soft tissues by components of a fixed appliance can be minimized if due care and attention is exercised during bonding, banding, and placement of wires and elastics. If chronic irritation of the gingiva does occur then a localized, acute inflammatory reaction will quickly follow. This may develop further into a region of gingival enlargement or a fibrous epulis that is superimposed upon a burrowing infrabony lesion.

Key Points

Orthodontic problems:
- gingivitis;
- enlargement;
- root resorption;
- gingival trauma.

11.11 AGGRESSIVE PERIODONTAL DISEASES

Aggressive periodontal diseases comprise a group of rare, but rapidly progressing infections that affect the primary and permanent dentitions. The disorders are associated with a more specific microbial challenge and an inherent defect in the host's immunological response. The nature of these diseases can lead to premature tooth loss at an early age. Prompt diagnosis is essential if treatment is to be successful, and the periodontal status must be monitored regularly to ensure that the treated disease remains quiescent.

Aggressive periodontal diseases were previously known as early-onset diseases, namely, prepubertal and juvenile periodontitis. A classification system for periodontal diseases and conditions published in 1999 effectively combined these two diseases into one—aggressive periodontitis (see Further Reading). This classification, which is used in this chapter, removed the arbitrary age limitations that were previously inferred by terms such as prepubertal, juvenile, and even adult periodontitis. It is now recognized that aggressive periodontitis can affect the primary and permanent dentitions both in localized and generalized forms.

11.11.1 Primary dentition (prepubertal periodontitis)

The disease may present immediately after the teeth have erupted. In the generalized form the gingiva appear fiery red, swollen, and haemorrhagic. The tissues become hyperplastic with granular or nodular proliferations that precede gingival clefting and extensive areas of recession. Gross deposits of plaque are inevitable as the soft tissue changes make it difficult to maintain oral hygiene. The disease progresses extremely rapidly, with primary tooth loss occurring as early as 3–4 years of age. The entire dentition need not be affected, however, as the bone loss may be restricted to one arch. Children with generalized disease are susceptible to recurrent general infections, principally otitis media and upper respiratory tract infections.

Localized disease progresses more slowly than the generalized form and bone loss characteristically affects only incisor–molar teeth. Plaque levels are usually low, consequently soft tissue changes are minimal with gingivitis and proliferation involving only the marginal tissues.

The predominant micro-organisms that have been identified are aggressive periodontopathogens: *Actinobacillus actinomycetemcomitans*, *Porphyromonas gingivalis*, *Fusobacterium nucleatum*, and *Eikenella corrodens*. This suggests that there is an infective component to the disease, although defects in the hosts' response have also been identified. Profound abnormalities in chemotaxis and phagocytosis of polymorphonuclear neutrophils and monocytes are frequently reported in these patients. These immunological defects are heritable risk factors that help to define phenotypically the disease entity. Conversely, they may also be associated with more serious and life-threatening conditions, and thus a full medical screen is indicated.

Oral hygiene instruction, scaling, and root planing should be undertaken at frequent intervals. Bacterial culturing of the pocket flora identifies specific periodontopathogens. If pathogens persist after oral debridement, an antibiotic such as metronidazole or amoxycillin (amoxicillin) should be given systemically after sensitivity testing, as a short course over 1–2 weeks. Generalized disease responds poorly to treatment. Some improvement has been achieved following a granulocyte transfusion in a patient with a defect in neutrophil function. Extraction of involved teeth has also produced an improvement in neutrophil chemotaxis, which suggests that the defect may be induced by certain organisms in the periodontal flora. Furthermore, in severe cases of generalized periodontitis, extraction of all primary teeth (and the provision of a removable prosthesis) can limit the disease to the primary dentition. Presumably, anaerobic pathogens are unable to thrive in the absence of teeth. When the permanent teeth erupt, bacterial culturing of the subgingival flora ensures that reinfection is detected early.

11.11.2 Permanent dentition (juvenile periodontitis)

In the permanent dentition, aggressive periodontitis involves severe periodontal destruction with an onset around puberty. The localized form occurs in otherwise healthy individuals, with destruction classically localized and around the first permanent molars and incisors, and not involving more than two other teeth. Generalized periodontitis also occurs in otherwise healthy individuals but involves more than 14 teeth, that is, being generalized to an arch or the entire dentition. Some reports have monitored children suffering from aggressive periodontitis of the primary dentition to find that, at around puberty, the disease became generalized to involve the entire dentition.

Epidemiology

Studies show a prevalence of about 0.1% in developed countries and about 5% in underdeveloped nations, although some variation may be due to different methods of screening and different criteria used to define the disease. The disease is clearly more prevalent in certain ethnic groups. In the United Kingdom an epidemiological study of 7266 schoolchildren in Coventry and Birmingham showed an overall prevalence of 0.02% in Caucasians, 0.2% in Asians, and 0.8% in the AfroCaribbean population. There was no difference in prevalence between males and females, which does not concur with the data of many earlier epidemiological studies of the disease which reported a female to male ratio of 3 : 1.

Clinical and radiographic features

The age of onset is between 11 and 15 years. The clinical features are pocket formation and loss of attachment associated with the permanent incisors and first molar teeth. The radiographic pattern of bone loss is quite distinctive. Bilateral angular bone defects are identified on the mesial and, or distal surfaces of molars (Fig. 11.12 (a) and (b)). Angular defects are sometimes seen around the incisors, although the very thin interproximal bone is resorbed more evenly to give a horizontal pattern of resorption. The bone loss around the molars can be detected on routine bitewing radiographs. The interpretation of the films must be made with a sound knowledge of the patient's dental history, however, as localized angular defects are found adjacent to teeth with overhanging or deficient interproximal restorations, and teeth that have tilted slightly (Fig. 11.13). The gingiva can appear healthy when the levels of plaque are low, but a marginal gingivitis will be present if a good standard of plaque control is not evident.

The generalized form may also present at puberty. Severe generalized bone loss is the characteristic feature (Fig. 11.14). The pattern may be a combination of angular and horizontal resorption producing an irregular alveolar crest. When patients have good plaque control the degree of bone resorption is not commensurate with the level of oral hygiene. The more generalized nature of the disease predisposes to multiple and recurrent abscess formation which is a common presenting feature.

Invariably, one of the presenting signs is tooth migration or drifting of incisors. Tooth movement is not necessarily a consequence of advanced disease as drifting may occur when only a fraction of a tooth's periodontal support is lost. Conversely, extensive bone loss can occur with no spontaneous movement of teeth and the subject may

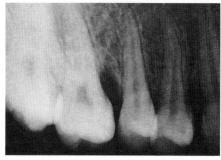

(a)

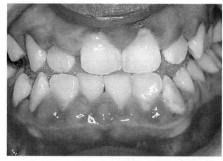

(b)

Fig. 11.12 (a) Clinical appearance of a 13-year-old girl with localized aggressive periodontitis. (b) Radiographic appearance of vertical bone loss on the mesial aspect of 6|. (Reproduced by kind permission of Mr D. G. Smith, Consultant in Restorative Dentistry, Newcastle upon Tyne).

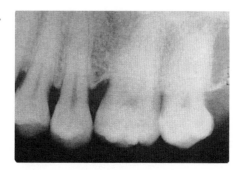

Fig. 11.13 Radiographic view of |7 that has erupted and tipped mesially into the |6 extraction site. The contour of the bone crest on the mesial of |7 gives the impression of a vertical bony defect.

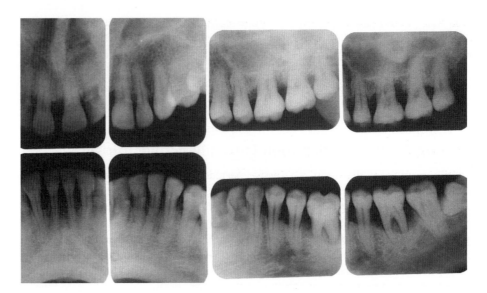

Fig. 11.14 Aggressive periodontitis with generalized bone loss in a 16-year-old male.

only be alerted to the problem when a minor traumatic episode, such as a blow to the mouth during a sporting activity, causes unexpected loosening of teeth.

Bacteriology and pathogenesis

The subgingival microflora comprises loosely adherent, Gram-negative anaerobes including *Eikenella corrodens*, *Capnocytophaga* spp., and *Prevotella intermedia*. The most frequently implicated organism is *Actinobacillus actinomycetemcomitans*, which has been found in over 90% of patients. Sufferers also have raised IgG titres to *A. actinomycetemcomitans*, but levels of the bacteria fall significantly following successful treatment of the condition.

> **Key Points**
>
> Permanent dentition (Juvenile periodontitis):
> * onset around puberty;
> * localized/generalized;
> * *Actinobacillus actinomycetemcomitans*;
> * neutrophil chemotaxis defect.

The extreme pathogenicity of *A. actinomycetemcomitans* is due to its ability to invade connective tissues and the wide range of virulence factors that it produces. These include a potent lipopolysaccharide that induces bone resorption, collagenase, an epitheliotoxin, a fibroblast-inhibiting factor, and a leucotoxin that kills neutrophils and so dampens the host's first line of defence against bacterial challenge.

About 70% of patients have defects in neutrophil chemotaxis and phagocytosis. The chemotactic defect is linked to reduced amounts of cell-surface glycoproteins and is transmitted as a dominant trait. About 50% of siblings of patients who have both aggressive periodontitis and chemotactic defects, also demonstrate impaired neutrophil function.

Treatment

A combined regimen of regular scaling and root planing with a 2-week course of systemic tetracycline therapy (250 mg, four times daily) has been used extensively in the management of this condition. *A. actinomycetemcomitans* is sensitive to tetracycline, which also has the ability to be concentrated up to 10 times in gingival crevicular fluid when compared with serum. More recently, a combination of metronidazole (250 mg) and amoxicillin (amoxycillin) (375 mg), three times a day for 1 week, in association with subgingival scaling, has also been found to be effective.

A more radical approach is to undertake flap surgery so that better access is achieved for root cleaning, and the superficial, infected connective tissues are excised. An antimicrobial regimen can also be implemented in conjunction with a surgical approach.

Key Points

Permanent dentition (juvenile periodontitis)—treatment:

- plaque control;
- mechanical debridement;
- systemic antimicrobials;
- periodontal surgery.

11.11.3 Genetic factors and aggressive diseases

The increased prevalence of aggressive periodontitis in certain ethnic groups and within families strongly suggests that susceptibility to these diseases may be influenced by a number of genetic determinants. Furthermore, genetic factors are implicated in the pathogenesis of the diseases as many affected patients have functionally defective neutrophils.

The mode of transmission has not been determined unequivocally. The apparent increased incidence in females suggests an X-linked dominant mode of inheritance with reduced penetrance. The association with females, however, may reflect epidemiological bias as females are more likely to seek dental attention. Large family studies of subjects with aggressive periodontitis suggest an autosomal-recessive pattern of inheritance.

The role of hereditary components in periodontal diseases has been supported by the link with specific tissue markers. The major histocompatibility complex (MHC) determines the susceptibility of subjects to certain diseases. Class I and II genes in the MHC encode for specific human leucocyte antigens (HLA I and II), which account for individual variation in immunoresponsiveness. There are clear associations between HLA serotypes and diabetes mellitus and rheumatoid arthritis. A strong link between an HLA serotype and aggressive diseases has still to be determined, although a mild association between the HLA-A9 antigen and aggressive periodontitis has been found.

Key Points

Genetic components of periodontitis:

- family associations;
- ethnic associations;
- major histocompatibility complex link;
- link with syndromes.

11.12 PERIODONTITIS AS A MANIFESTATION OF SYSTEMIC DISEASE

The genetic basis for aggressive periodontitis in particular is substantiated by the definite association between the condition and a number of rare inherited medical conditions and syndromes (Table 11.1). The pattern of inheritance reflects a single gene disorder, commonly involving inherited defects of neutrophils, enzyme reactions, or collagen synthesis.

11.12.1 Papillon–Lefèvre syndrome (PLS)

This syndrome is characterized by palmar–plantar hyperkeratosis, premature loss of primary and permanent dentitions, and ectopic calcifications of the falx cerebri. Some patients show an increased susceptibility to infection. The syndrome is an autosomal-recessive trait with a prevalence of about 1–4 per million of the population. Consanguinity of parents is evident in about one-third of cases.

Rapid and progressive periodontal destruction affects the primary dentition with an onset at about 2 years (Fig. 11.15). Exfoliation of all primary teeth is usual before the permanent successors erupt and patients may be edentulous by the mid to late teens. Cases of a late-onset variant of PLS have also been described in which the palmar–plantar and periodontal lesions are relatively mild and only become evident in the permanent dentition. An extensive family dental history supported by clinical, laboratory, and radiographic examinations confirms the diagnosis.

11.12.2 Neutropenias

The neutropenias comprise a heterogeneous group of blood disorders that are characterized by a periodic or persistent reduction in the number of circulating polymorphonuclear neutrophils. Neutropenias can be drug-induced or be secondary to severe bacterial or viral infections or autoimmune diseases such as lupus erythematosus. Cyclic neutropenia, benign familial neutropenias, and severe familial neutropenias are all heritable conditions transmitted as autosomal-dominant traits and diagnoses are often made during early childhood. The chronic benign neutropenia of childhood is diagnosed between 6 and 24 months of age and is characterized by frequent and multiple pyogenic infections of the skin and mucous membranes.

The periodontal problems associated with the neutropenias are very similar, and in many cases the patient presents with a localized or generalized aggressive periodontitis. Occasionally, the primary dentition may not be involved, and clinical signs do not appear until the permanent dentition has erupted. The gingiva are inflamed and oedematous; gingival recession, ulceration, and desquamation can also occur.

The treatment of a neutropenic-induced periodontitis involves local removal of plaque and calculus. Strict plaque control measures are difficult to achieve in younger children, so use of an antibacterial mouthrinse may prove useful.

11.12.3 Chediak–Higashi syndrome

This is a rare and very often fatal disease inherited as an autosomal-recessive trait. Clinical features include partial albinism, photophobia, and nystagmus. The patients suffer from recurrent pyogenic infections and malignant lymphoma—which is accompanied by neutropenia, anaemia, and a thrombocytopenia. The neutrophils show defects in migration, chemotaxis, and phagocytosis producing a diminished bactericidal capacity.

Periodontal changes associated with the syndrome include severe gingival inflammation and rapid, and extensive, alveolar bone resorption that can lead to premature exfoliation. The nature of the changes has not been fully established, but they may be plaque-induced, secondary to infection, or related to the underlying defect in neutrophil function.

11.12.4 Leucocyte–adhesion deficiency syndrome (LAD)

This autosomal-recessive trait is characterized clinically by a delayed separation of the umbilical cord, severe recurrent bacterial infections, impaired wound healing,

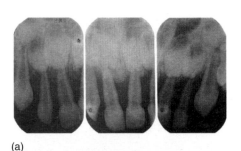
(a)

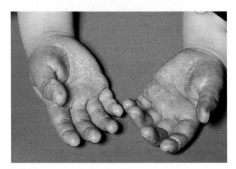
(b)

Fig. 11.15 Papillon–Lefèvre syndrome in a 3-year-old boy. (a) Radiographic appearance showing almost total bone loss around maxillary anterior teeth. (b) Hyperkeratosis of the palms of the hand.

formation of pus, and an aggressive gingivitis, which may be the presenting sign of the disorder. Consanguinity between the parents of affected children confirms the mode of the inheritance as autosomal-recessive.

The syndrome demonstrates the important role of leucocytes (and other white blood cells) in protecting the host against periodontal disease. Moderate phenotypes, however, may appear relatively disease-free, but then develop symptoms and progress 'downhill' extremely rapidly. The majority of patients do not survive beyond 30 years. The progressive periodontal condition is very difficult to control and is often of secondary importance to other life-threatening infections.

11.12.5 Ehlers–Danlos syndrome

The syndrome is an autosomal-dominant trait with nine variants that display defects in the synthesis, secretion, or polymerization of collagen. The variants of the syndrome exhibit extensive clinical heterogeneity and collectively represent the most common of the heritable disorders of connective tissues. The clinical findings are principally excessive joint mobility, skin hyperextensibility, and susceptibility to scarring and bruising of the skin and oral mucous membranes (Fig. 11.16). Defective type IV collagen supporting the walls of small blood vessels predisposes to persistent postextraction haemorrhage.

Gingival tissues are fragile and have a tendency to bleed on toothbrushing. The type VIII syndrome is associated with advanced periodontal disease. Periodontitis has also been linked with the type IV variant, although other variants do not appear to be affected. Ultrastructural changes also occur in the teeth, with abnormalities of the amelodentinal junction, vascular inclusions in dentine, fibrous degeneration of the pulp, and disorganization of cementum.

Type VIII patients require a thorough preventive periodontal programme as root debridement can cause extensive trauma to the fragile soft tissues. Periodontal surgery should be avoided because of the risk of haemorrhage and the potential problems encountered with suturing soft tissue flaps.

11.12.6 Langerhans' cell histiocytosis

Langerhans' cell histiocytosis (LCH) is a non-malignant granulomatous, childhood disorder that is characterized pathologically by uncontrolled proliferation and accumulation of Langerhans' cells, mixed with varying proportions of eosinophils and multinucleated giant cells. LCH replaced the term 'histiocytosis X' and the closely related syndromes eosinophilic granuloma, Hand–Schuller–Christian disease, and Letterer–Siwe disease. The clinical hallmark of LCH is the presence of lytic bone lesions that may be single or multiple. When lesions are widespread they can affect the pituitary gland and retro-orbital region, thus causing diabetes insipidus and exophthalmos, respectively. The disseminated form of LCH is extremely aggressive and has a poor prognosis. It is often diagnosed in the first 6 months of life before becoming widespread by about 3 years of age.

The periodontal manifestations of LCH may be the presenting signs, which include a marginal gingivitis, bleeding gingiva, abscess formation, pain, and drifting and mobility of the teeth. Radiographs show localized or generalized bone loss, characteristic osteolytic lesions, and 'floating teeth' with no alveolar bone support (Fig. 11.17).

A biopsy will confirm the diagnosis and a full radiographic screening determines the severity of the syndrome. Local lesions that are confined to bone respond well to curettage and excision. The mortality rate increases in the more widely disseminated forms of the syndrome and when overlying soft tissues are involved. Treatment is by radiotherapy and chemotherapy.

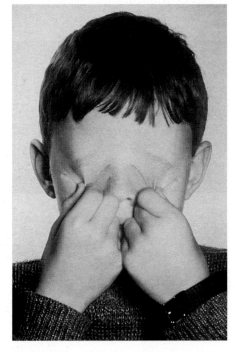

Fig. 11.16 Cutaneous hyperextensibility of the upper eyelids in a 9-year-old child with Ehlers–Danlos syndrome.

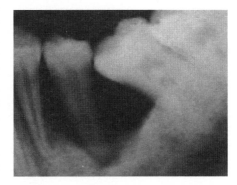

Fig. 11.17 Extensive bone loss around mandibular left premolars in a 15-year-old child with Langerhans cell histiocytosis. (Reproduced by kind permission of Dr I. L. Chapple, Professor of Periodontology, Birmingham, UK.)

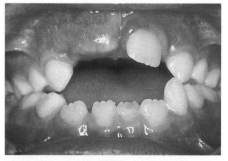

(a)

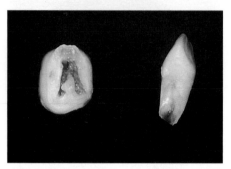

(b)

Fig. 11.18 (a) Premature loss of BA|AB in a 3½-year-old child with hypophosphatasia. The $\frac{1}{21|12}$ have already erupted. (b) Extensive root resorption led to exfoliation of |CD at 4 years of age. (Reproduced by kind permission of Dr I. L. Chapple, Professor of Periodontology, Birmingham, UK.)

11.12.7 Hypophosphatasia

Hypophosphatasia is a rare, inborn error of metabolism characterized by defective bone mineralization, a deficiency of alkaline phosphatase (ALP) activity, and an increased excretion of phosphoethanolamine in the urine. ALP plays a major part in the mineralization of hard tissues and so the absence of the enzyme predisposes to a range of bone and cartilage defects. The condition is an autosomal-recessive trait, although the inheritance pattern of some milder forms of hypophosphatasia may be autosomal-dominant.

> **Key Points**
> Prepubertal periodontitis/systemic diseases:
> * very rare;
> * autosomal mode of inheritance;
> * aggressive periodontal destruction.

The lesions of juvenile or childhood hypophosphatasia become apparent before 2 years of age. Bone defects are usually quite mild with bowing of the legs, proptosis, and wide-open fontanelles being prominent signs. Dental features are resorption of alveolar bone (in the absence of marked gingivitis), premature exfoliation of anterior deciduous teeth, hypoplasia or complete absence of cementum, and the presence of 'small teeth' that have enlarged pulp chambers as a consequence of defective mineralization (Fig. 11.18(a) and (b)). The aplastic or hypoplastic cementum and a weakened periodontal attachment is thought to render the patients susceptible to infection with periodontopathogens.

The diagnosis of hypophosphatasia is confirmed biochemically by low activity of serum ALP and a raised level of phosphoethanolamine in a 24-h urine sample.

11.12.8 Down syndrome

Children with Down syndrome (trisomy 21) do not suffer aggressive periodontal disease, However, there are a significant number of local and general risk factors that may exist as a result of the syndrome. Local factors that may serve to increase dental plaque retention are:

* Angles Class III malocclusions with crowding;
* Lack of an anterior lip seal;
* Anterior open bites.

General risk factors for periodontal disease are mainly centred on leucocyte defects and may include:

* Defects of polymorphonuclear leucocyte function (chemotaxis, killing, and phagocytosis);
* Reduced T-cell activity.

11.13 SUMMARY

1. Anatomical variation, which occurs during tooth eruption, and the maturation of the periodontal tissues can mimic signs of gingivitis, recession, and bone loss.

2. Herpetic gingivostomatitis is most frequently seen in children under 5 years of age, whereas necrotizing ulcerative gingivitis is more prevalent in young adults.

3. Although the prevalence of dental caries has declined in the UK and other European countries, the prevalence of plaque-induced gingivitis in children has not reduced over the last 20 years.

4. Chronic gingivitis in children appears to be a relatively stable lesion, which does not necessarily progress to periodontal destruction.

5. Gingival changes can also occur in children who are prescribed drugs to control epilepsy or following transplant surgery, during orthodontic therapy, as well as at sites of self-inflicted trauma.

6. Early signs of chronic periodontitis are sometimes seen during adolescence, and targeting this age group with a primary prevention strategy may help to reduce tooth loss in later life.

7. Extreme vigilance is necessary to diagnose aggressive periodontal diseases and those periodontal conditions that may be associated with systemic disease. Bleeding after gentle probing in the presence of apparently healthy gingiva indicates the need for further investigation.

11.14 FURTHER READING

Armitage, G. C. (1999). Development of a classification system for periodontal diseases and conditions. *Annals of Periodontology*, **4**, 1–6.
Heanue, M., Deacon, S. A., Deery, C., Robinson, P. G., Walmsley, A. D., Worthington, H. V., and Shaw, W. C. (2003). Manual versus powered toothbrushing for oral health. In *The Cochrane Library* (Issue 1). Oxford.
O'Brien, M. (1993). *Children's Dental Health in the UK, 1993*. Office of Population Censuses and Surveys, HMSO, London.
Sabiston, C. B., Jr (1986). A review and proposal for the etiology of acute necrotising gingivitis. *Journal of Clinical Periodontology*, **13**, 727–34. (*An overview of the epidemiology of NUG with an emphasis on a viral rather than a bacterial aetiology.*)
Schenkein, H. A. (1994). Genetics of early-onset periodontal diseases. In *Molecular pathogenesis of periodontal disease* (ed. R. Genco, S. Hamada, T. Lehner, J. McGhee, and S. Mergenhagen), pp. 373–86. ASM Press, Washington. (*An appraisal of the role that genetic factors play in the pathogenesis of juvenile and prepubertal periodontitis.*)
Seymour, R. A. (1993). Drug-induced gingival enlargement. *Adverse Drug Reactions and Toxicology Review*, **12**, 215–32. (*A general account of the drugs that induce gingival overgrowth.*)
Seymour, R. A. and Heasman, P. A. (1992). *Drugs, diseases and the periodontium*. Oxford Medical Publications, Oxford University Press, Oxford. (*Comprehensive accounts of early-onset diseases, systemic disease and the periodontium, and gingival overgrowth.*)

11.15 REFERENCES

Aass, A. M., Alabandar, J., Aasenden, R., Tollefsen, T. and Gjermo, P. (1988). Variation in prevalence of radiographic alveolar bone loss in subgroups of 14-year-old schoolchildren in Oslo. *Journal of Clinical Periodontology*, **15**, 130–3.
Bimstein, E., Treasure, E. T., Williams, S. M. and Dever, J. G. (1994). Alveolar bone loss in 5-year-old New Zealand children: its prevalence and relationship to caries prevalence, socio-economic status and ethnic origin. *Journal of Clinical Periodontology*, **21**, 447–50.
Clerehugh, V., Lennon, M. A. and Worthington, H. V. (1990). 5-year results of a longitudinal study of early periodontitis in 14- to 19-year-old adolescents. *Journal of Clinical Periodontology*, **17**, 702–8.
Hansen, B. F., Gjermo, P. and Bergwitz-Larsen, K. R. (1984). Periodontal bone loss in 15-year-old Norwegians. *Journal of Clinical Periodontology*, **11**, 125–31.
Hull, P. S., Hillam, D. G. and Beal, J. F. (1975). A radiographic study of the prevalence of chronic periodontitis in 14-year-old English schoolchildren. *Journal of Clinical Periodontology*, **2**, 203–10.

Keszthelyi, G. and Szabó, I. (1987). Attachment loss in primary molars. *Journal of Clinical Periodontology*, **14**, 48–51.

Lennon, M. A. and Davies, R. M. (1974). Prevalence and distribution of alveolar bone loss in a population of 15-year-old schoolchildren. *Journal of Clinical Periodontology*, **1**, 175–82.

Sjodin, B. and Matsson, L. (1994). Marginal bone loss in the primary dentition. A survey of 7–9-year-old children in Sweden. *Journal of Clinical Periodontology*, **21**, 313–19.

12

Traumatic injuries to the teeth

12 Traumatic injuries to the teeth

R. R. Welbury and J. M. Whitworth

12.1 EPIDEMIOLOGY

Dental trauma in childhood and adolescence is common (Fig. 12.1). At 5 years of age 31–40% of boys and 16–30% of girls, and at 12 years of age 12–33% of boys and 4–19% of girls will have suffered some dental trauma. Boys are affected almost twice as often as girls in both the primary and the permanent dentitions.

The majority of dental injuries in the primary and permanent dentitions involve the anterior teeth, especially the maxillary central incisors. Concussion, subluxation, and luxation are the commonest injuries in the primary dentition (Fig. 12.2), while uncomplicated crown fractures are commonest in the permanent dentition (Fig. 12.3). Prognosis of traumatic injuries has improved significantly in the last 20 years. This has been largely due to a greater understanding and knowledge of pulpal procedures.

12.2 AETIOLOGY

The most accident prone times are between 2 and 4 years for the primary dentition and 7 and 10 years for the permanent dentition. In the primary dentition co-ordination and judgement are incompletely developed and the majority of injuries are due to falls in and around the home as the child becomes more adventurous and explores its surroundings. In the permanent dentition most injuries are caused by falls and collisions while playing and running, although bicycles are a common accessory. The place of injury varies in different countries according to local customs but accidents in the school yard remain common. Sports injuries usually occur in teenage years and are commonly associated with contact sports. Injuries due to road traffic accidents and assaults are most commonly associated with the late teenage years and adulthood and are often closely related to alcohol abuse.

One form of injury in childhood that must never be forgotten is child physical abuse or non-accidental injury (NAI). More than 50% of these children will have orofacial injuries (Fig. 12.4).

Dental injuries can be the result of either direct or indirect trauma. Direct trauma occurs when the tooth itself is struck. Indirect trauma is seen when the lower dental arch is forcefully closed against the upper, for example, blow to chin. Direct trauma implies injuries to the anterior region while indirect trauma favours crown or crown–root fractures in the premolar and molar regions as well as the possibility of jaw fractures in the condylar regions and symphysis. The factors which influence the outcome or type of injury are a combination of: (1) energy impact; (2) resilience of impacting object; (3) shape of impacting object; and (4) angle of direction of the impacting force.

Increased overjet with protrusion of upper incisors and insufficient lip closure are significant predisposing factors to traumatic dental injuries. Injuries are almost twice as frequent among children with protruding incisors and the number of teeth affected in a particular incident for an individual patient also increase.

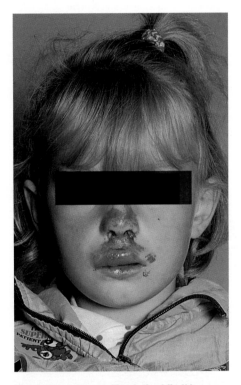

Fig. 12.1 A 7-year-old girl who fell off her bicycle and sustained orofacial injuries.

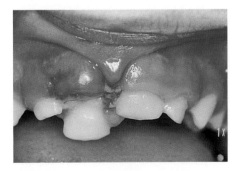

Fig. 12.2 A 3-year-old child with a combination of injuries to her upper anterior teeth.

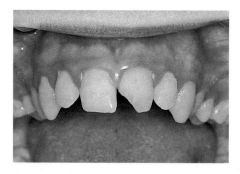

Fig. 12.3 A fracture of the upper left central incisor involving enamel and dentine.

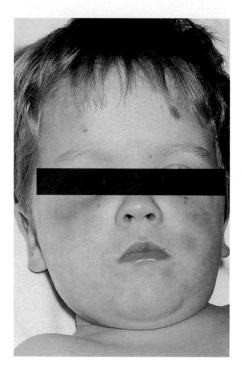

Fig. 12.4 A 3-year-old boy with bruises and abrasions resulting from non-accidental injury.

12.3 CLASSIFICATION

Table 12.1 summarizes the classification of dento-alveolar injuries based on the World Health Organization (WHO) system.

12.4 HISTORY AND EXAMINATION

A history of the injury followed by a thorough examination should be completed in any situation.

12.4.1 Dental history

1. When did injury occur? The time interval between injury and treatment significantly influences the prognosis of avulsions, luxations, crown fractures with or without pulpal exposures, and dento-alveolar fractures.
2. Where did injury occur? May indicate the need for tetanus prophylaxis.
3. How did injury occur? The nature of the accident can yield information on the type of injury expected. Discrepancy between history and clinical findings raises suspicion of physical abuse.
4. Lost teeth/fragments? If a tooth or fractured piece cannot be accounted for when there has been a history of loss of consciousness then a chest radiograph should be obtained to exclude inhalation.
5. Concussion, headache, vomiting or amnesia? Brain damage must be excluded and referral to a hospital for further investigation organized.
6. Previous dental history? Previous trauma can affect pulpal sensibility tests and the recuperative capacity of the pulp and/or periodontium. Alternatively are there suspicions of physical abuse? Previous treatment experience, age, and parental/child attitude will affect the choice of treatment.

12.4.2 Medical history

1. Congenital heart disease, a history of rheumatic fever or severe immunosuppression? These may be contra-indications to any procedure that is likely to require prolonged endodontic treatment with a persistent necrotic/infected focus. All congenital heart defects do not carry the same risks of bacterial endocarditis and the child's paediatrician/cardiologist should be consulted before a decision regarding endodontic treatment is made.
2. Bleeding disorders? Very important if soft tissues are lacerated or teeth are to be extracted.
3. Allergies? Penicillin allergy requires alternative antibiotics.
4. Tetanus immunization status? Referral for tetanus toxoid injection is necessary if there is soil contamination of the wound and the child has not had a 'booster' injection within the last 5 years.

12.4.3 Extraoral examination

When there are associated severe injuries a general examination is made with respect to signs of shock (pallor, cold skin, irregular pulse, hypotension), symptoms of head injury suggesting brain concussion, or maxillofacial fractures.

Facial swelling, bruises, or lacerations may indicate underlying bony and tooth injury. Lacerations will require careful debridement to remove all foreign material and suturing. Antibiotics and/or tetanus toxoid may be required if wounds are

Table 12.1   Classification of the nature of dentoalveolar injuries

Injuries to the hard dental tissues and the pulp	
Enamel infraction	Incomplete fracture (crack) of enamel without loss of tooth substance
Enamel fracture	Loss of tooth substance confined to enamel
Enamel–dentine fracture	Loss of tooth substance confined to enamel and dentine not involving the pulp
Complicated crown fracture	Fracture of enamel and dentine exposing the pulp
Uncomplicated crown–root fracture	Fracture of enamel, dentine, and cementum but not involving the pulp
Complicated crown–root fracture	Fracture of enamel, dentine, and cementum and exposing the pulp
Root fracture	Fracture involving dentine, cementum, and pulp. Can be subclassified into: apical, middle and coronal (gingival) third
Injuries to the periodontal tissues	
Concussion	No abnormal loosening or displacement but marked reaction to percussion
Subluxation (loosening)	Abnormal loosening but no displacement
Extrusive luxation (partial avulsion)	Partial displacement of tooth from socket
Lateral luxation	Displacement other than axially with comminution or fracture of alveolar socket
Intrusive luxation	Displacement into alveolar bone with comminution or fracture of alveolar socket
Avulsion	Complete displacement of tooth from socket
Injuries to supporting bone	
Comminution of mandibular or maxillary alveolar socket wall	Crushing and compression of alveolar socket. Found in intrusive and lateral luxation injuries
Fracture of mandibular or maxillary alveolar socket wall	Fracture confined to facial or lingual/palatal socket wall
Fracture of mandibular or maxillary alveolar process	Fracture of the alveolar process which may or may not involve the tooth sockets
Fracture of mandible or maxilla	May or may not involve the alveolar socket
Injuries to gingiva or oral mucosa	
Laceration of gingiva or oral mucosa	Wound in the mucosa resulting from a tear
Contusion of gingiva or oral mucosa	Bruise not accompanied by a break in the mucosa, usually causing submucosal haemorrhage
Abrasion of gingiva or oral mucosa	Superficial wound produced by rubbing or scraping the mucosal surface

contaminated. Limitation of mandibular movement or mandibular deviation on opening or closing the mouth indicate either jaw fracture or dislocation.

Crown fracture with associated swollen lip and evidence of a penetrating wound suggests retention of tooth fragments within the lip. Clinical and radiographic examination should be undertaken (Fig. 12.5(a)–(d)).

12.4.4 Intraoral examination

This must be systematic and include the recording of:

1. Laceration, haemorrhage, and swelling of the oral mucosa and gingiva (Fig. 12.6). Any lacerations should be examined for tooth fragments or other foreign material. Lacerations of lips or tongue require suturing but those of the oral mucosa heal very quickly and may not need suturing.

2. Abnormalities of occlusion, tooth displacement, fractured crowns, or cracks in the enamel.

The following signs and reactions to tests are particularly helpful:

1. *Mobility.* Degree of mobility is estimated in a horizontal and a vertical direction. When several teeth move together 'enblock' a fracture of the alveolar process is suspected. Excessive mobility may also suggest root fracture or tooth displacement.

2. *Reaction to percussion.* In a horizontal and vertical direction and compared against a contralateral uninjured tooth. A duller note may indicate root fracture.

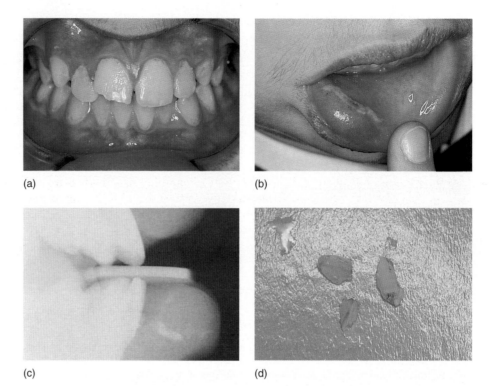

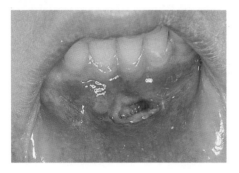

Fig. 12.5 (a) A 12-year-old child presented with an enamel and dentine fracture of the upper right, permanent central incisor. (b) The lower lip was swollen with a mucosal laceration. (c) A lateral radiograph confirmed the presence of tooth fragments in the lip. (d) Fragments were retrieved under local anaesthesia from the lip.

Fig. 12.6 Degloving injury to the lower labial sulcus that required exploration to remove grit.

3. *Colour of tooth.* Early colour change associated with pulp breakdown is visible on the palatal surface of the gingival third of the crown.

4. *Reaction to sensitivity tests.* Thermal tests with warm gutta percha or ethyl chloride (e.c.)are widely used. However, an electric pulp tester (e.p.t.) in the hands of an experienced operator is more reliable. Nevertheless, sensibility testing, especially in children is notoriously unreliable and should never be assessed in isolation from the other clinical and radiographic information. Neither negative nor positive responses should be trusted immediately after trauma. A positive response does not rule out later pulpal necrosis and a negative response while indicating pulpal damage does not necessarily indicate a necrotic pulp. The negative reaction is often due to a 'shock wave' effect damaging apical nerve supply. The pulp in such cases may have a normal blood supply. In all sensibility testing always include and document the reaction of uninjured contralateral teeth for comparison. In addition, all neighbouring teeth to the obviously injured teeth should be regularly assessed as they have probably suffered concussion injuries.

12.4.5 Radiographic examination

Periapical

Reproducible 'long cone technique' periapicals are the best for accurate diagnosis and clinical audit. Two radiographs at different angles may be essential to detect a root fracture. However, if access and co-operation are difficult then one anterior occlusal radiograph rarely misses a root fracture. Periapical films positioned behind lips can be used to detect foreign bodies.

Occlusal

To detect root fractures when used intaorally, and foreign bodies within the soft tissues when held by patient/helper at the side of the mouth in a lateral view (Fig. 12.5(c)).

Orthopantomogram

Essential in all trauma cases where underlying bony injury is suspected.

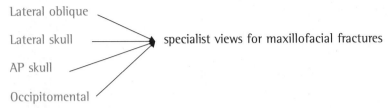

Lateral oblique

Lateral skull $\longrightarrow$ specialist views for maxillofacial fractures

AP skull

Occipitomental

In the patients clinical notes the clinical and radiographic examinations at each visit can be combined into a simple aide-memoir in the form of a 'trauma stamp' (Fig. 12.7). Information that is collected in this standardized way is easily accessible when making clinical decisions and comparing responses at review appointments.

Tooth eg.	12	11	21	22
Color				
Mobility				
t.t.p.				
e.c				
e.p.t				
Radiograph				

Fig. 12.7 The 'trauma stamp'.

12.4.6 Photographic records

Good clinical photographs are useful to assess outcome of treatment and for medico-legal purposes. Written consent must be obtained and in the case of digital images, uncropped originals held in an appropriately secure format and location.

> **Key Points**
>
> • Develop a systematic approach to history and examination

12.5 INJURIES TO THE PRIMARY DENTITION

During its early development the permanent incisor is located palatally to and in close proximity with the apex of the primary incisor. With any injury to a primary tooth there is risk of damage to the underlying permanent successor.

Most accidents in the primary dentition occur between 2 and 4 years of age. Realistically, this means that few restorative procedures will be possible and in the majority of cases the decision is between extraction or maintenance without performing extensive treatment. A primary incisor should always be removed if its maintenance will jeopardize the developing tooth bud.

A traumatized primary tooth that is retained should be assessed regularly for clinical and radiographic signs of pulpal or periodontal complications. Radiographs may even detect damage to the permanent successor. Soft tissue injuries in children should be assessed weekly until healed. Tooth injuries should be reviewed every 3–4 months for the first year and then annually until the primary tooth exfoliates and the permanent successor is in place.

Traumatic injuries that occur prior to eruption of primary teeth can also interfere with their development.

12.5.1 Uncomplicated crown fracture

Either smooth sharp edges or restore with an acid-etch restoration if co-operation is satisfactory.

12.5.2 Complicated crown fracture

Normally, extraction is the treatment of choice. However, pulp extirpation and canal obturation with zinc oxide cement, followed by an acid-etch restoration is possible with reasonable co-operation.

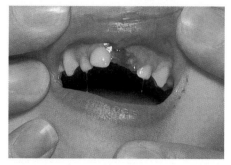

(a)

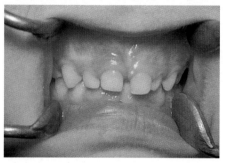

(b)

Fig. 12.8　(a) A 4-year-old boy with complete intrusion of the upper right incisor. (b) 6 months post-trauma, the tooth has spontaneously re-erupted.

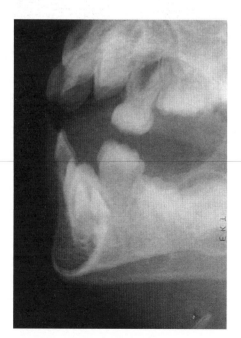

Fig. 12.9　Severe intrusion of an upper primary central incisor necessitating extraction.

12.5.3 Crown-root fracture

The pulp is usually exposed and any restorative treatment is very difficult. The tooth is best extracted.

12.5.4 Root fracture

Without displacement and with only a small amount of mobility the tooth should be kept under observation. If the coronal fragment becomes non-vital and symptomatic then it should be removed. The apical portion usually remains vital and undergoes normal resorption. Similarly with marked displacement and mobility only the coronal portion should be removed.

12.5.5 Concussion, subluxation, and luxation injuries

Associated soft tissue damage should be cleaned by the parent twice daily with 0.2% chlorhexidine solution using cotton buds or gauze swabs until it heals.

Concussion

Often not brought to a dentist until the tooth discolours.

Subluxation

If slight mobility then the parents are advised on a soft diet for 1–2 weeks and to keep the traumatized area as clean as possible. Marked mobility requires extraction.

Extrusive luxation

Marked mobility requires extraction.

Lateral luxation

If the crown is displaced palatally the apex moves buccally and hence away from the permanent tooth germ. If the occlusion is not gagged then conservative treatment to await some spontaneous realignment is possible. If the crown is displaced buccally then the apex will be displaced towards the permanent tooth bud and extraction is indicated in order to minimize further damage to the permanent successor.

Intrusive luxation

This is the most common type of injury. The aim of investigation is to establish the direction of displacement by thorough radiological examination. If the root is displaced palatally towards the permanent successor then the primary tooth should be extracted to minimize the possible damage to the developing permanent successor. If the root is displaced buccally then periodic review to monitor spontaneous re-eruption should be allowed (Fig. 12.8(a) and (b)). Review should be weekly for a month then monthly for a maximum of 6 months. Most re-eruption occurs between 1 and 6 months and if this does not occur then ankylosis is likely and extraction is necessary to prevent ectopic eruption of the permanent successor (Fig. 12.9).

Exarticulation (Avulsion)

Replantation of avulsed primary incisors is not recommended due to the risk of damage to the permanent tooth germs. Space maintenance is not necessary following the loss of a primary incisor as only minor drifting of adjacent teeth occurs. The eruption of the permanent successor may be delayed for about 1 year as a result of abnormal thickening of connective tissue overlying the tooth germ.

12.6 SEQUELAE OF INJURIES TO THE PRIMARY DENTITION

12.6.1 Pulpal necrosis

Necrosis is the commonest complication of primary trauma. Evaluation is based upon colour and radiography. Teeth of a normal colour rarely develop periapical inflammation but conversely mildly discoloured teeth may be vital. A mild grey colour occurring soon after trauma may represent intrapulpal bleeding with a pulp that is still vital. This colour may recede, but if it persists then necrosis should be suspected. Radiographic examination should be 3 monthly to check for periapical inflammation (Fig. 12.10(a) and (b)). Failure of the pulp cavity to reduce in size is an indicator of pulpal death. Teeth should be extracted whenever there is evidence of periapical inflammation, to prevent possible damage to the permanent successor.

12.6.2 Pulpal obliteration

Obliteration of the pulp chamber and canal is a common reaction to trauma (Fig. 12.11). Clinically, the tooth becomes yellow/opaque. Normal exfoliation is usual but occasionally periapical inflammation may intervene and therefore annual radiography is advisable.

12.6.3 Root resorption

Extraction is advised for all types of root resorption where there is evidence of infection (Fig. 12.12).

12.6.4 Injuries to developing permanent teeth

Injuries to the permanent successor tooth can be expected in between 12% to 69% of primary tooth trauma and 19% to 68% of jaw fractures. Intrusive luxation causes most disturbances but avulsion of a primary incisor will also cause damage if the apex moved towards the permanent tooth bud before the avulsion. Most damage to

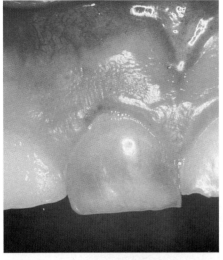

(a)

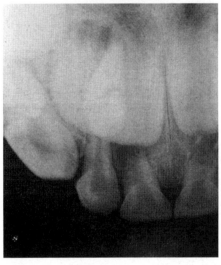

(b)

Fig. 12.10 (a) Severe discolouration of the upper right primary central incisor. (b) Radiographic evidence of periapical pathology. Extraction was necessary.

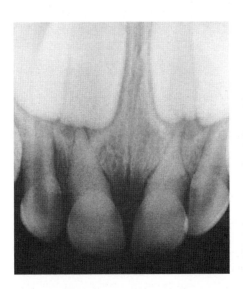

Fig. 12.11 Pulp canal obliteration and external surface resorption of upper primary central incisors after a luxation injury.

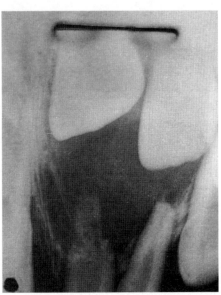

Fig. 12.12 External inflammatory resorption of previously injured primary incisors.

the permanent tooth bud occurs under 3 years of age during its developmental stage. However, the type and severity of disturbance are closely related to the age at the time of injury. Changes in the mineralization and morphology of the crown of the permanent incisor are commonest but later injuries can cause radicular anomalies. Injuries to developing teeth can be classified as follows:

1. White or yellow-brown hypomineralization of enamel. Injury at 2–7 years (Fig. 12.13(a)–(c)).

2. White or yellow-brown hypominerlaization of enamel with circular enamel hypoplasia. Injury at 2–7 years (Fig. 12.14).

3. Crown dilaceration. Injury at about 2 years (Fig. 12.15(a)–(c)).

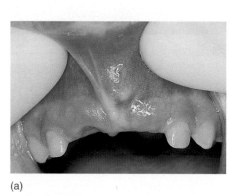

(a)

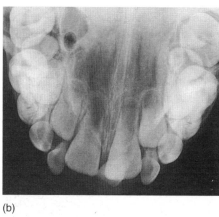

(b)

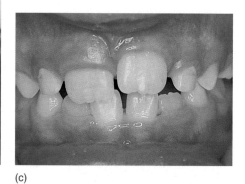

(c)

Fig. 12.13 (a)–(c) Investigation of delayed eruption of the permanent upper central incisors revealed an intruded upper left primary central incisor on radiograph. Following removal of the retained primary incisor the permanent successor erupted spontaneously with a white hypoplastic spot on the labial surface.

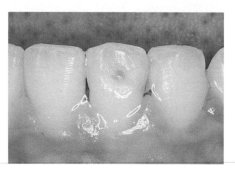

Fig. 12.14 Brown hypoplastic area on the lower left permanent central incisor resulting from trauma to the primary predecessor.

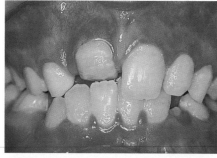

(a)

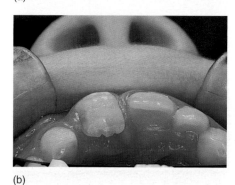

(b)

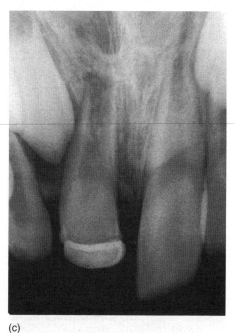

(c)

Fig. 12.15 (a)–(c) Severe crown dilaceration of the upper right permanent central incisor which erupted spontaneously.

4. Odontoma-like malformation. Injury at <1–3 years.
5. Root duplication. Injury at 2–5 years.
6. Vestibular or lateral root angulation and dilaceration. Injury at 2–5 years (Fig. 12.16(a) and (b)).
7. Partial or complete arrest of root formation. Injury at 5–7 years (Fig. 12.17(a) and (b)).
8. Sequestration of permanent tooth germs.
9. Disturbance in eruption.

The term dilaceration describes an abrupt deviation of the long axis of the crown or root portion of the tooth. This deviation results from the traumatic displacement of already formed hard tissue in relation to developing soft tissue.

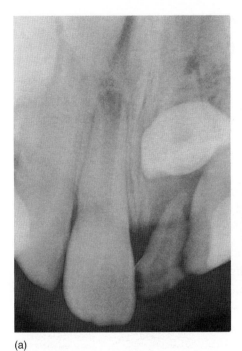

(a)

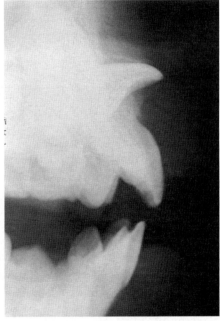

(b)

Fig. 12.16 (a) and (b) Unerupted, dilacerated, upper left permanent central incisor resulting from an accident sustained by a 3-year-old child.

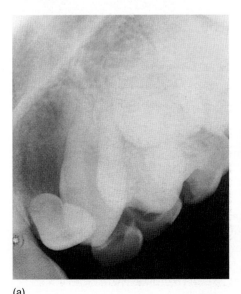

(a)

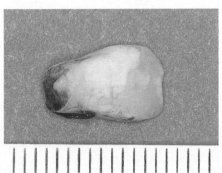

(b)

Fig. 12.17 (a) and (b) Failure of root formation of the upper left permanent lateral incisor in a 5-year-old child with a history of intrusive trauma to the primary predecessor.

The term angulation describes a curvature of the root resulting from a gradual change in the direction of root development, without evidence of abrupt displacement of the tooth germ during odontogenesis. This may be vestibular, that is, labiopalatal, or lateral, that is, mesiodistal.

Evaluation of the full extent of complications following injuries must await complete eruption of all permanent teeth involved. However, most serious sequelae (disturbances in tooth morphology) can usually be diagnosed radiographically within the first year post-trauma.

Eruption disturbances may involve delay due to connective tissue thickening over a permanent tooth germ, ectopic eruption due to lack of eruptive guidance, and impaction in teeth with malformations of crown or root.

Key Points

In primary tooth trauma:
- Risk of damage to permanent successors is high—warn parents
- Intrusive injuries carry the highest risk to the permanent successors

12.6.5 Treatment of injuries to the permanent dentition

Yellow-brown hypomineralization of enamel with or without hypoplasia

1. Acid-pumice microabrasion.
2. Composite resin restoration: localized, veneer, or crown.
3. Porcelain restoration: veneer or crown (anterior); fused to metal crown (posterior). Conservative approaches are preferred whenever possible.

Crown dilaceration

1. Surgical exposure + orthodontic realignment.
2. Removal of dilacerated part of crown.
3. Temporary crown until root formation complete.
4. Semi or permanent restoration.

Vestibular root angulation

Combined surgical and orthodontic realignment.

Other malformation

Extraction is usually the treatment of choice.

Disturbance in eruption

Surgical exposure + orthodontic realignment.

Injuries to supporting bone

Most fractures of the alveolar socket in primary dentition do not require splinting due to rapid bony healing in small children. Jaw fractures are treated in the conventional manner, although stabilization after reduction may be difficult due to lack of sufficient adjacent teeth.

12.7 INJURIES TO THE PERMANENT DENTITION

Most traumatized teeth can be treated successfully. Prompt and appropriate treatment improves prognosis. The aims and principles of treatment can be broadly categorized into:

1. Emergency:
   (a) retain vitality of fractured or displaced tooth;
   (b) treat exposed pulp tissue;
   (c) reduction and immobilization of displaced teeth;
   (d) antiseptic mouthwash, $+/-$ antibiotics and tetanus prophylaxis.
2. Intermediate:
   (a) + pulp therapy;
   (b) minimally invasive crown restoration.
3. Permanent:
   (a) apexogenesis/apexification;
   (b) root filling + root extrusion;
   (c) + gingival and alveolar collar modification;
   (d) semi or permanent coronal restoration.

Trauma cases require painstaking follow up to identify any complications and institute the correct treatment. The 'trauma stamp' is invaluable in this. In the review period the following schedule is a guide: 1 week; 1, 3, 6, and 12 months; and then annually for 4–5 years.

12.7.1 Injuries to the hard dental tissues and the pulp

Enamel infraction

These incomplete fractures without loss of tooth substance and without proper illumination are easily overlooked. Review is necessary as above as the energy of the blow may have been transmitted to the periodontal tissues or the pulp.

Enamel fracture

No restoration is needed and treatment is limited to smoothing of any rough edges and splinting if there is associated mobility. Periodic review as above.

Enamel–dentine (uncomplicated) fracture

Immediate treatment is necessary and the pulp requires protection against thermal osmotic irritation and from bacteria via the dentinal tubules. Restoration of crown morphology also stabilizes the position of the tooth in the arch.

Emergency protection of the exposed dentine can be achieved by:

1. A composite resin (acid etched) or Compomer bandage
2. Glass ionomer cement within an orthodontic band or incisal end of a stainless-steel crown if there is insufficient enamel available for acid-etch technique.

Intermediate restoration of most enamel–dentine fractures can be achieved by:

1. Acid-etched composite either applied freehand or utilizing a celluloid crown former. The majority of these restorations can be regarded as semi-permanent/permanent. Larger fractures can utilize more available enamel surface area for bonding by employing a complete celluloid crown former to construct a 'direct'

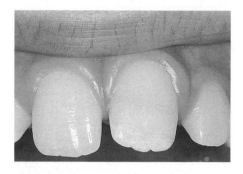

Fig. 12.18   An upper left permanent central incisor 3 years after reattachment of a fractured incisal fragment.

composite crown. At a later age this could be reduced to form the core of a full or partial coverage porcelain crown preparation.

2. Reattachment of crown fragment. Few long-term studies have been reported and the longevity of this type of restoration is uncertain. In addition, there is a tendency for the distal fragment to become opaque or require further restorative intervention in the form of a veneer or full coverage crown (Fig. 12.18). If the fracture line through dentine is not very close to the pulp then the fragment may be reattached immediately. If, however, it runs close to the pulp then it is advisable to place a suitably protected calcium hydroxide dressing over the exposed dentine for at least 1 month while storing the fragment in saline, which should be renewed weekly.

Technique

1. Check the fit of the fragment and the vitality of the tooth.
2. Clean fragment and tooth with pumice-water slurry.
3. Isolate the tooth with rubber dam.
4. Attach fragment to a piece of sticky wax to facilitate handling.
5. Etch enamel for 30 s on both fracture surfaces and extend for 2 mm from fracture line on tooth and fragment. Wash for 15 s and dry for 15 s.
6. Apply bonding agent +/− dentine primer according to manufacturer's instructions and light cure for 10 s.
7. Place appropriate shade of composite resin over both surfaces and position fragment. Remove gross excess and cure 60 s labially and palatally.
8. Remove any excess composite resin with sandpaper discs.
9. Remove a 1-mm gutter of enamel on each side of fracture line both labially and palatally to a depth of 0.5 mm using a small round or pear-shaped bur. The finishing line should be irregular in outline.
10. Etch the newly prepared enamel, wash, dry, apply composite, cure, and finish.

Enamel–dentine–pulp (complicated) crown fracture

The most important function of the pulp is to lay down dentine which forms the basic structure of teeth, defines their general morphology, and provides them with mechanical strength and toughness. Dentine deposition commences many years before permanent tooth eruption and when a tooth erupts the pulp within still has work to do in completing root development. Newly erupted teeth have short roots, their apices are wide and often diverging, and the dentine walls of the entire tooth are thin and relatively weak (Fig. 12.19(a)). Provided the pulp remains healthy, dentine deposition and normal root development will continue for 2–3 years after eruption in permanent teeth (Fig. 12.19(b)). Loss of pulp vitality before a tooth has reached maturity may leave the tooth vulnerable to fracture, and with an unfavourable crown–root ratio. In addition endodontic treatment of non-vital, immature teeth can also present technical difficulties which may compromise the long-term prognosis of the tooth.

The major concern after pulpal exposures in immature teeth is the prevention of physical, chemical, and microbial invasion and the preservation of pulpal vitality in order to allow continued root growth. The radicular pulp has enormous capacity to remain healthy and undergo repair if all infected and inflamed coronal tissue is removed and an appropriate wound dressing and sealing coronal restoration is applied. Pulp amputation by partial pulpotomy or complete coronal pulpotomy is often the treatment of choice but pulp capping can be considered in certain circumstances.

Vital pulp therapy

- Pulp capping
- Pulpotomy ⟨ partial
                complete

Non-vital pulp therapy

- Pulpectomy

VITAL PULP THERAPY—PULP CAPPING

The procedure must be done within 24 h of the incident. The tooth should be isolated with rubber dam and no instruments should be inserted into the exposure site. Any bleeding should be controlled with sterile cotton wool which may be moistened with saline or sodium hypochlorite, and not with a blast of air from the 3 in 1 syringe which may drive debris and micro-organisms into the pulp. A layer of setting calcium hydroxide cement is gently flowed onto the exposed pulp and surrounding dentine quickly overlaid with a 'bandage' of adhesive material. for example, compomer pending definitive aesthetic restoration at a later date. A successful direct pulp cap will preserve the remaining pulp in health and should promote the deposition of a bridge of reparative dentine to seal off the exposure site.

Review after a month, then 3 months, and eventually at 6 monthly intervals for up to 4 years in order to assess pulp vitality. Periodic radiographic review should also be arranged to monitor dentine bridge formation, root growth, and to exclude the development of necrosis and resorption. On the radiograph check the following:

- root is growing in length;
- root canal is maturing (narrowing);
- Compare with antimere.

If growth is not occuring the pulp should be assumed to be non-vital.

VITAL PULP THERAPY—PULPOTOMY

In pulpotomy a portion of exposed vital pulp is removed to preserve the radicular vitality and allow completion of apical root development (apexogenesis) and further deposition of dentine on the walls of the root. This procedure is the treatment of choice following trauma where the pulp has been exposed to the mouth for more than 24 h.

Operative procedure (Fig. 12.20)

- Under local anaesthesia and rubber dam, pulp tissue is excised with a diamond bur running at high speed under constant water cooling. This causes least injury to the underlying pulp and is preferred to hand excavation or the use of slow-speed steel burs.
- Microbial invasion of an exposed, vital pulp is usually superficial and generally only 2–3 mm of pulp tissue should be removed (partial pulpotomy [Cvek]).
- Excessive bleeding from the residual pulp which cannot be controlled with moist cotton wool, or indeed no bleeding at all, indicates that further excision is required to reach healthy tissue (coronal pulpotomy).
- Removal of tissue may occasionally extend more deeply into the tooth (full coronal pulpotomy) in an effort to preserve the apical portion of the pulp and safeguard apical closure.
- Gently rinse the wound with sterile saline or sodium hypochlorite (1–2%)and remove any shredded tissue. All remaining tags of tissue in the coronal portion must be removed as they may act as a nidus for re-infection, and a pathway for coronal leakage.

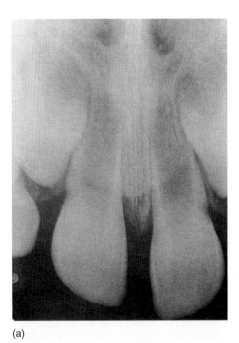

(a)

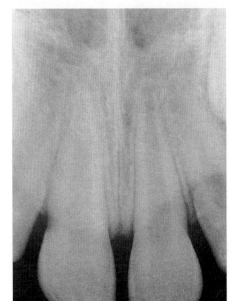

(b)

Fig. 12.19 Maturation of permanent incisors. (a) Immature incisors showing short roots with incomplete, wide-open apices. The lateral walls of the roots are thin and structurally weak. (b) The same teeth 2 years later, the roots are now almost complete following continued dentine deposition by healthy pulp.

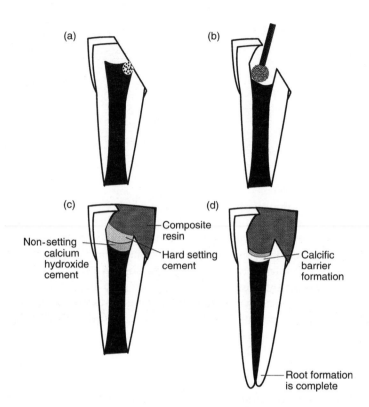

Fig. 12.20 Pulp amputation (apexogenesis procedure) of a permanent incisor. (a) Complicated fracture of an immature incisor with microbial invasion of the coronal pulp. The pulp has been exposed to the mouth for more than 24 h. (b) Access to the coronal pulp and amputation of coronal pulp tissue with a diamond bur running at high speed with constant water cooling. (c) Dressing the pulpal wound to promote calcific repair. Non-setting calcium hydroxide cement is flowed on to the pulp, then overlaid with a hard cement, and the tooth restored with composite resin. (d) The same tooth after 12 months showing calcific barrier formation. The calcific barrier was directly inspected in this case, (not always required), and a new layer of setting calcium hydroxide cement placed on the barrier before definitive restoration. The remaining pulp has stayed healthy and deposited dentine to complete root formation.

- Apply a calcium hydroxide dressing to the pulp to destroy any remaining micro-organisms and to promote calcific repair. In superficial wounds, a setting calcium hydroxide cement may be gently flowed onto the pulp surface, but if the excision was deep, it is often easier to prepare a stiff mixture of calcium hydroxide powder (analytical grade) in sterile saline or local anaesthetic solution, which is carried to the canal in an amalgam carrier and gently packed into place with pluggers.

- Overlay the calcium hydroxide dressing with a hard cement to prevent its forceful injection into the pulp by chewing forces and a final adhesive restoration which will seal the preparation against the re-entry of micro-organisms.

REVIEW

- after a month,
- 3 months,
- 6 monthly intervals for up to 4 years in order to assess pulp vitality,
- periodic radiographic review should also be arranged to monitor dentine bridge formation, root growth, and to exclude the development of necrosis and resorption. If vitality is lost, non-vital pulp therapy should be undertaken whether or not there is a calcific bridge (see below),
- success rates for partial (Cvek) pulpotomies are quoted at 97%. Those for coronal pulpotomies at 75%.

Elective pulpectomy and root canal treatment of a vital pulp may be considered at a later date only if the root canal is required for restorative purposes.

Key Point

Pulpotomy procedures

- Give a better prognosis than pulp capping for small exposures exposed for more than 24 h,
- are not recommended if there are signs and symptoms of radicular pathosis.

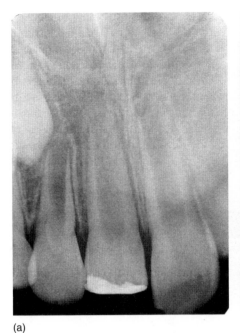
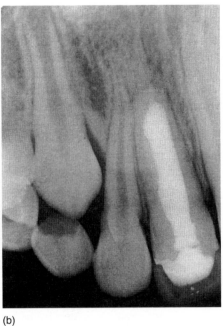

(a)   (b)

Fig. 12.21 Root-end closure (apexification). (a) Immature, permanent central incisor devitalized by trauma. (b) The same tooth 18 months later. Canal debridement and calcium hydroxide therapy has allowed the development of an apical calcific barrier. The canal has been densely obturated with thermoplastic gutta percha and sealer.

NON-VITAL PULP THERAPY—PULPECTOMY

Premature loss of pulp vitality leaves a thin and relatively weak tooth structure which should not be weakened further by excessive dentine removal during canal preparation. The open and often diverging apices of immature permanent teeth create technical difficulties for the controlled condensation of root filling materials, and a root end closure (apexification) procedure is usually required to produce an apical calcific barrier against which filling materials may be packed (Fig. 12.21). The most important pre-condition for calcific barrier formation is the elimination of micro-organisms from the root canal system by thorough canal debridement and the long-term application of a non-toxic, antimicrobial medicament such as non-setting calcium hydroxide.

Traditional root end closure of this sort may take 9–24 months before definitive canal obturation and restoration is possible.

Operative procedure (Fig. 12.22)

- Access with a high-speed, medium tapered fissure bur. In the pulp chamber use safe-ended burs to remove the entire roof without the danger of overcutting or perforation.
- Remove loose debris from the pulp chamber with hand instruments, accompanied by copious, gentle irrigation with sodium hypochlorite solution (1–2%).
- Gates Glidden drills may be used to improve access to canals for instruments and irrigant. They should not be used deep in the canals of immature teeth where they may overcut and create a strip perforation.
- Canal preparation involves two processes: *cleaning* with irrigants to free the root canal system of organic debris, micro-organisms and their toxins; and *shaping* with enlarging instruments, to modify the form of the existing canal to allow the placement of a well-condensed root filling. In canals which are often as wide as this, little dentine removal and shaping is needed. Sodium hypochlorite solution (1–2%) as an irrigant will continue dissolving organic debris and killing micro-organisms deep in the canal.
- Working apically, files are directed around the canal walls with a light rasping action to remove adherent debris. Instrumentation is frequently punctuated by high-volume, low-pressure irrigation to flush out debris.

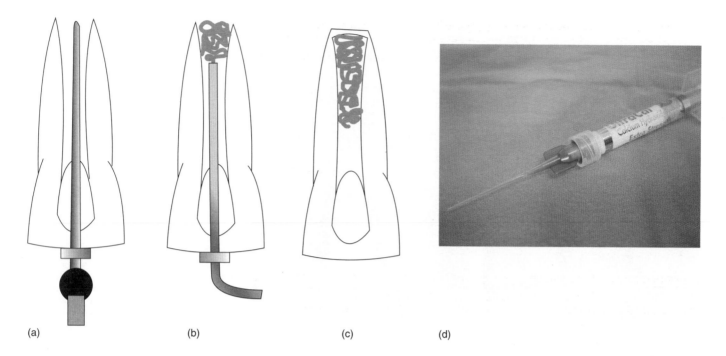

(a)   (b)   (c)   (d)

Fig. 12.22 (a) Following irrigation and gentle debridement in a crown-to-apex direction, the working length is determined. (b) Non-setting calcium hydroxide paste is syringed into the canal via a flexible tip. (c) The same tooth 18 months later. A calcific barrier is apparent, and the tooth is ready for definitive obturation and restoration. (d) The flexible tip system (Ultracal).

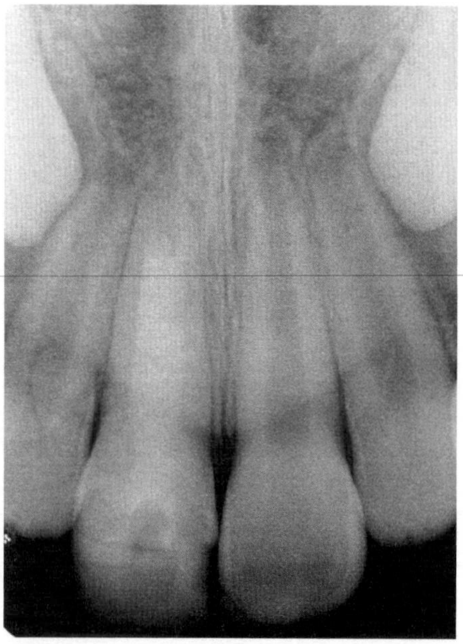

- Irrigant is delivered either by pre-measured, 27 gauge needle and syringe or with the aid of sonic/ultrasonic energy. The latter involves flooding the canal with irrigant before inserting a small (size 16–20) file attached to a sonic/ultrasonic unit to stir the irrigant in the canal. Wall contact with the file should be avoided, as the action is liable to cause turbulence in the irrigant which scrubs the walls of debris.

- Provisional working length should be 2–3 mm from the radiographic apex, estimated from an undistorted pre-operative periapical film. A working length radiograph is then taken to establish a definitive working length 1 mm short of the radiographic root apex. Further gentle filing and irrigation is then continued to the definitive working length.

- Dry canal with pre-measured paper points to avoid inadvertent over-extension and damage to the periapical tissues.

- Fill canal with a relatively fluid proprietary calcium hydroxide paste such as Ultracal (Optident, UK. This may be syringed into the canal via a disposable flexible tip (Fig. 12.22d) or alternatively spun into the canal with a spiral paste filler. The antimicrobial and mild tissue solvent activity of non-setting calcium hydroxide will continue to cleanse the canal, and its high pH is believed to encourage calcific root end closure.

- A radiograph may be taken to ensure a dense fill to each root terminus (Fig. 12.23).

- Seal access cavity tightly between appointments to prevent the leaching of calcium hydroxide, and critically, to prevent the re-entry of micro-organisms from the mouth which would disturb the process of root end closure. A 3 mm thickness of glass ionomer cement or composite resin is adequate to provide a bacteria-tight seal. Cotton-wool fibres should not be allowed to remain at the cavo-surface of the cavity.

REVIEW

- 3 monthly to monitor root end closure. At each appointment the calcium hydroxide dressing is carefully washed from the canal and the presence of a calcified barrier assessed by gently tapping a pre-measured paper point at the working length.

- Radiographs should be taken to assess the progress of barrier formation.

Fig. 12.23 Radiograph to confirm dense obliteration of the prepared canal with non-setting calcium hydroxide paste.

- If the canal is closed, obturation may proceed. If calcific barrier formation is not complete, the canal should be redressed for a further 3 months. Calcific barrier formation is usually complete within 9–18 months, but could take up to 2 years.

Key Point

Root-end closure

- Gives predictable results if infection is controlled and canal sealed bacteria-tight;
- Infection is controlled by irrigation and disinfection;
- Canal is enlarged enough only to allow irrigant access and dense obturation;
- Adds nothing to the strength of the tooth;
- Coronal restoration is critical to long-term success.

Techniques for obturation

Obturation with gutta percha and sealer prevent the re-entry of oral micro-organisms to the apical tissues. Cold lateral condensation of gutta percha and sealer may provide satisfactory results in regular, apically converging canals, but in irregular and diverging canals, a thermoplastic gutta percha technique is required to improve adaptation. The use of single cone techniques cannot be recommended in any circumstance.

Manual obturation in apically divergent canal (Fig. 12.24(a)–(c)).

- Select a master point and try into the canal. This is usually the widest point which will reach the canal terminus, and may be inverted in the widest canals.
- Dry the canal and lightly coat its walls with a slow setting sealer.
- Soften the tip of the master point by passage through a bunsen burner flame. Insert the point to the apical limit of the canal and press gently against the calcific barrier to adapt the softened gutta percha.
- Cold lateral condensation with a spreader to within 1 mm of the apical limit of the canal adding accessory gutta percha cones lightly coated with sealer. Continue condensation until the spreader can advance no more than 2 or 3 mm into the canal.
- Check radiograph to assess the quality of fill before removing excess gutta percha with a hot instrument and vertically condensing the warm gutta percha at the canal entrance. Further cold or warm condensation may be undertaken at this stage if required to obtain a uniformly dense obturation.

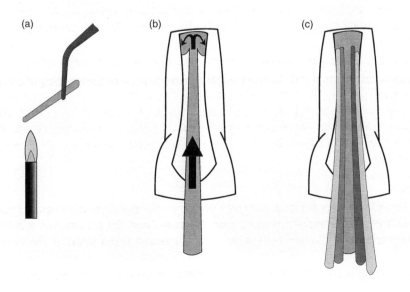

(a)   (b)   (c)

Fig. 12.24 Obturation following root-end closure in an apically diverging canal. (a) The widest gutta percha point that will reach the apical terminus of the canal is warmed by passage of its tip through a flame. (b) Without delay, the point is introduced to the canal (the canal is already lightly coated with sealer), and advanced to adapt against the apical barrier. (c) Additional points are now packed around the master point with cold or warm condensation until the canal is densely filled.

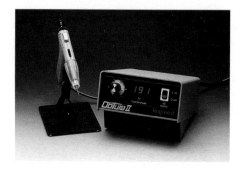

Fig. 12.25 Obtura II. Low-temperature, injection-moulded, thermoplastic gutta percha.

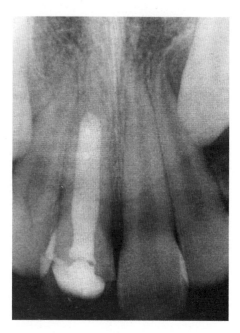

Fig. 12.26 Rapid, dense obturation of a wide and irregularly shaped canal with injection-moulded, thermoplastic gutta percha and sealer.

Thermoplastic obturation (Figs 12.25 and 12.26).

Warm gutta percha techniques offer the possibility of extremely rapid and dense obturation of the most irregularly shaped spaces.

- Dry the canal and lightly coat its walls with a slow setting sealer;
- Inject thermoplastic gutta percha into the apical portion of the canal and condense;
- Radiograph to check apical GP is in the correct place;
- Back-fill with GP and seal access cavity with an adhesive restoration.

While allowing dense and controlled canal obturation, the root-end closure procedure adds nothing to the canal wall thickness or mechanical strength of immature teeth. The final restoration should therefore be planned to optimize the durability of the remaining tooth structure. Dentine bonded composite resins may be particularly helpful in this regard, especially if extended several millimetres into the root canal to provide internal splinting. The advent of light-transmitting fibre posts opens new potential for rehabilitation and also provides a ready patency for canal re-entry if needed. Periodic clinical and radiographic review should be arranged.

Alternatives to the root-end closure procedure

- Recently the potential has arisen to seal open apices with mineral trioxide aggregate (MTA). Based on Portland building cement it is packed into the canal with pre-measured pluggers and sets to form a hard, sealing, biocompatible barrier within 4 h. Moist cotton wool is placed into the canal to promote setting and the material is checked after at least 24 h before filling the remainder of the canal with gutta percha and sealer, or with composite and a fibre post. Clinical studies are ongoing, but this material seems likely to allow root end closure in 1 or 2 visits which will demand less patient compliance (Fig. 12.27).

- When pulp vitality is lost in an almost fully formed tooth, it may be possible to avoid lengthy root-end closure procedures by creating an apical stop against which a root filling may be packed. Following crown to apex preparation as described above, endodontic hand files may be used in gentle watch-winding or balanced-force motion at working length to shave an apical seat for canal obturation. Alternatively,

Fig. 12.27 (a) Immature apex tooth 11. (b) Apical 'plug' of MTA and backfill with thermoplastic GP. (Courtesy of Professor M.S.Duggal.)

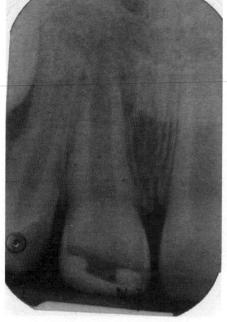

(a)

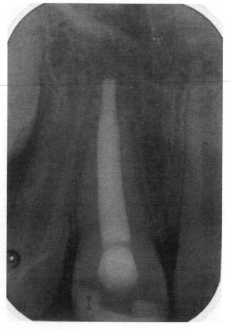

(b)

MTA can be packed into the apical 1–2 mm of the canal with pluggers to provide an immediate apical seal.

- Endodontic surgery with root-end filling is becoming less popular as a means of treatment in the case of non-closure. However, it may be considered to address problems of serious, irretrievable overfill which may arise if the calcific barrier was erroneously diagnosed as complete, or if the barrier was broken by heavy-handed obturation.

Uncomplicated crown-root fracture

After removal of the fractured piece of tooth these vertical fractures are commonly a few millimetres incisal to the gingival margin on the labial surface but down to the cemento-enamel junction palatally. Prior to placement of a restoration the fracture margin has to be brought supragingival either by gingivoplasty or extrusion (orthodontically or surgically) of the root portion.

Complicated crown-root fracture

As above with the addition of endodontic requirements. If extrusion is planned then the final root length must be no shorter than the final crown length otherwise the result will be unstable. Root extrusion can be successful in a motivated patient and leads to a stable periodontal condition.

Root fracture

Root fractures occur most frequently in the middle or the apical third of the root. The coronal fragment may be extruded or luxated. If displacement has occurred the coronal fragment should be repositioned as soon as possible by gentle digital manipulation and the position checked radiographically. Optimal repositioning favours both healing with hard tissue and reduces the risk of pulpal necrosis. Mobile root fractures need to be splinted to encourage repair of the fracture. With the possible exception of coronal third fractures which may require longer splinting periods, it appears that a period of 4 weeks with a semi-rigid or functional splint is sufficient to ensure healing. A functional splint is one that includes one abutment teeth on either side of the fractured tooth. Splinting for longer periods may be required in individual cases. The splint should allow colour observations and sensitivity testing and access to the root canal if endodontic treatment is required. The splint design and placement techniques are discussed in the next section on 'splinting'.
Three main categories of repair are recognized:

1. repair with calcified tissue: invisible or hardly discernible fracture line (Fig. 12.28(a)–(c));
2. repair with connective tissue: narrow radiolucent fracture line with peripheral rounding of the fracture edges (Fig. 12.29);
3. repair with bone and connective tissue: a bony bridge separates the two fragments (Fig. 12.30).

In addition to these changes in the fracture area, pulp canal obliteration is commonly seen. Fractures in the cervical third of the root will repair as long as no communication exists between the fracture line and the gingival crevice. If such a communication exists then splinting is not recommended and an early decision must be made either: to extract the coronal fragment and retain the remaining root; internally splint the root fracture; or extract the two fragments.

EXTRACTION OF CORONAL FRAGMENT AND ROOT RETENTION

The remaining radicular pulp should be removed and the canal temporarily dressed prior to obturating with gutta percha. Three options are now available for the root

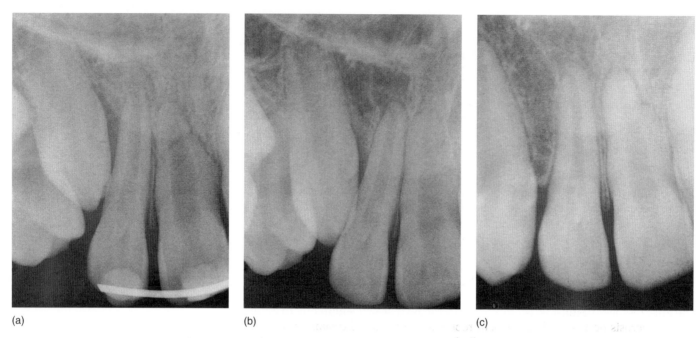

(a)   (b)   (c)

Fig. 12.28 (a) An apical third root fracture of the upper right permanent central incisor with a rigid splint. (b) Appearance of the fracture 15 months later. (c) Good calcified tissue repair evident 3 years' post-trauma.

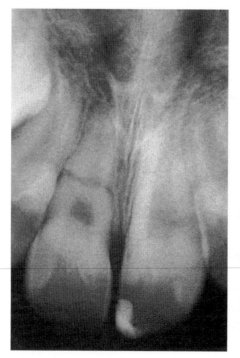

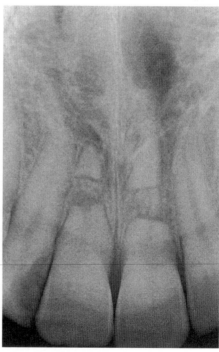

Fig. 12.29 Middle third root fracture of the upper right permanent central incisor with connective tissue repair.

Fig. 12.30 Middle third root fracture of both permanent central incisors with bony repair and sclerosis of the apical fragments.

treated radicular portion:

1. Post, core, and crown restoration if access is adequate.

2. Extrusion of root either surgically or orthodontically if the fracture extends too subgingivally for adequate access. Rapid orthodontic extrusion over 4–6 weeks aiming to move the root a maximum of 4 mm is the best option. This is achieved by cementing a 'J' hook made from 0.7-mm stainless steel wire into the canal and using elastic traction applied over an arch wire cemented between one

abutment tooth on either side of the injured tooth. Retention for one month at the end of movement is advised to prevent relapse (Fig. 12.31). If aesthetics are a particular concern then an orthodontic bracket can be bonded to a temporary crown made over the 'J' hook. The temporary crown length will need to be reduced as extrusion occurs (Fig. 12.32(a)–(d)).

3. Cover the root with a mucoperiosteal flap. This will maintain the height and width of the arch and will facilitate later placement of a single tooth implant.

INTERNAL SPLINTING

Fractures arising in the coronal and middle third of the root often result in excessive mobility of the coronal fragment and techniques have been described to internally splint the coronal and apical portions together with a rigid root filling material. Internal splints have ranged from hedstroem files to nickel–chromium points, screwed and cemented into position. These approaches are in effect single cone root filling procedures, and cannot be relied upon to give a long-term safeguard against the re-entry of oral micro-organisms to the canal and fracture line. Most are doomed to failure and other restorative options are preferred.

PULPAL NECROSIS IN ROOT FRACTURE

Pulpal necrosis occurs in about 20% of root fractures and is the main obstacle to adequate repair. The initial amount of displacement of the coronal portion rather than the level of the fracture or the presence of an open or closed apex is the most significant factor in determining future pulpal prognosis. Most cases of necrosis are diagnosed within 3 months of a root fracture. A persistent negative response to electric stimulation is usually confirmed on radiography by radiolucencies adjacent to the fracture line. The apical fragment almost always contains viable pulp tissue and invariably scleroses. Rarely it may require surgical removal.

In apical and middle third fractures any endodontic treatment is usually confined to the coronal fragment only. A barrier is achieved on the coronal aspect of the fracture line by preparation of a stop with non-setting calcium hydroxide or MTA, and the coronal canal is obturated with gutta percha. After completion of endodontic treatment, repair and union between the two fragments with connective tissue is a consistent finding.

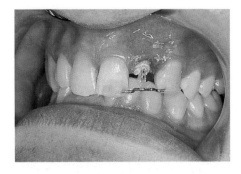

Fig. 12.31 Extrusive force being applied via a 'J' hook cemented into the root canal of the upper left permanent lateral incisor.

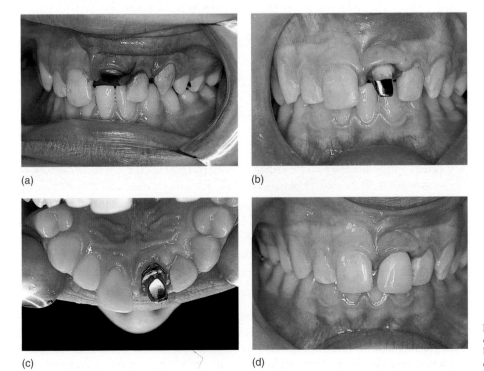

(a)

(b)

(c)

(d)

Fig. 12.32 (a) Initial presentation of a high coronal root fracture which extended palatally below alveolar bone. (b) and (c) Post, core, and diaphragm after root extrusion.

In coronal third fractures that develop necrosis either the radicular portion can be retained (see above), both portions extracted, or the fracture internally splinted (see above).

12.7.2 Splinting

Trauma may loosen a tooth either by damaging the periodontal ligament (p.l.) or fracturing the root. Splinting immobilizes the tooth in the correct anatomical position so that further trauma is prevented and healing can occur. Different injuries require different splinting regimens. A functional splint involves one, and a rigid splint two, abutment teeth either side of the injured tooth.

Regimens

P.L. INJURIES

Sixty per cent of p.l. healing has occurred after 10 days and it is complete within a month. The splinting period should be as short as possible and the splint should allow some functional movement to prevent replacement root resorption (ankylosis). As a general rule exarticulation (avulsion) injuries require 7–10 days and luxation injuries 2–3 weeks of functional splinting.

ROOT FRACTURES

These require 4 weeks of functional splinting. Individual cases may require longer splinting. Excessive mobility leads to the fracture site becoming filled with granulation tissue.

DENTOALVEOLAR FRACTURES

These require 3–4 weeks of rigid splinting.

Types and methods of constructing splints

COMPOSITE RESIN/ACRYLIC AND WIRE SPLINT

This method uses either a composite resin or a temporary crown material. The composite resin is easier to place but the acrylic resin is easier to remove. Although acrylic resin does not have the bond strength to enamel as the composite resin it is suitable for all types of functional splinting (Fig. 12.33).

Technique for a functional resin–wire splint:

1. Bend a flexible orthodontic wire to fit the middle third of the labial surface of the injured tooth and one abutment tooth either side.
2. Stabilize the injured tooth in the correct position with soft red wax palatally.
3. Clean the labial surfaces. Isolate, dry, and etch middle of crown of teeth with 37% phosphoric acid for 30 s, wash, and dry.
4. Apply 3-mm diameter circle either of unfilled then filled composite resin or of acrylic resin, to the centre of the crowns.
5. Position the wire into the filling material then apply more composite or acrylic resin.
6. Use a brush lubricated with unfilled composite resin to mould and smooth the composite. Acrylic resin is more difficult to handle and smoothing and excess removal can be done with a flat plastic instrument.
7. Cure the composite for 60 s. Wait for the acrylic resin to cure.
8. Smooth any sharp edges with sandpaper discs.

Figure 12.33 shows an example of a functional splint. For a rigid splint use the same technique but incorporate two abutment teeth on either side of the injured tooth. These splints should not impinge on the gingiva and should allow assessment of colour change and sensitivity testing.

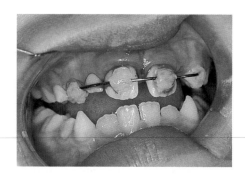

Fig. 12.33 Composite resin and wire splint for a luxation injury of both upper permanent central incisors.

ORTHODONTIC BRACKETS AND WIRE

For displacement injuries and exarticulations these splints have the advantage of allowing a more accurate reduction of the injury by gentle forces (Fig. 12.34(a and b)).

FOIL/CEMENT SPLINT

A temporary splint made of soft metal (cooking foil) and cemented with quick setting zinc oxide-eugenol cement is an effective temporary measure either during the night when it is difficult to fit a composite-wire splint as a single-handed operator or while awaiting construction of a laboratory made splint.

Technique:

1. Cut metal to size, long enough to extend over two or three teeth on each side of the injured tooth and wide enough to extend over the incisal edges and 3–4 mm over the labial and palatal gingiva.
2. Place foil over teeth and mould it over labial and palatal surfaces. Remove any excess.
3. Cement the foil to the teeth with quick setting zinc oxide–eugenol cement.

LABORATORY SPLINTS

(1) acrylic;
(2) thermoplastic.

These are used where it is impossible to make a satisfactory splint by the direct method, for example, a 7–8 year old with traumatized maxillary incisors, unerupted lateral incisors, and either carious or absent primary canines. Both methods require alginate impressions and very loose teeth may need to be supported by wax, metal foil, or wire ligature so they are not removed with the impression.

1. *Acrylic.* There is full palatal coverage and the acrylic is extended over the incisal edges for 2–3 mm of the labial surfaces of the anterior teeth. The occlusal surfaces of the posterior teeth should be covered to prevent any occlusal contact in the anterior region. This also aids retention and Adams Cribs may not be required. The splint should be removed for cleaning after meals and at bedtime.
2. *Thermoplastic.* The splint is constructed from polyvinylacetate–polyethylene (PVAC–PE) copolymer in the same way as a mouthguard with extension onto the mucosa. It should be removed like the acrylic splint after meals and at bedtime. However, with more severely loosened teeth it could be retained at night.

Both forms of laboratory splint allow functional movement and therefore promote normal periodontal healing. They are not suitable for root fractures as they compromise oral hygiene.

12.7.3 Injuries to the periodontal tissues

Concussion

The impact force causes oedema and haemorrhage in the p.l. and the tooth is tender to percussion (t.t.p.). There is no rupture of p.l. fibres and the tooth is firm in the socket.

Subluxation

In addition to the above there is rupture of some p.l. fibres and the tooth is mobile in the socket, although not displaced (Fig. 12.35). The treatment for both these injuries is:

(1) occlusal relief;
(2) soft diet for 7 days;

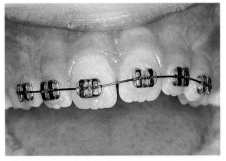

(a)

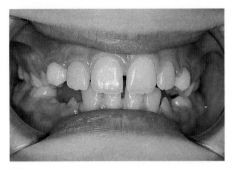

(b)

Fig. 12.34 (a) and (b) Gentle reduction and splinting of luxated upper right permanent central incisor.

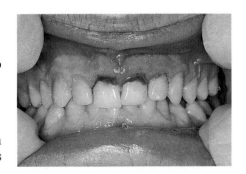

Fig. 12.35 Subluxated upper permanent central incisors.

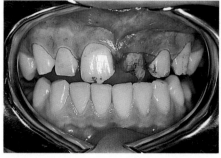

(a)

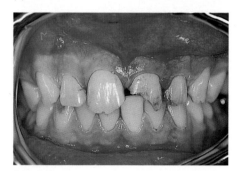

(b)

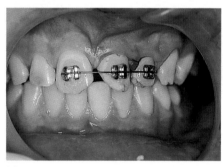

(c)

Fig. 12.36 (a) Palatally luxated upper left permanent incisor with other associated injuries. (b) Upper left permanent central incisor repositioned atraumatically. (c) Non-rigid orthodontic splint in place.

Table 12.2 Five-year pulpal survival after injuries involving the periodontal ligament

Type of injury	Open apex (%)	Closed apex (%)
Concussion	100	96
Subluxation	100	85
Extrusive luxation	95	45
Lateral luxation	95	25
Intrusive luxation	40	0
Replantation	30	0

(3) immobilization with a splint if teeth have fully formed apices or if t.t.p. is significant;

(4) chlorhexidine 0.2% mouthwash, twice daily.

Figures for pulpal survival 5 years after injury (Table 12.2) show that there is minimal risk of pulpal necrosis. In addition, in over 97% of cases there is no evidence of any resorption.

Extrusive luxation

There is a rupture of p.l. and pulp.

Lateral luxation

There is a rupture of p.l, pulp, and the alveolar plate (Fig. 12.36(a)). The treatment for both these injuries is:

(1) atraumatic repositioning with gentle but firm digital pressure (Fig. 12.36(b));

(2) local anaesthetic is required if there is an alveolar plate injury;

(3) non-rigid functional splint for 2–3 weeks (Fig. 12.36(c));

(4) antibiotics, for example, amoxycillin 250 mg three times daily (<10 years old 125 mg three times daily) for 5 days;

(5) chlorhexidine 0.2% mouthwash twice daily while splint is in position;

(6) soft diet 2–3 weeks.

Antibiotics may have a beneficial effect in promoting repair of the p.l. They do not appear to affect pulpal prognosis.

After 2–3 weeks the teeth are radiographed. If there is no evidence of marginal breakdown the splint can be removed. If marginal breakdown is present then it should be retained for a further 2–3 weeks.

For both these injuries the decision whether to progress to endodontic treatment depends on the combination of clinical and radiographic signs at regular review (Fig. 12.7). Five-year pulpal survival figures (Table 12.2) show that prognosis is significantly better for open apex teeth but nevertheless a proportion of mature closed apex teeth will retain vitality. In addition, over 4% of mature teeth involved in luxation injuries will exhibit on radiographs a natural healing phenomenon known as 'transient apical breakdown' (t.a.b.) which can mimic apical inflammation. Ambivalent clinical and radiographic signs should be given the 'benefit of the doubt' until the next review.

With more significant damage to the p.l. in both extrusive and lateral luxation injuries there is an increased risk of root resorption. Thirty-five per cent of mature teeth that have undergone lateral luxation show subsequent evidence of surface resorption.

In some cases of lateral luxation the displacement cannot be reduced with gentle finger pressure. It is not advisable to use more force as this can further damage the periodontal ligament. Orthodontic appliances, either a removable or a sectional fixed appliance can be used to reduce the displacement over a period of a few weeks (Fig. 12.37(a–c)).

Intrusive luxation

These injuries are the result of an axial, apical impact and there is extensive damage to p.l, pulp, and alveolar plate(s).

Two distinct treatment categories exist: the open and closed apex. Both categories can be discussed depending on whether the intrusive injury is: mild(<3 mm); moderate (3–6 mm); or severe (>6 mm).

OPEN APEX

- Mild intrusion <3 mm. Excellent eruptive potential. Treat conservatively and review. If no movement in 2–4 months move orthodontically.
- Moderate Intrusion 3–6 mm. Disimpact (with forceps if necessary) and either allow to erupt spontaneously for 2–4 months before extruding orthodontically or apply orthodontic forces early.
- Severe intrusion >6 mm. Orthodontic repositioning may be impossible and disimpaction followed by surgical repositioning under either LA, LA/sedation, or GA is appropriate. Functional splint for 2–3 weeks.

Monitor pulpal status clinically and radiographically at regular intervals during the first 6 months after injury, and then 6 monthly, and start endodontics if necessary: Non-setting calcium hydroxide in root canal does not preclude against orthodontic movement. Once apexification has occurred and orthodontic movement has ceased (Fig. 12.38(a–c)) obturate canal with gutta percha.

CLOSED APEX

- Mild intrusion <3 mm. Orthodontic extrusion is probably indicated straight away although some authors have advocated conservative treatment. The danger of a tooth ankylosing in an intruded position should always be borne in mind and in this respect active treatment is preferable to a conservative approach.
- Moderate intrusion 3–6 mm. Orthodontic extrusion is indicated straight away.
- Severe intrusion >6 mm. Surgical repositioning. Functional splint for 2–3 weeks.

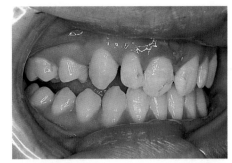
(a)

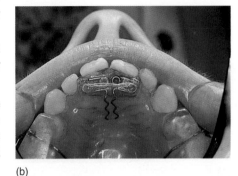
(b)

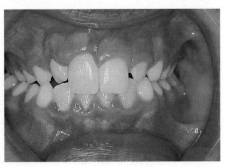
(c)

Fig. 12.37 (a) Delayed presentation of palatally luxated upper permanent central incisors in traumatic occlusion. (b) and (c) An upper removable appliance used to procline the upper incisors over 2 months.

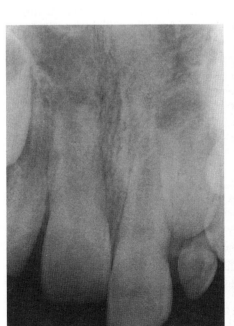
(a)

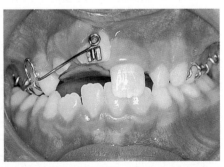
(b)

(c)

Fig. 12.38 (a) A 7-year-old child with intrusion of the upper right permanent central incisor which failed to re-erupt spontaneously. (b) and (c) Orthodontic extrusion of the upper right central incisor.

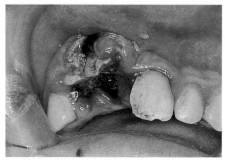

(a)

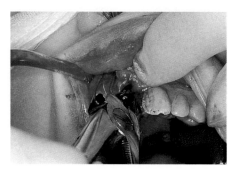

(b)

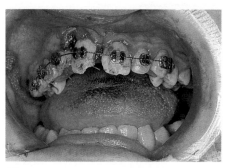

(c)

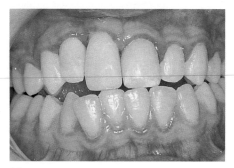

(d)

Fig. 12.39   (a) A severe intrusive injury in a 15-year-old girl. (b) Surgical extrusion of the upper right permanent incisors. (c) Orthodontic splinting. (d) Completed composite restorations.

Table 12.3   Periodontal ligament healing after intrusive luxation injuries

Type of healing	Open apex (%)	Closed apex (%)
Normal	33	0
Inflammatory resorption	41	35
Replacement resorption (ankylosis)	10	31
Surface resorption	16	34

Elective pulp extirpation will be necessary for all significant intrusive luxation injuries in closed apex teeth (Table 12.3) at about 10 days.

Maintain non-setting calcium hydroxide in root canal during orthodontic movement before obturation with gutta percha (Fig. 12.39 (a–d)).

If endodontic treatment is commenced within 2 weeks after any injury to the p.l. then the initial intracanal dressing should be with an antibiotic/steroid (Ledermix, Lederle) paste. This may help to reduce the incidence of inflammatory resorption.

At the initial examination both open and closed apex teeth should receive antibiotics, chlorhexidine mouthwash, and a soft diet.

The risk of pulpal necrosis in these injuries is high, especially in the closed apex (Table 12.2). The incidence of resorption and ankylosis sequelae is also high (Table 12.3)

Key Point

In p.l.injuries

*   The incidence of pulpal necrosis is higher in closed apex teeth;
*   The incidence of resorption increases with severity of injury.

Avulsion and replantation

Replantation should nearly always be attempted even though it may offer only a temporary solution due to the frequent occurrence of external inflammatory resorption (e.i.r.). Even when resorption occurs the tooth may be retained for years acting as a natural space maintainer and preserving the height and width of the alveolus to facilitate later implant placement.

Successful healing after replantation can only occur if there is minimal damage to the pulp and the p.l. The extra-alveolar dry time (e.a.d.t.), the type of extra-alveolar storage medium, and the total extra-alveolar time (e.a.t.), that is, the time the tooth has been out of the mouth are critical factors. The first question that must be known is 'what is the e.a.d.t. of the tooth? If the e.a.d.t. is not greater than 1 h then the suggested protocol for replantation can be divided into: advice on phone; immediate treatment in surgery; and review.

Replantation of teeth with a dry storage time of less than 1 h

ADVICE ON PHONE (TO TEACHER, PARENT, ETC.)

1.   Don't touch root—hold by crown.
2.   If tooth is dirty, wash briefly (10 s) under cold running water.
3.   Replace into socket or transport in milk to surgery.
4.   If replaced bite gently on a handkerchief to retain it and come to surgery.

The best transport medium is the tooth's own socket. Understandably non-dentists may be unhappy to replant the tooth and milk is an effective iso-osmolar medium. Saliva, the patient's buccal sulcus, or normal saline are alternatives.

IMMEDIATE SURGERY TREATMENT

1. Do not handle root. If replanted remove tooth from socket.
2. Rinse tooth with normal saline. Note state of root development. Store in saline.
3. Local analgesia.
4. Irrigate socket with saline and remove clot and any foreign material.
5. Push tooth gently but firmly into socket.
6. Non-rigid functional splint for 7–10 days.
7. Check occlusion.
8. Baseline radiographs: periapical or anterior occlusal. Any other teeth injured?
9. Antibiotics, chlorhexidine mouthwash, soft diet as previously.
10. Check tetanus immunization status.

REVIEW

1. Radiograph—prior to splint removal at 7–10 days.
2. Remove splint 7–10 days.
3. Endodontics—commence prior to splint removal for categories (b) and (c):
   (a) open apex. e.a.t. <30–45 min. Observe.
   (b) open apex. e.a.t. >30–45 min. Endodontics.
      (i) initial intracanal dressing—antibiotic/steroid (Ledermix, Lederle) paste.
      (ii) subsequent intracanal dressings—non-setting calcium hydroxide paste.
      (iii) replace calcium hydroxide 3 monthly until apical barrier (up to maximum of 2 years.
      (iv) obturate canal with GP
   (c) Closed apex. Endodontics.
      (i) initial intracanal dressing antibiotic/steroid (Ledermix, Lederle) paste;
      (ii) subsequent intracanal dressing with non-setting calcium hydroxide paste;
      (iii) obturate with gutta percha at 6 months as long as no progressive resorption.
4. Radiographic review: 1, 3, and 6 monthly for 2 years then annually.
5. If resorption is progressing unhalted keep non-setting calcium hydroxide in the tooth until exfoliation, changing it 6 monthly.

The immature tooth with an e.a.t. of less than 30–45 min may undergo pulp revascularization (Table 12.2). However, these teeth require regular clinical and radiographic review because once e.i.r. occurs it progresses rapidly.

Replantation of teeth with a dry storage time of greater than 1 h

The consensus opinion is that teeth with very immature apices should not be replanted. The incidence of resorption, ankylosis, and subsequent loss is high due to the high rate of bone remodelling in this age group.

Mature teeth with a dry storage time of greater than 1 h will have a non-vital p.l. The necrotic p.l. and the pulp should be removed at chairside with pumice and water on a bristle brush prior to rinsing with normal saline. The root canal is then obturated with gutta percha and the tooth replanted and splinted for a longer period of up to 6 weeks. The aim of this treatment is to produce ankylosis allowing the tooth to be maintained as a natural space maintainer, perhaps for a limited period only.

Pulpal and periodontal status in p.d.l. injuries

Pulpal necrosis is the most common complication and is related to the severity of the periodontal injury (Table 12.2). Immature teeth have a better prognosis than mature teeth due to the wide apical opening where slight movements can occur without disruption of the apical neurovascular bundle. Necrosis can be diagnosed in most cases within 3 months of injury but in some cases may not be evident for at least 2 years. A combination of clinical and radiological signs are often required to diagnose necrosis.

SENSITIVITY TESTING

The majority of injured teeth test negatively to e.p.t. immediately following trauma. Most pulps that recover test positively within months but responses have been reported as late as 2 years after injury. A negative test alone therefore should not be regarded as proof of necrosis. Postpone endodontics until at least one other clinical and/or radiographic sign is present.

TOOTH DISCOLOURATION

Initial pinkish discolouration may be due to subtotal severance of apical vessels leading to penetration of haemoglobin from such ruptures into the dentine tubules. If the vascular system repairs then most of this discolouration will disappear. If the tooth becomes progressively grey then necrosis should be suspected. A grey colour that appears for the first time several weeks or months after trauma, signifies decomposition of necrotic pulp tissue and is a decisive sign of necrosis. Colour changes are usually most apparent on the palatal surface of the injured teeth.

TENDERNESS TO PERCUSSION

This may be the most reliable isolated indicator of pulpal necrosis.

PERIAPICAL INFLAMMATION

Radiological periapical involvement secondary to pulp necrosis and infection can be seen as early as 3 weeks after trauma. In mature teeth transient apical breakdown (t.a.b.) may be mistaken for periapical inflammation and may be present up to 2–3 months after trauma. It represents the response to an ingrowth of new tissue into the pulp canal.

ARREST OF ROOT DEVELOPMENT

If necrosis involves the epithelial root sheath before root development is complete, then no further root growth will occur (Fig. 12.17(a) and (b)). In an injured pulp necrosis may progress from coronal to apical portion and hence residual apical vitality may result in formation of a calcific barrier across a wide apical foramen. Failure of the pulp chamber and root canal to mature and reduce in size on successive radiographs compared with contralateral uninjured teeth is also a reliable indicator of necrosis.

12.7.4 Resorption

Root resorption is a serious and destructive complication which may follow trauma to primary and permanent teeth. Primary teeth which develop pathological resorptive lesions are not good candidates for conservative treatment and should be extracted. Permanent teeth on the other hand may often be successfully treated provided tissue destruction has not advanced to an unrestorable state.

Two general forms of pathological root resorption are recognized, inflammatory and replacement.

INFLAMMATORY ROOT RESORPTION

Internal and external root surfaces injured as a result of trauma are rapidly colonized by multinuclear giant cells. If giant cells are continuously stimulated, most commonly by microbial products from an infected root canal or periodontal pocket, progressive inflammatory root resorption may follow with catastrophic consequences. Inflammatory root resorption may be classified according to its site of origin as external root resorption, cervical resorption (a special form of external resorption), or internal root resorption.

EXTERNAL INFLAMMATORY ROOT RESORPTION

Teeth affected by external inflammatory root resorption are invariably non-vital with infected pulp canals. Resorptive activity is initiated by damage to p.l. in trauma but propagated by infected root canal contents seeping to the external root surface through patent dentinal tubules, and may be extremely aggressive. However, if the infected canal contents are removed, the propagating stimulus is lost and the lesion will predictably arrest.

1. *Diagnosis.* External inflammatory root resorption is usually detected as a chance radiographic finding, and is characterized by change of the external contour of the root, which is often surrounded by a bony lucency (Figs 12.40 and 12.41). Sometimes it may present as a radiolucency overlying the root, and can be distinguished from internal resorption by its asymmetrical shape, by the superimposed contour of the intact root canal walls, and by the fact that it moves in relation to the root canal on periapical films of different horizontal angle.

2. *Treatment.* Provided the tooth is still restorable, external inflammatory root resorption should be treated without delay. Following access cavity preparation, the root canal should be cleaned and shaped, taking care not to weaken the root excessively, or to risk perforation into the resorbed area. It is common practice to dress the root canal with non-setting calcium hydroxide paste and to monitor the tooth for several months prior to definitive obturation to ensure that the lesion has arrested. Nevertheless, control of intracanal infection is the key determinant of success, and there is good evidence to suggest that if the canal is adequately prepared, it may be filled without protracted calcium hydroxide treatment.

Periodic clinical and radiographic review should be arranged.

CERVICAL RESORPTION

Cervical resorption is an unusual form of external inflammatory root resorption, initiated by damage to the root surface in the cervical region, and propagated either by infected root canal contents, or by the periodontal microflora. From a very small entry point, the resorptive process may extend widely before penetrating the pulp chamber (Fig. 12.42 (a and b)).

1. *Diagnosis.* Extensive intracoronal extension may occasionally present cervical resorption as a clinically visible pink spot. More commonly, it is identified on routine radiographs as a characteristically sited radiolucency (Fig. 12.42).

2. *Treatment.* If the tooth is non-vital, conventional root canal therapy should be undertaken to eliminate the propagating stimulus. Arrangements should then be made to open the resorptive defect in a similar manner to cavity preparation, and to curette away all traces of inflammatory tissue before restoring the resultant defect (Fig. 12.43). Often, a flap must be raised to adequately eliminate resorptive tissue and contour the subgingival restoration.

If the tooth is vital, and the pulp has not been invaded, treatment may be limited to opening and curetting the resorption lacuna before placing a setting calcium hydroxide lining and restoring the defect with an appropriate material.

Periodic clinical and radiographic review should again be arranged.

INTERNAL INFLAMMATORY ROOT RESORPTION

Internal inflammatory root resorption is seen in the canals of traumatized teeth which are undergoing progressive pulp necrosis. Infected material in the non-vital,

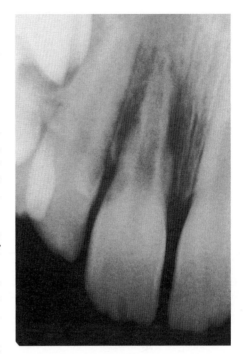

Fig. 12.40 External inflammatory resorption.

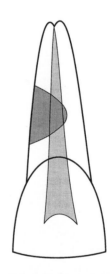

Fig. 12.41 External inflammatory root resorption. Usually presents as an asymmetrical radiolucency on the lateral surface of the root. If the lesion overlies the root canal, its lateral walls are usually still visible.

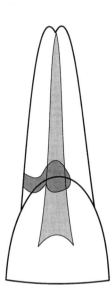

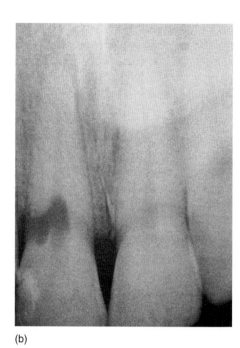

(a)   (b)

Fig. 12.42 Cervical resorption. (a) Resorption commences from a small entry point below the gingival crevice, and often spreads widely within the crown before the root canal is invaded. The lateral walls of the pulp chamber are often superimposed over the defect. (b) Periapical radiograph showing a typical clinical case.

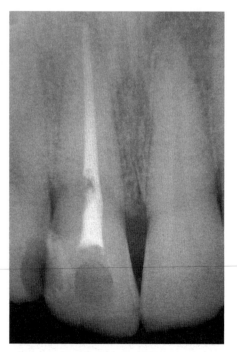

Fig. 12.43 Cervical resorption following endodontic treatment of the necrotic pulp and surgical repair of the external defect.

coronal part of the canal is believed to propagate resorption by the underlying vital tissue, and rapid tissue destruction follows.

1. *Diagnosis.* Large resorptive defects affecting the coronal third of the canal may present as a pink discoloration of the affected tooth. More commonly, it is detected as a chance finding on routine radiographic examination. Radiographically, internal resorption presents as a rounded, symmetrical radiolucency, centred on the root canal. The contours of the root canal walls are rarely superimposed (Figs. 12.44 and 12.45).

2. *Treatment.* Internal resorption should be considered to be a form of irreversible pulpitis and treated without delay. Following standard access cavity preparation, the pulp chamber and coronal portion of the canal is usually found to contain necrotic debris. However, deeper penetration of the canal often provokes torrential haemorrhage as the vascular, resorptive tissue is entered.

Root canal preparation is undertaken in the usual manner, and following apical enlargement, haemorrhage from the canal is greatly reduced as the blood supply to the resorptive tissue is severed. Instrumentation of the expanded, resorbed area is difficult, and can be greatly enhanced by the use of sonic or ultrasonic devices which are able to throw irrigant into uninstrumented areas. The antimicrobial and tissue solvent actions of sodium hypochlorite make it the irrigant of choice in such cases.

As in the case of external inflammatory resorption, it is usual to dress the canal with non-setting calcium hydroxide following debridement. This may be highly advantageous in the internal resorption case where the antimicrobial and mild tissue solvent actions of calcium hydroxide may be exploited further to clean the resorbed area.

Obturation may then be undertaken with gutta percha and sealer, usually employing a thermoplastic technique to allow satisfactory condensation and adaptation in the resorbed area (Fig. 12.46). Where internal reinforcement is indicated, dual curing composite resin and fibre posts may offer some advantages over full canal filling with gutta percha and sealer.

REPLACEMENT RESORPTION

Replacement resorption is a distinct form of root resorption which follows serious luxation or avulsion injury that has caused damage to the investing periodontal ligament. A classic scenario is the avulsed tooth, which has been stored dry, or p.l. removed before replantation, with resultant death of periodontal fibroblasts on much of the root surface. If more than 20% of the periodontal ligament is damaged or lost and the tooth is subsequently reimplanted, bone cells are able to grow into contact with the root surface more quickly than the remaining periodontal fibroblasts are able to recolonize the root surface and intervene between tooth and bone. The consequence is that the root now becomes involved in the normal remodelling process of the bone in which it is implanted, and is gradually replaced by bone over the course of the following years. In young children where the rate of bone remodelling is high, the root may be entirely lost within 3–4 years. In adolescents, it may be 10 years or more before the tooth is lost.

1. *Diagnosis.* The absence of a ligamentous joint between the tooth and its supporting bone (ankylosis) means that even when root resorption is advanced, the tooth will appear rock solid. A bright, metallic tone will also be noted if the tooth is percussed. Radiographically, the root will appear ragged in outline, with no obvious periodontal ligament space separating it from the surrounding bone (Fig. 12.47).

2. *Treatment.* There is no effective treatment for ankylosis but the rate of progression is relatively slow and the tooth can be maintained for 10 years or more. However, such teeth can be a problem in the growing child as they may cease to 'move' or 'grow' with the rest of the jaws and cannot be moved orthodontically. There is no effective treatment for established replacement resorption and parents and carers should be advised of the inevitable course of events.

From an endodontic point of view, it is important to reiterate that if pulp extirpation is undertaken within 2 weeks of reimplantation then the initial root canal dressing should be an antibiotic/steroid (Ledermix, Lederle) preparation which should be replaced subsequently with non-setting calcium hydroxide, no sooner than 2 weeks after tooth reimplantation. The antibiotic/steroid paste may help to reduce subsequent resorption.

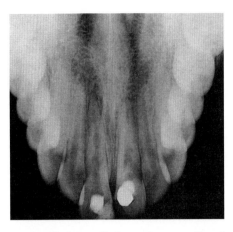

Fig. 12.44 Internal inflammatory resorption of both upper central incisors.

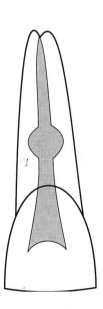

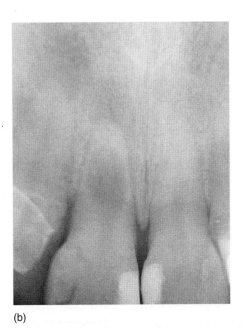

(a) (b)

Fig. 12.45 Internal inflammatory root resorption. (a) Symmetrical expansion of the root canal walls in a permanent central incisor. (b) Periapical radiograph showing a typical clinical case.

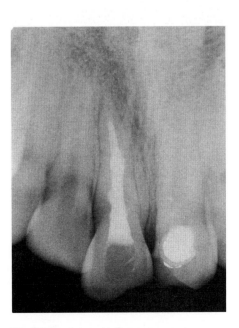

Fig. 12.46 Internal inflammatory root resorption. Maxillary central incisor demonstrating internal resorptive defects at two levels. The canal was cleaned, shaped, and obturated with thermoplasticized gutta percha and sealer.

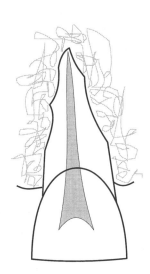

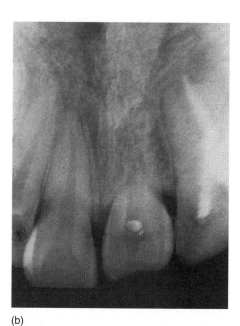

(a)   (b)

Fig. 12.47 Replacement resorption. (a) Roots affected by replacement resorption have ragged outlines, and merge with the surrounding bone to which they are fused. (b) Periapical radiograph showing advanced replacement resorption. Clinically, the tooth is rock solid.

If endodontic treatment was not undertaken soon after reimplantation and the tooth subsequently loses vitality, conventional root canal therapy may be undertaken in order to address any painful periapical pathosis and to avoid the additional insult of inflammatory resorption which would lead to more rapid loss of root substance. A resorbable root filling material such as root canal sealer alone or reinforced zinc oxide eugenol cement may be preferred to gutta percha in some cases.

Where resorption is progressive then consideration should be given to autotransplantation of either an upper second premolar or lower first or second premolar if any of these teeth were to be removed as part of an orthodontic treatment plan. If autotransplantation is completed while the root of the premolar is about two-thirds formed then there is a good chance of revascularisation and further root growth (Fig 12.48 (a and b)). If the autotransplanted tooth has a mature apex then revasculariztaion is unlikely and the tooth should be exptirpated at splint removal and the canal dressed with antibiotic/steroid (Ledermix/Lederle) initially, then non-setting calcium hydroxide. The tooth can be obturated with gutta percha when there is no evidence of progressive resorption.

Key Points

Pathological root resorption

- inflammatory: external (including cervical)and internal;
- inflammatory may arrest if cause is removed;
- replacement resorption is not amenable to treatment;
- maintain a resorbing tooth for as long as possible. It is the best space maintainer!

12.7.5 Pulp canal obliteration

There is progressive hard tissue formation within the pulp cavity leading to a gradual narrowing of the pulp chamber and root canal and partial or total obliteration. There is a reduced response to vitality testing and the crown appears slightly yellow/opaque. The exact initiating factor which produces this response from the odontoblasts is unknown. It is more common in immature teeth and in luxation injuries rather than in concussion and subluxation injuries. Although radiographs may suggest complete calcification there is usually a minute strand of pulpal tissue remaining. Pulpal obliteration has been described as 'natures own root filling'and although the late development of necrosis and infection in the thin thread of pulpal tissue in the sclerosed canal has been reported, it is less common than the endodontic complications that would be necessary to treat it. The obturation of an 'obliterating' canal is not justification for pre-eruptive root canal treatment in the absence of signs of pulp breakdown.

12.7.6 Injuries to the supporting bone

The extent and position of the alveolar fracture should be verified clinically and radiographically. If there is displacement of the teeth to the extent that their apices have risen up and are now positioned over the labial or lingual/palatal alveolar plates ('apical lock') then they will require extruding first to free the apices prior to repositioning. The segment of alveolus with teeth requires only 3–4 weeks of rigid splintage (composite-wire type) with two abutment teeth either side of the fracture, together with antibiotics, chlorhexidine, soft diet, and tetanus prophylaxis check (Fig. 12.49(a)–(c)). Pulpal survival is more likely if repositioning occurs within 1 h of the injury. Root resorption is rare.

12.8 CHILD PHYSICAL ABUSE

A child is considered to be abused if he or she is treated in a way that is unacceptable in a given culture at a given time (Fig. 12.4). Child physical abuse or non-accidental injury (NAI) is now recognized as an international issue and has been reported in many countries. Each week 2–3 children in Britain and 80 children in the

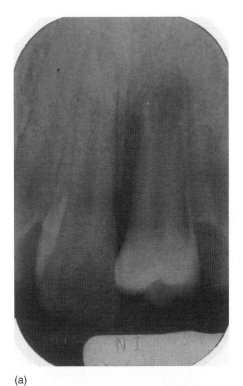

(a)

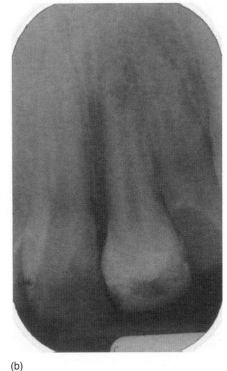

(b)

Fig. 12.48   (a) Autotransplanted premolar in 21 position. (b) Continued growth and revascularization of autotransplanted premolar Courtesy of Professor M.S. Duggal.

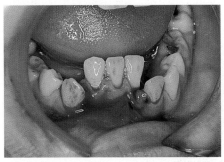

(a)

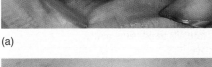

(b)

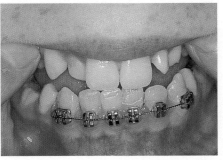

(c)

Fig. 12.49   (a) Dentoalveolar fracture of the lower labial segment. (b) Fracture reduced into the correct occlusion. (c) Splint in situ prior to removal.

United States will die as a result of abuse or neglect. At least one child per 1000 in Britain suffers severe physical abuse; for example, fractures, brain haemorrhage, severe internal injuries or mutilation, and in the United States more than 95% of serious intracranial injuries during the first year of life are the result of abuse. Although some reports will prove to be unfounded the common experience is that proved cases of child abuse are four to five times as common as they were a decade ago. Physical abuse is not a full diagnosis, it is merely a symptom of disordered parenting. The aim of intervention is to diagnose and cure the disordered parenting. It has been estimated in the United States that 35–50% of severely abused children will receive serious re-injury and 50% will die if they are returned to their home environment without intervention. In some cases the occurrence of physical abuse may provide an opportunity for intervention. If this opportunity is missed, there may be no further opportunity for many years.

More than 50% of cases diagnosed as physical abuse have extra and intraoral facial trauma and so the dental practitioner may be the first professional to see or suspect abuse. Injuries may take the form of contusions and ecchymoses (Fig. 12.50), abrasions and lacerations, burns, bites, dental trauma (Fig. 12.51), and fractures. The incidence of common orofacial injuries are shown in Table 12.4.

The following 11 points should be considered whenever doubts and suspicions are aroused.

1. Could the injury have been caused accidentally and if so how?
2. Does the explanation for the injury fit the age and the clinical findings?
3. If the explanation of cause is consistent with the injury, is this itself within normally acceptable limits of behaviour?
4. If there has been any delay seeking advice are there good reasons for this?
5. Does the story of the accident vary?
6. The nature of the relationship between parent and child.
7. The child's reaction to other people.
8. The child's reaction to any medical/dental examinations.
9. The general demeanour of the child.
10. Any comments made by child and/or parent that give concern about the child's upbringing or life-style.
11. History of previous injury.

Dental professionals should be aware of any established system in their locality which is designed to cope with these cases. In the United Kingdom each Local Authority Social Services Department is required to set up an 'Area Child Protection Committee' which are coordinated by 'Designated Doctors' in Primary Care Trusts. Dental professionals are advised how to refer and to whom, if they are concerned.

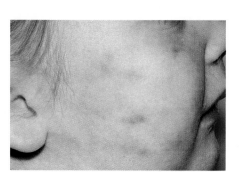

Fig. 12.50 Characteristic parallel bruising of a slap mark. (Reproduced with the kind permission of Munksgaard.)

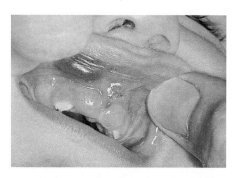

Fig. 12.51 Torn labial frenum in a young child not yet learning to walk could be an indicator of a non-accidental injury. (Reproduced with the kind permission of Munksgaard.)

Table 12.4   The incidence of common orofacial injuries in physical abuse

	Type of injury	Incidence (%)
Extraoral	Contusions and ecchymoses	66
	Abrasions and lacerations	28
	Burns and bites	4
	Fractures	2
Intraoral	Contusions and ecchymoses	43
	Abrasions and lacerations (including frenal tears)	29
	Dental trauma	29

12.9 SUMMARY

1. Boys experience dental trauma almost twice as often as girls.

2. Maxillary central incisors are the most commonly involved teeth.

3. Regular clinical and radiographic review is necessary to limit unwanted sequelae, institute appropriate treatment, and improve prognosis.

4. Injuries to the developing permanent dentition occur in half of all trauma to the primary dentition.

5. Splinting for avulsion, luxation, and root fractures should be functional to allow physiological movement and promote normal healing of the p.l. Splinting for dentoalveolar fractures should be rigid.

6. In all luxation injuries the prognosis for pulpal healing is better with an immature apex.

7. Root resorption increases with the severity of damage to the p.l.

8. The prognosis for replantation of avulsed teeth is best if it is undertaken within 1 h of the injury, with a hydrated p.l.

9. Orofacial injuries are found in at least 50% of cases of physical abuse.

10. Successful endodontics demands the co-operation of a comfortable child. Effective local anaesthesia should be provided if there is any risk of pain during treatment.

11. From indirect pulp capping to non-vital pulp therapy, control of microbial infection is the key determinant of endodontic treatment success. A well-fitting rubber dam should be in place wherever possible, and all stages of all endodontic procedures should be conducted with due regard to the elimination of infection and the prevention of its recurrence.

12. Root canal systems in young teeth are cleaned principally by antimicrobial and tissue-solvent irrigants and medicaments, not by exuberant dentine removal. Dentine removal, especially in fragile primary and young permanent teeth, should be rational and restricted to that required for effective irrigation and successful obturation only.

12.10 FURTHER READING

Andreasen, J. O. and Andreasen, F. M. (1994). Textbook and color atlas of traumatic injuries to the teeth (3rd edn). Munksgaard, Copenhagen. (*An excellent reference book with colour slides of each clinical procedure*)

Andreasen, J. O., Borum, M. K., Jacobsen, H. L., and Andreasen F. M. (1995). Replantation of 400 avulsed permanent incisors. *Endodontics and Dental Traumatology* **II**, 51–89. (*The largest published series on avulsed permanent incisors*)

Cohen, S. and Burns, R. C. (2001). *Pathways of the Pulp* (8th edn). Mosby, St Louis. (*The definitive endodontic reference book*)

European Society of Endodontology (1994). Consensus Report of the European Society of Endodontology on quality guidelines for endodontic treatment. *International Endodontic Journal*, **27**, 115–24. (*A synopsis of current terminology and good practice in endodontics*)

Kinirons M. J. (1998). Treatment of traumatically intruded permanent incisor teeth. *International Journal of Paediatric Dentistry*, 8, 165–8 (*UK National Clinical Guideline*).

Welbury R. R. (1994). Child Physical Abuse (Non Accidental Injury) In Textbook and color atlas of traumatic injuries to the teeth (ed. J. O. and F. M. Andreasen) (3rd edn). Munksgaard, Copenhagen. (*A reference of prevalence and orofacial signs in non-accidental injury*).

12.11 REFERENCE

Andreasen, J. O., Andreasen, F. M., Mejàre, I., Cvek, M. (2004). Healing of 400 intra-alveolar root fractures; Effect of treatment factors such as treatment delay, repositioning, splinting type and period and antibiotics. *Dental Traumatology*, 20, 203–11.

Anomalies of tooth formation and eruption

13 Anomalies of tooth formation and eruption

P. J. M. Crawford and M. J. Aldred

At the outset, we would wish to record both our personal and professional gratitude to the late Professor GB (Gerry) Winter. He always encouraged our work and was generous in his comments and sharing of material. Above all, he was an enthusiast and a champion of his patients. He is missed.

13.1 INTRODUCTION

Both the primary and permanent dentitions may be affected by variations in the number, size, and form of the teeth, as well as the structure of the dental hard tissues. These variations may be exclusively genetically determined, brought about by either local or systemically acting environmental factors, or possibly from a combination of both genetic and environmental factors acting together. The same interplay of influences may affect the eruption and exfoliation of primary teeth, as well as the eruption of permanent teeth. This chapter considers a range of conditions involving abnormalities of the number, size, form, and structure of teeth and their eruption.

It is important to be aware of the psycho-social aspect when meeting children and families affected by these conditions. We have too often heard stories of social isolation of even very young children as a result of their missing or discoloured teeth. In the case of discoloured teeth, parents have told us that they have been 'taken to task' by other adults for 'not looking after' their child's teeth—when the discolouration was intrinsic and unavoidable.

While investigating inherited conditions, it is important to enquire both sides of the family tree equally. Not only does this ensure that the investigation is complete, but it may also help to alleviate the sense of 'guilt' felt by an affected parent.

Wherever possible, we try to avoid the use of the word 'normal' in our clinical care although the word will be used in this text. Clinically we would speak—when offering restorative treatment for example— of making a smile 'ordinary', or 'boring'. The vast majority of children with these conditions want to become 'one of the crowd'. We have found this approach successful in our practices; our readers may choose this or one of many other approaches in order to further the care of these children.

We have been questioned repeatedly about the possibility of genetic treatment for some of these inherited conditions. We are not aware of any progress in this direction at present, outside the laboratory.

13.2 MISSING TEETH

Hypodontia is the term most often applied to a situation where a patient has missing teeth as a result of their failure of development. Anodontia describes the total lack of teeth of one or both dentitions. Oligodontia is a term used to describe a situation where multiple—usually more than six—teeth are missing.

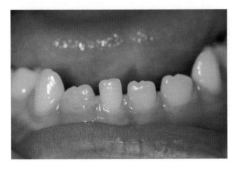

Fig. 13.1 Hypodontia, absent 41, retained 81.

13.2.1 Prevalence

In the primary dentition, missing teeth occur more commonly in the maxilla and typically the maxillary lateral incisor is the tooth involved. Various studies have shown the prevalence of missing primary teeth to be between 0.1 % and 0.9 % of Caucasian populations, with males and females affected equally. Developmentally missing permanent teeth are seen in both the maxilla and mandible (Fig. 13.1). In Caucasian populations the third molars are the most commonly missing teeth, followed by the mandibular second premolar, the maxillary lateral incisor, and the maxillary second premolar. A female to male ratio of 4 : 1 has been reported. Missing third molars occur in 9–30% of individuals. If the third molars are excluded, the prevalence in the permanent varies between 3.5 % and 6.5 % according to the study quoted.

Key Points

- Hypodontia
- 0.1–0.9% in the primary dentition;
- 3.5–6.5% in the permanent dentition;
- Missing permanent teeth are seen in 30–50% of patients who have missing primary teeth.

13.2.2 Aetiology

The cause of an isolated missing tooth is often unclear; this may be genetic in origin or associated with some environmental insult during development. Missing teeth have been reported in association with multiple births, low birth weight, and increased maternal age. Rubella and thalidomide embryopathies may also be associated with missing teeth.

Single gene disorders have been associated with missing teeth. Multiple missing teeth, as well as teeth with small crowns, may be seen in a number of syndromes including X-linked hypohidrotic ectodermal dysplasia (Fig. 13.2), autosomal dominant and autosomal recessive cases of ectodermal dysplasia and autosomal recessive chondroectodermal dysplasia (Ellis-van Creveld syndrome). Down syndrome (trisomy 21) is also associated with hypodontia.

Hypodontia and microdontia involving the maxillary lateral incisor occurs in clefts involving the lip and palate.

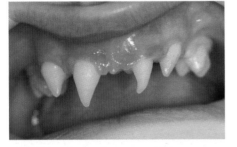

Fig. 13.2 Hypohidrotic ectodermal dysplasia; erupted permanent teeth.

X-linked hypohidrotic ectodermal dysplasia is characterized in males by thin sparse hair, dry skin, absence of sweating and therefore heat intolerance, and multiple missing teeth. These children are at risk due to their inability to cool themselves and may die in infancy if undiagnosed. This condition, while rare, is of particular importance as the dental professional be the first to come to a diagnosis, and thus to introduce families to support mechanisms. In heterozygous females the changes are milder and may be restricted to the teeth, although a distinctive facial profile (slight retrusion of the maxilla) may be recognized. Most commonly, one or both maxillary lateral incisors and/or the second premolars are missing. In some patients one maxillary lateral incisor may be of peg form. The responsible gene is the *ED1* gene on the X chromosome which encodes the protein ectodysplasin-A.

Autosomal dominant inheritance of missing teeth is seen in families with mutations in the *MSX1* gene on chromosome 4. Missing third molars and second premolars are the most common finding. These families may also have clefting segregating with the missing teeth. Mutations in the *MSX1* gene are also seen in the tooth-nail (Witkop) syndrome.

A pattern of autosomally dominant inheritance of missing teeth, particularly molars, is seen as a result of mutations in the *PAX9* gene on chromosome 14.

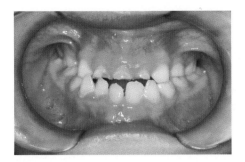

Fig. 13.3 Median maxillary central incisor syndrome.

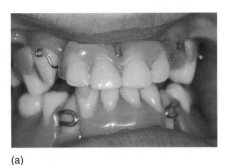

(a)

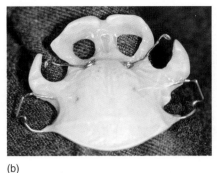

(b)

Fig. 13.4 Hypohidrotic ectodermal dysplasia; erupted permanent teeth masked by 'porthole' denture with canine retractors during eruption.

Some patients having a solitary median maxillary central incisor have been found to have mutations in the sonic hedgehog (*SHH*) gene on chromosome 7 (Fig. 13.3).

13.2.3 Treatment

The care of children with multiple missing teeth can be complex and ideally requires multidisciplinary input from paediatric dentists, orthodontists, and prosthodontists as well as genetic counselling. Missing teeth and small teeth often present together, so masking of conical or similarly distinctive teeth with composite is strongly advised. In cases of anodontia, full dentures are required. These can be provided, albeit with likely limited success, from about 3 years of age, with the possibility of implant support for prostheses provided in adulthood. (Fig. 13.4(a) and (b)). Multiple missing teeth can be treated by the use of partial dentures, with implants as part of the treatment protocol at a later age. Implant placement is best left until skeletal maturity. Dentures will need to be replaced as the jaws grow. Progressive provision of dentures with annual replacements during the school holidays ('the long vacation'), mimicking the developing dentition at the child's age, can do much to minimize the stigma of these conditions. Although, ultimately, dentures can be retained by implants, the lack of development of the alveolar bone may prove to be a limiting factor.

13.3 EXTRA TEETH

Extra teeth (supernumerary teeth) have been reported to occur in 0.2–0.8% of Caucasians in the primary dentition and 1.5–3% in the permanent dentition in the same populations. There is a male to female ratio of approximately 2 : 1. Patients with supernumerary primary teeth have a 30–50% chance of these being followed by supernumerary permanent teeth. Teeth which resemble those of the normal series are referred to as supplemental teeth (Fig. 13.5) while those of less typical, often reduced, form–sometimes further described as tuberculate or conical–can be termed accessory supernumerary teeth.

Supernumerary teeth are most often located in the anterior maxilla in the midline, or immediately adjacent to the midline, and are then referred to as a mesiodens. Supernumerary teeth in the molar regions adjacent or distal to the normal sequence of teeth are referred to as paramolars or distomolars respectively.

In some cases the supernumerary teeth may be an odontome.

Supernumerary teeth are more common in the maxilla than the mandible, with a ratio of about 5 : 1. Apart from those in the midline, they may be present bilaterally and symmetrically, hence the presence of a supernumerary in one part of the jaws should lead to consideration of further supernumeraries elsewhere. Supernumerary teeth may fail to erupt and may delay eruption of a permanent tooth which is

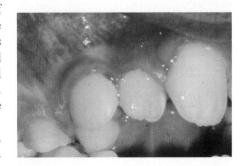

Fig. 13.5 Supplemental tooth 12.

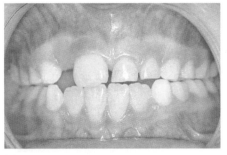

(a)

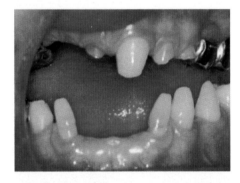

(b)

Fig. 13.6 Supernumerary tooth delaying the exfoliation of teeth 61, 62, and the eruption of tooth 21.

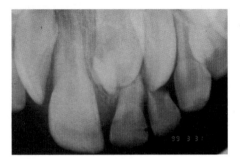

Fig. 13.7 Hypodontia concurrent with microdontia.

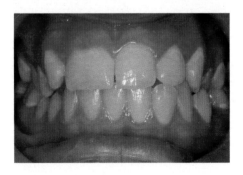

Fig. 13.8 Megadont tooth 11, absent tooth 12.

developing deeper within the jaw. This commonly occurs in the case of a mesiodens. (Fig. 13.6(a) and (b)).

There is a significant association between supernumerary teeth and invaginated teeth (see Section 13.5.3). There is also an association with palatal clefts, with approximately 40 % of patients with a cleft of the anterior palate having supernumerary teeth.

Multiple supernumerary teeth are seen in cleidocranial dysplasia as well as in other syndromes such as oral-facial-digital syndrome type 1 and Gardner syndrome. The management of supernumerary teeth is discussed in Chapter 14.

> **Key Points**
>
> Supernumerary teeth
> - 0.2–0.8% of the primary dentition;
> - 1.5–3.5% of the permanent dentition;
> - 2 : 1 male to female ratio;
> - 5 : 1 maxilla to mandible ratio.

13.4 ABNORMALITY OF TOOTH SIZE

13.4.1 Crown size

There is a degree of subjectivity regarding what constitutes normal ('ordinary') tooth size (and shape). Teeth which are obviously larger than normal are referred to as megadont or macrodont whereas teeth which are smaller than normal are termed microdont. Crown size is often related to root size, so teeth with large crowns often have large (broad) roots, teeth with small crowns tend to have small (slender) roots. Microdontia can be associated with hypodontia as in the example of X-linked hypohidrotic ectodermal dysplasia, where a heterozygous female might have one missing lateral incisor and a peg-shaped crown of the contralateral maxillary lateral incisor (Fig. 13.7).

Megadont teeth

Megadont maxillary incisors can occurs as a result of fusion of adjacent tooth germs or as a result of an attempt at separation of a single tooth germ to form two separate teeth. It is important in these circumstances to count the number of teeth to determine which of these possibilities has occurred, as this will influence treatment planning. The permanent maxillary central incisors are most often affected (Fig. 13.8) followed by the mandibular second premolars. Isolated megadontia has been estimated to occur in approximately 1% of patients in the permanent dentition. The condition may be symmetrical. Generalized megadontia has been reported in association with pituitary gigantism, in unilateral facial hyperplasia and in hereditary gingival fibromatosis.

Microdontia

Microdont primary teeth are uncommon, with a reported prevalence of 0.2–0.5%. In the permanent dentition the prevalence is approximately 2.5% for individual teeth, with generalized microdontia occurring in approximately 0.2% of individuals. Females are more often affected than males, with the maxillary lateral incisor being most commonly affected, having a peg-shaped or conical crown. (Fig. 13.9). As noted in the previous section (13.2), there is an association between microdontia and hypodontia.

13.4.2 Root size

Root length appears to be subject to some racial variation, with shorter roots being seen in people of Oriental background and larger roots in patients of African origin.

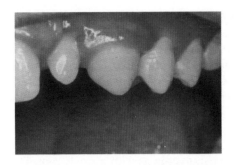

Fig. 13.9 Isolated microdontia affecting 22 in a female. Gingival architecture suggestive of occult cleft.

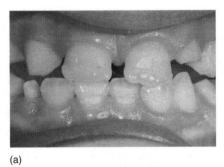

(a)

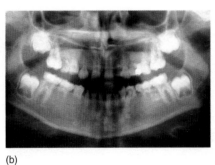

(b)

Fig. 13.10 Disturbed dental development—anti-leukaemic therapy.

Large root size

Larger than normal roots are most typically seen affecting the permanent maxillary central incisors, with a population prevalence in one Swedish study of 2.3%. Males were four times more likely to be affected than females.

Small root size

Short-rooted teeth in the primary dentition may be associated with other dental abnormalities. Short roots may also be seen in a number of conditions affecting the dentine and/or pulp. These will be considered in a later section.

Short roots may be seen affecting the permanent maxillary central incisors. The shortening affects approximately 2.5% of children and some 15% of these may have shortened roots on other teeth, most often premolars and/or canines. The cause is often unknown, though this can occur as a result of orthodontic treatment.

In regional odontodysplasia (Section 13.7.1) there is typically abnormal root formation as well as abnormalities of the crowns of the teeth.

Irradiation of the jaws, or chemotherapy, during the period of root formation may lead to truncation of the roots of teeth whose roots were developing at the time of treatment (Fig. 13.10(a) and (b)).

13.4.3 Treatment

As with hypodontia, the active cooperation of paediatric dentist, orthodontist, and restorative dentist should be encouraged to optimize treatment planning for young people affected by these conditions from an early age.

A megadont maxillary central incisor can be cosmetically unaesthetic and treatment decisions may need to be considered soon after (or, in some cases, before) eruption of the tooth. The options include acceptance, remodelling of the tooth, extraction of the tooth with orthodontic treatment if necessary, and subsequent masking of the space with a bridge, denture, or implant (Fig. 13.11).

A microdont tooth, particularly if this affects the maxillary lateral incisors, may be modified by acid-etch composite material being added to the tooth to reproduce the typical contours of the crown. (Fig. 13.12). In adult life, porcelain veneers may also be used or the tooth can be crowned.

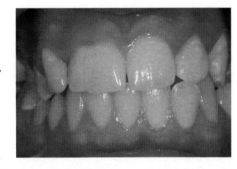

Fig. 13.11 Megadont tooth 11. Minimal adjustment of tooth form 11, 13, from original state in Fig. 13.8

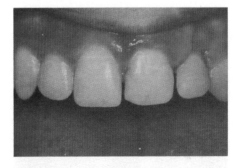

Fig. 13.12 Isolated microdontia affecting 22 in a female. Restored with composite.

13.5 ABNORMALITY OF TOOTH FORM

13.5.1 Abnormality of crown form

Fusion and gemination

Some cases of megadont crowns are as a result of fusion of adjacent tooth germs (fusion), or attempts at developmental separation of a single tooth germ to produce

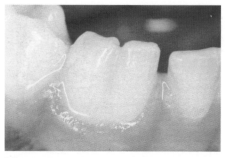

(a)

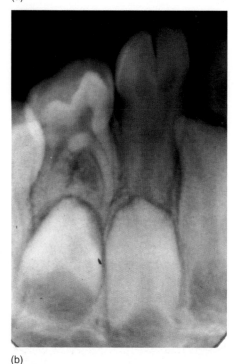

(b)

Fig. 13.13   Clinical and radiographic appearance of geminated lower primary lateral incisor/canine.

two separate teeth (gemination) and a variety of terms have been used for such situations. The term 'double teeth' has been applied to cover both situations. It is important to count the number of teeth present clinically and, with the aid of radiographs to determine whether fusion or gemination is more likely to have occurred. The prevalence of such abnormalities ranges from 0.5% to 1.6% of Caucasian populations studied in the primary dentition. The permanent dentition is less commonly affected (prevalence 0.1–0.2%). Males and females are affected equally. A genetic basis has been suggested but not confirmed.

The clinical manifestation may vary from a minor notch on the incisal edge of an abnormally wide incisor crown to two separate crowns with a single root. The crowns and root may be in continuity along their entire length or may be almost separate; some pulp intercommunication is often present. The most typical areas affected are the anterior segments of the arches in the primary dentition, with the mandible more commonly affected than the maxilla (Fig. 13.13(a) and (b)). There may be an association with hypodontia, so that a larger than normal tooth of the primary series together with a missing tooth in that series may represent an intermediate stage between the presence or absence of a tooth.

Physiological root resorption of primary fused or geminated teeth may be delayed and this may lead to delayed eruption of the permanent successors.

Treatment

When this condition affects the primary dentition no treatment *per se* is required. It is important, however, to consider the possibility of abnormalities of the number and/or form of the permanent dentition in the area. One problem which can occur is that caries can develop at the interface between the two crown segments (Fig. 13.14). This can be prevented by an etch-retained restoration to fill in the defect, which will also improve the cosmetic appearance. In the permanent dentition, the final decision on whether to retain, extract, surgically divide or otherwise treat such teeth will depend on many factors including space available within the arch, the morphology of the pulp chambers and/or root canals and the degree of attachment between the two parts of the tooth or teeth.

> **Key points**
> Double teeth
> - 0.1–1.6% in the primary dentition;
> - 0.1–0.2% in the permanent dentition;
> - No sex predilection;
> - Permanent anomalies in 30–50 % of primary cases.

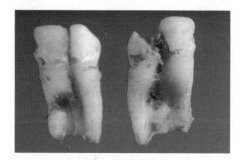

Fig. 13.14   Caries in extracted geminated teeth.

13.5.2 Accessory cusps

Extra cusps are not uncommon in the human dentition and may occur in both the primary and permanent dentition, most commonly affecting molar teeth. In the primary dentition the most common accessory cusps are seen either on the mesiobuccal aspects of the maxillary first molar or the mesiopalatal aspect of the maxillary second molar, the latter being similar to the cusp of Carabelli seen on the first permanent molar. The latter is a relatively frequent finding on the mesiopalatal aspect of the crown of the maxillary first molars, is typically bilateral and may be seen in 10–60% of various populations. Permanent incisor teeth may have an additional cusp arising from the lingual cingulum, often referred to as a 'talon cusp'. This affects the maxillary central incisor most commonly. Talon cusps may interfere with the occlusion and may be aesthetically unpleasing. (Fig. 13.15 (a) and (b)). As with double teeth, caries may occur in the groove between the cusp and palatal surface of the incisor. Other incisor evaginations have been reported. (Fig. 13.16(a and b)). Permanent canines may also have a prominent lingual cusp, perhaps indicating a tendency towards a premolar tooth form. Additional cusps may uncommonly be seen on premolars.

Treatment

The talon cusp may require action for both aesthetic and occlusal reasons. Selective grinding, repeated over a period of time, will reduce the height of the cusp and allow deposition of reactionary dentine on the pulpal surface of the dentine. Single visit sectioning of the cusp from the tooth followed by elective pulpotomy can also be considered.

13.5.3 Invaginated teeth

This term refers to the presence of an invagination in the crown of the tooth, forming an infolding lined by enamel within the crown of the tooth, sometimes extending into the root. An invagination of enamel epithelium into the dental papilla during development leads to the formation of the abnormality. The terms invaginated tooth or dens invaginatus can be used; other terms commonly applied (but not necessarily correctly) are dens in dente, gestant composite odontome, and dilated composite odontome.

The maxillary lateral incisor is the most commonly affected tooth (Fig. 13.17 (a) and (b)). The maxillary central incisors are less commonly affected and, occasionally, the canines are affected. In its mildest form an invaginated tooth is typically a maxillary lateral incisor with a deep cingulum pit on the palatal aspect of the crown. In its more extreme form the invagination is associated with a grossly abnormal crown form and root form (Fig. 13.18). In these gross examples the crown is tuberculate with the invagination appearing on the cusp of the abnormal tooth. Radiographs show the extent of the invagination chamber. Enamel, which may be extremely thin and may even be absent, can be seen lining this chamber. The pulp may be displaced and surround the invagination cavity, appearing radiographically as narrow slits around the dentine forming the wall of the invagination. Sometimes the root is significantly expanded.

Invagination of primary teeth is uncommon but in the permanent dentition has been estimated to affect between 1% and 5% of different groups. Males are more commonly affected than females, with a ratio of 2 : 1. Invaginations may also differ in different racial groups, with people of Chinese ethnicity being reportedly more commonly affected.

Invaginated teeth may cause problems because of the development of caries and pulpal pathology. This can occur soon after tooth eruption, with the child presenting an acute abscess or facial cellulitis. In such cases the radiograph will invariably demonstrate incomplete root formation as well as periapical rarefaction (Fig. 13.17 (a) and (b)). The presence of one invaginated tooth should lead to consideration of the contralateral tooth and/or adjacent teeth being affected. Invaginations are often bilateral,

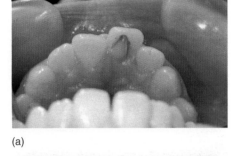
(a)

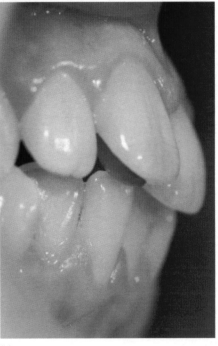
(b)

Fig. 13.15 Evagination—talon cusp with plaque accumulation and interfering with the occlusion.

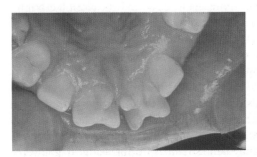
(a)

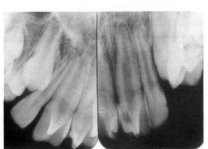
(b)

Fig. 13.16 Evaginations—triform and cruciform teeth, 11, 21.

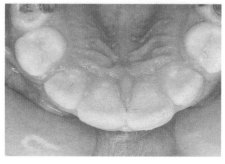

(a)

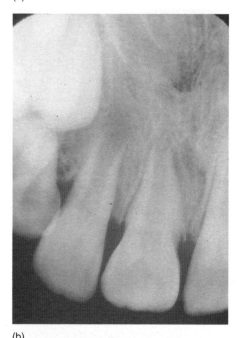

(b)

Fig. 13.17 Infected, palatal invagination, tooth 12.

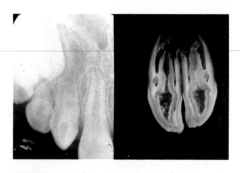

Fig. 13.18 Infected, invaginated odontome, tooth 12.

though not necessarily symmetrical. Some patients with invaginated teeth may also have supernumerary teeth and therefore full radiographic examination is warranted.

Treatment

If invaginations are identified at an early stage after eruption of the tooth then etch-retained resin sealants can be placed to prevent bacteria entering the invagination and subsequent development of caries. Acute infective episodes, particularly when associated with cellulitis, should be treated with appropriate antibiotic therapy as well as incision and drainage of any pointing abscess. The tooth should be opened, or extracted if the long-term prognosis is poor. This tends to be the case with the more gross examples where the crown and root form are abnormal. In less extreme forms endodontic treatment, firstly involving apexification, can be considered.

13.5.4 Evaginated teeth

Evaginated teeth, or dens evaginatus, most commonly affect the premolar teeth. Permanent molar teeth may also be affected. Typically there is a small tubercule on the occlusal surface of the premolar in the central part of the fissure pattern. The condition is more common in patients of Chinese descent and has been estimated to occur in 1–4% of the group. The evaginations are typically fractured off or worn down by virtue of normal wear, leading to pulpal exposure, pulpal pathology, and periapical involvement.

Treatment

Careful radiographic evaluation is necessary to determine the extent of any pulpal extension into the evagination. Restricted and repeated grinding of the tubercule can be undertaken to promote reactionary dentine deposition on the pulpal aspect of the evagination. However, this approach may only be applicable in a small number of cases and, more commonly, removal of the tubercule and a limited pulpotomy are required.

13.6 ABNORMALITY OF ROOT FORM

13.6.1 Taurodontism

The term taurodontism (literally—bull-like teeth, resembling a bull's neck) is used to describe molar teeth in which the body of the tooth is enlarged vertically at the expense of the roots. The normal constriction of a tooth at the level of the amelocemental junction is frequently reduced or absent in affected teeth. The mechanism leading to taurodontism is the late invagination (or failure) of Hertwig's root sheath, which maps out the shape of root formation. The furcation is displaced apically. Varying degrees of taurodontism are seen, with the most extreme example being when only a single root is present rather than separate roots. Taurodont teeth may also be described as pyramidal, cuneiform, or fused. The root canal morphology may have implications when endodontic treatment or extraction is required.

Taurodontism is most commonly recognized in the permanent dentition. Although the term is traditionally applied only to molars, in some patients with taurodontism of the molar teeth the pulps of single-rooted teeth may be larger than normal. The prevalence of taurodontism varies according to the criteria used. In British schoolchildren a prevalence of 6% for mandibular first permanent molars has been reported. Higher prevalences have been recorded in certain racial groups such as the Bantu in South Africa. In some families taurodontism seems to follow an autosomal dominant pattern of inheritance. Taurodontism has also been considered to be an atavistic trait. It is found in association with amelogenesis imperfecta, the tricho-dento-osseous syndrome, ectodermal dysplasias, and a number of other syndromes. Taurodontism is also more common in X-chromosomal aneudoploidy.

13.6.2 Accessory roots

Accessory roots may occur in almost any tooth. In the primary dentition this most commonly affects the molars but the primary canines and maxillary incisors can also be affected. In the permanent dentition, accessory roots are occasionally seen in maxillary incisors, mandibular canines, premolars, and molars. These accessory roots are often situated on the distolingual aspect of the tooth, may vary in shape, and may be difficult to identify radiographically. Accessory roots have been reported to occur in 1–9% of the primary dentition and from 1% to 45% of the permanent dentition. There is an association between accessory roots and large cusps of Carabelli on the maxillary first permanent molar and with accessory cusps on maxillary second and third molars. In some cases the presence of accessory roots reflects macrodontia.

13.7 ABNORMALITY OF TOOTH STRUCTURE

13.7.1 All tissues

Arrested development of tooth-germs

Arrested development of tooth-germ formation may occur following such external influences as trauma, ionizing radiation, osteomyelitis, or chemotherapy. The teeth affected and the particular tissues affected will be dependent upon the nature and timing of the insult. In teeth whose crowns are developing, this may result in enamel defects and corresponding dentine defects may be seen on microscopic sections should the tooth ultimately be extracted (Fig. 13.10(a) and (b)). If roots are developing at the time of the insult these may appear stunted.

Locally, one or more permanent tooth-germs may be affected by infection from an overlying primary predecessor. Such teeth are termed Turner teeth and typically have areas of enamel hypoplasia and/or enamel hypomineralization. The mandibular premolars are most commonly affected (Fig. 13.19).

Regional odontodysplasia

This is an uncommon developmental anomaly, typically affecting the primary teeth and corresponding permanent successors within a segment of the dentition. The anterior teeth are more commonly affected than the posterior teeth and the defect may cross the midline. The term 'ghost teeth' is sometimes applied to reflect the radiographic appearance seen. Affected patients may present with abscesses prior to the eruption of the teeth. The abnormal teeth have poorly developed crowns with enamel and dentine changes, large pulp chambers, and open apices. The permanent teeth may be less severely affected than the primary predecessors (Fig. 13.20(a) and (b)).

Treatment

The removal of teeth affected by regional odontodysplasia is often necessary. As this is often the case in the primary dentition, consideration then needs to be given to management of the affected permanent successors. While there are reports of the effective use of etch-retained restorations in these cases, the teeth are often slow to erupt, with a distinctive local gingivitis, and the pulpal morphology is such that infection is a frequent outcome. Root development may be slow but restoratively

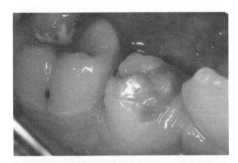

Fig. 13.19 Turner tooth. Hypoplastic lower premolar—previous infection in primary tooth.

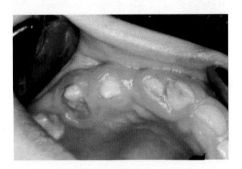

(a)

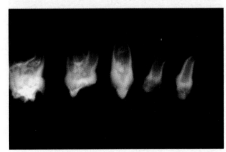

(b)

Fig. 13.20 Regional odontodysplasia—clinical and radiographic appearance.

useful. A case-by-case approach to treatment planning is required. Block removal of unerupted teeth with surrounding bone is not required.

13.7.2 Enamel defects

Enamel defects may be caused by genetic or environmental factors, acting alone or in combination. Where less enamel matrix than normal is produced the resulting enamel will be thinner (hypoplasia). If there is a defect in mineralization of the enamel matrix proteins then the result will be poorly mineralized enamel (hypomineralization—sometimes subdivided into hypocalcification for more severe defects and hypomaturation for milder changes). In many cases there will be a combination of both hypoplasia and hypomineralization, although sometimes the defect will be perceived clinically as predominantly one or the other. When enamel hypoplasia is seen the enamel may be uniformly thin, or grooved or pitted. In hypomineralization the enamel will typically be discoloured, usually a yellow-brown colour. This is particularly so where the defect is severe (hypocalcification) whereas in a less severe presentation (hypomaturation) the enamel may be almost normal but appear mottled or even only slightly opaque rather than translucent.

> **Key Points**
> - Enamel defects;
> - Hypoplasia—deficient matrix;
> - Hypomineralisation—poor mineralisation.

Amelogenesis imperfecta

Amelogenesis imperfecta is the term applied to generalized enamel defects affecting all (or predominantly all) of the teeth of both the primary and permanent dentitions. It is of genomic origin and thus there may be a family history of similar defects in other family members. Although the term strictly relates to enamel defects only, in some patients there may be subtle or substantial changes in other dental tissues and cranio-facial structures, or the condition may involve more widespread abnormalities as part of a syndrome. Dentally, there may be failures of eruption with resorption of the unerupted teeth. A case may be made for regular radiographic review of these patients (Fig. 13.21).

Amelogenesis imperfecta is seen in single gene mutations with autosomal dominant, autosomal recessive, and X-linked patterns of inheritance. Apparently sporadic cases are also seen—it is not clear whether these represent new mutations, or whether these will then be passed on to future offspring (Fig. 13.22). AI is relatively uncommon, but there are marked population differences in prevalence. In parts of Sweden the condition is relatively common (one in approximately 700 of the population). In one study in the United States the prevalence was found to be approximately 1 in 14,000.

The classification of amelogenesis imperfecta has traditionally been based on the phenotype—the clinical appearance. Following this system, patients are allocated according to the perceived defect—hypoplasia, hypocalcification, or hypomaturation. Some classifications have an additional category of hypomaturation–hypoplasia with taurodontism to reflect the fact that some families show a combination of thin and/or poorly mineralized enamel as well as taurodontism. However, it is important to realize, both from a diagnostic and from a classification point of view, that not all individuals within a family may show the same finding. As a result, phenotype classifications become problematic when different members of the same family are grouped into different categories. Furthermore, this classification system fails when there is uncertainty as to which is the presumed predominant defect. It is

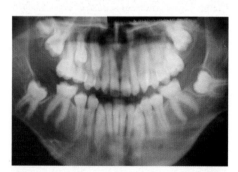

Fig. 13.21 Sporadic case; Amelogenesis imperfecta; hypomineralized with anterior open bite. Shows failure of eruption teeth 17, 15, 13, 27, 37, 47.

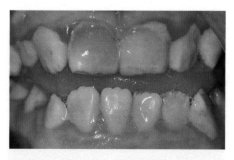

Fig. 13.22 Sporadic case; Amelogenesis imperfecta; hypomineralized; anterior open bite. The poor oral hygiene and staining are typical when, as here, the teeth are sensitive to thermal and mechanical stimuli.

possible that the inheritance pattern will be forgotten in attempting to categorize individuals.

For this reason an alternative classification system has been suggested where the mode of inheritance (autosomal dominant, autosomal recessive, X-linked or apparently sporadic) is considered before the clinical phenotype. This classification also allows for the fact that there may be some overlap between the clinical defects in the same or different members of a family. The full classification scheme includes the genomic and biochemical identity of the defect; however, for practical purposes, a simplified use of this modern classification might, for example, define a patient's presentation as 'autosomal dominant hypoplastic amelogenesis imperfecta'.

Autosomal dominant amelogenesis imperfecta

In autosomal dominant AI there is typically a clear pattern of inheritance with individuals in successive generations being affected (Fig. 13.23). Because the mutant gene is on one of the autosomes there is a 50% chance of an affected individual passing this on to each offspring. Males and females are equally affected. The primary and permanent dentitions are generally both involved, although the permanent dentition may be the more severely affected of the two (Fig. 13.24). There is a wide range of presentations (phenotypes). The enamel may be thin and hard with normal translucency but may be difficult to discern on radiographs because of its limited thickness. In some cases the enamel may be both hypoplastic and hypomineralized, in which case the enamel is thin and discoloured with a loss of normal translucency. Some patients may have enamel of normal thickness which is poorly mineralized, and yet others may have enamel of normal thickness which lacks the normal translucency and is therefore regarded as showing features of hypomaturation. Occasionally, subtle enamel defects may only be identified on histopathological examination of extracted teeth. In some families taurodontism is seen. Anterior open bite may occur in autosomal dominant amelogenesis imperfecta as well as in other inheritance patterns. The mechanism producing the sometimes associated anterior open bite has not yet been elucidated.

Aetiology

The enamelin gene on chromosome 4 has been shown to be mutated in some families with autosomal dominant amelogenesis imperfecta. Other genes involved in normal enamel formation have been implicated in autosomal dominant amelogenesis imperfecta. Patients with tricho-dento-osseous syndrome, an autosomal dominant syndrome characterized by amelogenesis imperfecta with taurodontism as well as curly hair and bone changes, have been found to have mutations in the *DLX3* gene on chromosome 17.

Autosomal recessive amelogenesis imperfecta

Autosomal recessive conditions are typically seen when there is parental consanguinity, so that that the parents may be first cousins (Fig. 13.25). There may be cultural reasons for this or, alternatively, consanguinity may be seen in isolated communities with little outside contact and where there is consequently a limited gene pool. In other recessive conditions, such as cystic fibrosis, these restrictions do not apply and the relative prevalence of the condition is related to the frequency of gene carriers in the population. Where the parents are close relatives, both carrier adults will be unaffected but there will be a one in four chance of offspring inheriting two copies of the mutant gene.

Autosomal recessive mutations causing amelogenesis imperfecta seem to be uncommon apart from Polynesia, where, presumably, the mutation is relatively common. Such individuals may have enamel hypoplasia and/or enamel hypomineralization and the

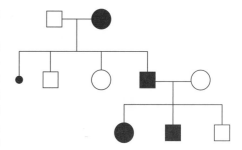

Fig. 13.23 Pedigree chart. Autosomal dominant inheritance of AI.

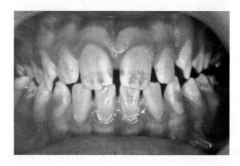

Fig. 13.24 Autosomal dominant AI. All teeth affected similarly.

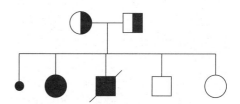

Fig. 13.25 Pedigree chart. Autosomal recessive inheritance of AI.

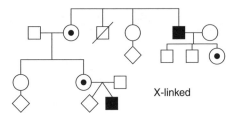

X-linked

Fig. 13.26 Pedigree chart. X-linked inheritance—no male to male transmission.

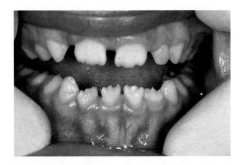

Fig. 13.27 X-linked; AI; Male; thin, smooth enamel.

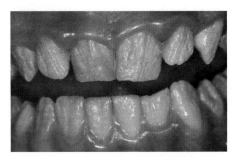

Fig. 13.28 X-linked; AI; female; ridged, predominantly hypoplastic enamel.

designator 'pigmented enamel' has been applied. A gene on chromosome 2 has been linked to autosomal recessive amelogenesis imperfecta associated with ocular defects.

X-linked amelogenesis imperfecta

X-linked amelogenesis imperfecta is characterized by a difference in the appearance of the teeth of affected males and females. The majority of families studied to date have an alteration in the amelogenin gene on the short arm of the X chromosome. Affected males cannot pass on the condition to their sons (by virtue of passing on their Y chromosome to their sons) but their daughters (to whom they necessarily pass on their X chromosome) will all inherit the mutant gene. Such daughters will always show some dental features although these might be subtle in some cases. These heterozygous females can pass on the mutant gene to children of either sex. (Fig. 13.26).

The enamel in both sexes may be hypoplastic, hypomineralized, or show elements of both features. The appearance seen will be the result of the exact nature of the change in the amelogenin gene and the sex of the patient.

Males, by virtue of having a single X chromosome, will be more severely and uniformly affected. The enamel may be thin (hypoplastic—reduced in quantity) or discoloured (with affected mineralisation) or a combination of both (Fig. 13.27). Females within the same family who inherit the affected gene will show a vertical pattern of markings of the enamel, either vertical ridges and grooves (the equivalent of the male, uniform hypoplasia), with or without discolouration or loss of translucency of the enamel (where the mineralization is affected) (Fig. 13.28).

Aetiology

The amelogenin gene, which encodes the enamel protein amelogenin, is located on the short arm of the X chromosome. Mutations in the gene are responsible for most cases of X-linked amelogenesis imperfecta but there also appears to be another gene on the long arm of the X chromosome which is responsible for similar clinical appearances in another family.

Genetic enamel defects associated with generalized disorders

Widespread enamel defects can be seen in a number of conditions with extraoral manifestations. These include conditions such as epidermolysis bullosa, tuberous sclerosis, oculo-dento-osseus dysplasia, as well as the amelogenesis imperfecta associated with tricho-dento-osseous syndrome. The exact genomic relationship between these and other conditions and amelogenesis imperfecta remains to be established in most cases.

Key Points

Amelogenesis imperfecta
- Inheritance,
- Autosomal dominant,
- Autosomal recessive,
- X-linked,
- Apparently sporadic.

Phenotype

Hypoplastic $+/-$ hypomineralization (hypocalcification to hypomaturity)

Pure hypoplasia or hypomineralization are probably rare
Profound hypomineralization leads to teeth so soft that they are reduced in size although this is, in fact, a later change.

Molar-incisor hypoplasia

In recent years reports have been published of children with mineralization defects of the first permanent molars and, sometimes, the permanent incisors. This has been referred to as molar-incisor hypomineralization or hypoplasia and also as 'cheese molars' because of the friable nature of the enamel of the molar tooth enamel. Although the condition would seem to have a chronological distribution (Fig. 13.29 (a) and (b)) , close inspection will often show 'un-matched' teeth to be affected—teeth that would have been forming at the same time do not present with symmetrical affliction. Only one molar, or perhaps three of the four, may be affected. The defects in the incisors—which are usually less severe and most likely to show isolated mottling—will likewise be irregularly distributed. (Fig. 13.30 (a,b, and c)). To the best of our knowledge, this is the first publication of such a familial association.

The cause of this anomaly, and even whether it represents a new phenomenon, is uncertain. It has been suggested that there might be a genetic predisposition combining with an environmental insult that produces these changes, but this has yet to be substantiated.

Treatment

The condition is problematic for both patients and practitioners. The destruction of the molar teeth in particular, although probably a post-eruptive change, presents in many cases at a time when children are not acclimatized to dental treatment. Treatment options should include a careful analysis of the occlusion, since many of the molar teeth are severely compromised, and the child may benefit in the long term by their elective loss as part of a comprehensive treatment plan. For the 2 years between the eruption of the first permanent molar teeth and the commonly recommended time for their removal, management may be difficult. It is clear that many children with this condition are apprehensive patients for dental treatment. This is likely to be because, in its early stages, practitioners adopt a minimalist approach with the attempted use of fissure sealants and adhesive restorations. These are often applied without local anaesthesia, are painful in the process, and frequently unsuccessful anyway. Preformed metal crowns applied under local anaesthesia provide a useful measure in these cases.

The incisor defects are not noticeably uncomfortable and should be managed with the techniques described in Chapter 10.

'Environmentally determined' enamel defects

Enamel defects may arise as a result of an 'environmental' insult. Within this sense we include both a systemic upset and the result of a local factor involving a developing tooth (as discussed previously in Section 13.7).

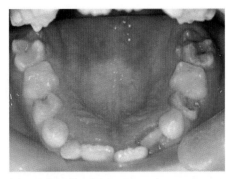
(a)

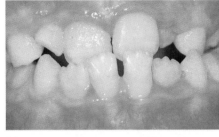
(b)

Fig. 13.29 Molar-incisor hypomineralization (MIH) with features of chronological disturbance but no relevant medical history.

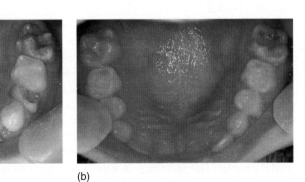

(a)   (b)

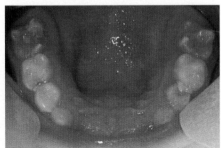

(c)

Fig. 13.30   MIH in a sister and two brothers.

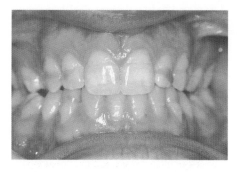

Fig. 13.31   Hypoplasia in a 'chronological distribution'.

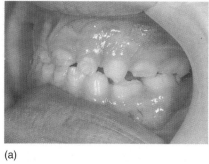

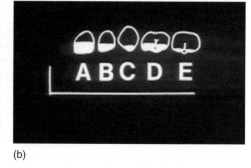

(a)   (b)

Fig. 13.32   Primary dentition—pre-term hypoplasia.

Where there is a systemic insult the teeth will be affected in a chronological pattern, so that a band of abnormal enamel is seen in horizontal distribution at some part on the tooth crown. Typically this results in a groove in the enamel of affected teeth. The term chronological hypoplasia is often used to describe such cases (Fig. 13.31). A knowledge of the timing of commencement of formation of the teeth will aid in understanding the timing of such an insult.

Systemic (chronological) enamel defects

Enamel formation in utero may be affected by a wide range of maternal and foetal conditions. These will include endocrine disturbances (hypoparathyroidism), infections (rubella), drugs (thalidomide), nutritional deficiencies, and haematological and metabolic disorders (Rhesus incompatibility). In such cases, the enamel covering the incisal portions of the crowns of the primary incisors will typically be affected in the pattern shown in Fig. 13.32(a) and (b). Similar changes may be seen in pre-term, low birth weight, infants. It is not yet clear whether this is associated with the use of intubation for these children in the neonatal period although the latter has been identified as a local cause affecting forming incisors only.

When there is a systemic upset or marked physiological changes occur at birth or in the neonatal period, corresponding enamel defects may be seen in the primary dentition. Illness in the neonatal period may also affect the tips of the first permanent molars as these commence development at around birth.

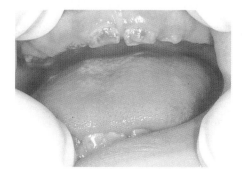

Fig. 13.33   Primary teeth; both jaws affected by icterus gravis neonatorum (Rhesus disease), upper teeth with superadded 'bottle caries'.

Enamel defects may also arise as a result of acute or chronic childhood illnesses (Fig. 13.33). This will include hypothyroidism and hypoparathyroidism, chronic renal disease, and gastrointestinal disorders producing malabsorption, such as coeliac disease. The use of tetracycline during pregnancy and childhood is to be avoided because of deposition of the tetracycline in developing dental matrices, producing a distinctive blue/grey discolouration of the teeth, sometimes in a chronologically banded distribution (Fig. 13.34).

In the past, exanthematous fevers caused by measles and other infections were associated with a disturbance of normal enamel formation and a corresponding chronological hypoplasia affecting the crowns of developing teeth. Modern medical care has now made this uncommon, unless such changes may occur in the case of babies and infants who develop pneumonia.

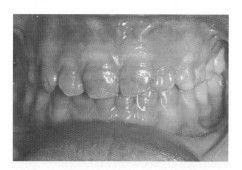

Fig. 13.34   Tetracycline staining associated with horizontal, hypoplastic banding representing repeated childhood illness and its treatment.

Enamel formation is also sensitive to chemical agents, such as fluoride. Excessive intake of fluoride, either from naturally occurring sources such as drinking water with fluoride levels over 1–2 ppm, or from over use of fluoride supplements or fluoride toothpastes, can cause enamel mottling. In its mildest form fluorosis appears as an opacity of the enamel. The condition is dose-dependant, with increasing intake of fluoride being associated with more marked opacity, areas of discolouration of the enamel as well as pitting, and more extensive hypoplastic defects (Fig. 13.35(a)). Confusion

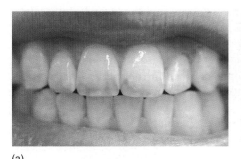
(a)

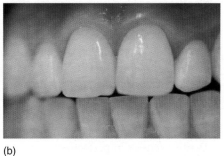
(b)

Fig. 13.35 Disturbed dental development, fluorotic mottling:pre-and post-microabrasion.

between fluorosis and amelogenesis imperfecta can occur. One distinguishing feature may be that amelogenesis imperfecta does not show a chronological distribution and that fluorosis, depending on the timing of the excessive intake, does. Local, fluorotic lesions may respond very well to the microabrasion technique (Fig. 13.35(b)).

Local factors

As well as the possibility of damage to the forming teeth that may be caused by dental injuries (Fig. 13.36) (see Chapter 12), pressure on the premaxilla from the use of an oro-tracheal tube may cause damage to the developing primary incisor teeth. Children with a cleft lip and palate often have enamel defects of the maxillary incisors. Sometimes this may be related to surgical treatment rather than the effect of the cleft *per se*.

Treatment

The treatment of children with enamel defects requires more consideration than simply mechanical treatment of the teeth. Children with amelogenesis imperfecta, in particular, may be subject to teasing. This is a serious issue and requires the most sensitive handling by professionals. Affected adult family members will often describe their own childhood in lurid and painful terms. Many children will not admit to this from the outset and need to be given 'permission' (with their parent's knowledge) to contact the practitioner at a later date to revisit these issues.

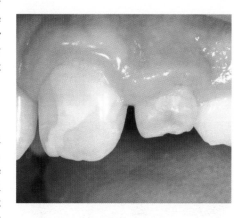

Fig. 13.36 Disturbed dental development—previous primary tooth injury.

Typically, as well as the aesthetics, there may be thermal, contact or osmotic sensitivity of the teeth. Oral hygiene may be poor and irremediable as a result (Fig. 13.22). The occlusion may be compromised by lack of vertical dimension as a result of thinner enamel than normal, or there may be loss of enamel because of poorly mineralized enamel matrix. Some practitioners advocate the early preventive use of full coverage restorations in the primary dentition for these children.

Localized defects are much more amenable to simple measures.

13.7.3 Dentine defects

As with enamel defects, dentine defects may be of genetic origin or caused by environmental effects.

Genetically determined dentine defects

DENTINOGENESIS IMPERFECTA

Dentinogenesis imperfecta is an autosomal dominant inherited condition. It may occur in isolation or in association with osteogenesis imperfecta. This represents two conditions, rather than a spectrum of effect. The term hereditary opalescent dentine is sometimes applied because of the typical opalescent hue of the teeth.

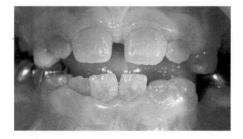

Fig. 13.37 Dentinogenesis imperfecta—early mixed dentition.

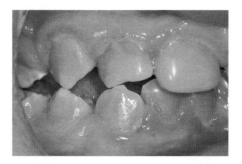

Fig. 13.38 Dentinogensis imperfecta; 18-year-old-male; composite additions teeth 12, 11, 42, 41. Typical dark dentine colouration; short clinical crowns.

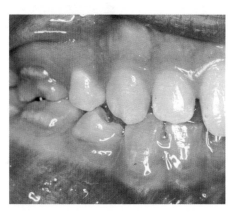

Fig. 13.39 Dentinogenesis imperfecta; variable expression in one individual.

Dentinogenesis imperfecta, both the typical variant and the 'Brandywine isolate' variant in the eastern United States, has been mapped to chromosome 4 and the *DSPP* gene has been shown to be mutated in several families (some of whom also have had hearing defects). In some of the Brandywine isolate families, occasional individuals have teeth which are indistinguishable from the more typical form of dentinogenesis imperfecta; it is therefore likely that this represents an allelic variant of the same genetic condition.

Similarly, the diagnosis of coronal dentinal dysplasia has been proposed but this also seems likely to be a variant of dentinogenesis imperfecta.

Dentinogenesis imperfecta occurring in association with osteogenesis imperfecta is a result of mutations in one of the two collagen type 1 genes on chromosome 7 or 17. The dentine defects may be very apparent or rather subtle, in some cases requiring electron-microscopy for their identification.

Dentine (sometimes with enamel) changes can also be seen in some types of Ehlers Danlos syndrome involving mutations in the collagen 1 genes.

Dentinogenesis imperfecta occurring in the absence of osteogenesis imperfecta is inherited as an autosomal dominant trait. The primary and permanent dentitions are usually affected. The teeth are opalescent with a greyish or brownish colour (Figs 13.37, 13.38). There may be some variation in the severity of the appearance in different members of the same family. Some variability may also be seen in the severity of affliction of individual teeth in any one individual (Fig. 13.39). The enamel may chip away from the dentine to expose the dentine and the crowns may suffer from attrition so that the teeth are worn down to the level of the gingivae (Fig. 13.40). This situation is most commonly seen to affect the primary dentition. In the primary dentition the pulps may be large and hence pulpal exposure may occur early. In many cases, the pulps of the teeth tend to be obliterated, hence pulpal exposure and abscess formation tend to occur later than might otherwise be expected. The chipping of the enamel has often been claimed to result from a smooth enamel–dentine junction but some studies have demonstrated that the contour of the enamel–dentine junction is not a factor, with the weakness being within the dentine.

Radiographically the crowns appear relatively bulbous, the roots are shortened and may be thinner than normal. The pulp chambers may be large initially, particularly in the primary dentition, but more typically the pulps are obliterated as a result of deposition of dentine in a rather haphazard manner (Fig. 13.41(a) and (b)). This

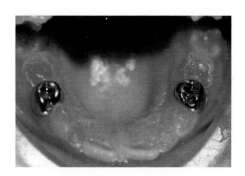

Fig. 13.40 Dentinogenesis imperfecta showing tooth wear 55, 65.

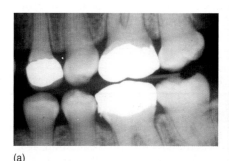

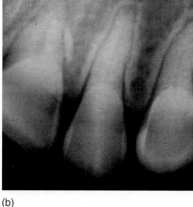

(a)   (b)

Fig. 13.41 Dentinogenesis imperfecta radiograph showing bulbous molar crowns, and obliterated pulp chambers.

can be seen in histopathological sections where the mantle dentine adjacent to the enamel–dentine junction is essentially normal but the deeper dentine is grossly abnormal.

OSTEOGENESIS IMPERFECTA

Osteogenesis imperfecta arises as a result of a mutation in one of the two collagen type 1 genes. Although it used to be regarded as having autosomal dominant and autosomal recessive modes of inheritance, it is now believed that autosomal dominant mutations are the norm but that the severity varies in different individuals and families. Cases such as those previously thought to be autosomal recessive are now considered most likely to arise as a result of gonadal mosaicism.

The condition is characterized by bone fragility so that children may have a history of fractures (from such mild trauma as walking into furniture), blue sclera, deafness (though this does not usually develop until the third decade of life), and lax ligaments around joints. There may or may not be dentinal changes, or these may be so subtle that they are not apparent clinically or radiographically.

> **Key Points**
>
> Dentinogenesis imperfecta
>
> * Autosomal dominant condition—isolated trait or associated with osteogenesis imperfecta or other collagen abnormalities.

DENTINAL DYSPLASIA

Dentinal dysplasia was first described in the 1920s; 'rootless teeth' is an alternative, descriptive, title. The condition is an autosomal dominant trait with both dentitions being affected. The teeth may be clinically normal but root formation is abnormal to varying degrees. Some teeth may have extremely short blunt roots, others taper markedly towards the apex (Fig. 13.42). The pulp is partially obliterated, appearing in the molar teeth as a small demilune. Under the microscope the coronal dentine is normal but the root dentine is not, with masses of abnormal dentine obliterating the pulp space. The microscopic appearance has been likened to boulders in a flowing stream. The short roots may cause problems because of mobility and this may lead to the condition being identified.

The above condition is often referred to as dentinal dysplasia type I to distinguish it from a condition referred to by some as dentinal dysplasia type II (coronal dentinal dysplasia). The latter is most likely to represent an allelic variant of dentinogenesis imperfecta as genetic linkage studies have shown it to map to the same region of chromosome 4 as dentinogenesis imperfecta and a mutation in the *DSPP* gene has also been identified in one family diagnosed as having dentinal dysplasia type II.

It remains to be seen whether dentinal dysplasia (type I) is also allelic to dentinogenesis imperfecta.

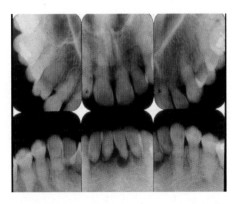

Fig. 13.42 Radicular dentinal dysplasia.

VITAMIN D-RESISTANT RICKETS

Vitamin D-resistant rickets is an X-linked inherited condition. Affected males tend to be short in stature with bowed legs and other skeletal changes. They may present dentally with abscesses forming in the absence of caries. Of the dental hard tissues, the dentine is most markedly affected with interglobular dentine being the chief histopathological finding. Radiographically the pulp spaces are larger than normal and pulpal extensions of the pulp horns may be exposed as a result of attrition of the teeth (Fig. 13.43) Heterozygous females tend to be more mildly affected and may not exhibit any dental manifestations.

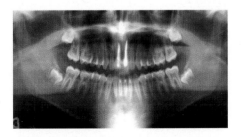

Fig. 13.43 Vitamin D resistant Ricketts. DPT of male showing large pulp chambers, less dense dentine adjacent to EDJ.

'Environmentally determined' dentine defects

Local trauma may interfere with dentine formation. This may be permanently recorded in the dentine as a prominent incremental line. Systemic influences including nutritional deficiencies, tetracycline administration, and chemotherapeutic agents such as anti-cancer therapy involving cytotoxic drugs can also affect the formation of dentine.

Treatment

As with enamel defects there may be severe psycho-social problems as a result of the appearance of the teeth. Many of the arguments presented in the consideration of enamel conditions will apply to dentine also. In dentinogenesis imperfecta, management is focused on the prevention of tooth wear, the maintenance of the vertical dimension and improvement of the appearance (Chapter 10). In rickets, the treatment should be similarly directed but cases presenting late may require acute management of dental abscesses on the teeth as a result of pulp death.

13.7.4 Cementum defects

The cementum can be affected in a number of genetic disorders. The consequences of alterations in cementum can have profound effects on the fate of the dentition.

There are a number of rare but significant conditions associated with the early loss of primary teeth. Any case of early or spontaneous loss of teeth is a cause for further investigation. In one of these, hypophosphatasia (both autosomal dominant and autosomal recessive inheritance are known), there may be premature exfoliation of the primary teeth or loss of the permanent teeth. The serum alkaline phosphatase level is low; phosphoethanolamine is excreted in the urine. Histopathological examination in hypophosphatasia will show aplasia or marked hypoplasia of the cementum. There may also be abnormal dentine formation with a wide predentine zone and the presence of interglobular dentine (similar to vitamin D-resistant rickets).

Treatment

Local measures such as scrupulous oral hygiene may slow the loss of teeth in cases of hypophosphatasia but the prime focus of treatment may be the replacement of teeth of the primary and permanent dentitions as they are lost.

13.8 DISTURBANCES OF ERUPTION

Considerable variations exist in the timing of eruption of the permanent dentition. There may be some racial variation and eruption may also be influenced by environmental factors such as nutrition and illness. Eruption times of permanent teeth in females tend to be slightly ahead of the corresponding eruption times in males; this becomes a more marked difference with the later erupting teeth.

13.8.1 Premature eruption

Some families report that early tooth eruption is a family feature. Children with high birth weight have been reported to have earlier eruption of their primary teeth than children with normal or low birth weights. Early eruption of the permanent dentition may occur in children with precocious puberty and children with endocrine abnormalities, particularly those of the growth or thyroid hormones.

Natal and neonatal teeth

Teeth present at birth are known as natal teeth and those that erupt within the first month of life as neonatal teeth. Approximately one in 2000–3000 live births are so affected. The mandibular central incisor is the most common natal or neonatal tooth. Occasionally maxillary (central) incisors or the first molars may appear as natal teeth. The vast majority of cases represent premature eruption of a tooth of the normal sequence. It has been suggested that this condition is a result of an ectopic position of the tooth-germ during foetal life.

Natal or neonatal teeth may also be seen in association with some syndromes including pachyonychia congenita, Ellis-van Creveld syndrome, and Hallermann-Streiff syndrome.

Natal or neonatal teeth are often mobile because of limited root development and may be a danger to the airway if they are inhaled. The crowns may be abnormal in form and the enamel may be poorly formed or thinner than normal. The mobility of the tooth frequently also causes inflammation of the surrounding gingivae. Trauma to the ventral surface of the tongue may cause ulceration (Fig. 13.44) and difficulty during feeding may occur if the infant is breastfed.

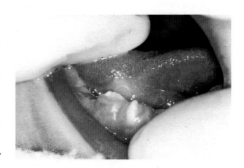

Fig. 13.44 Natal teeth 71, 81. Ulceration of ventral surface of tongue.

Treatment

Local measures such as smoothing of the sharp edges of the tooth with a rubber cone in a dental handpiece may help resolve the ulceration. In a number of cases, if the tooth is markedly loose it should be extracted as it is unlikely to form a useful part of the dentition. Firm application of Spencer–Wells forceps to the tooth crown is advised, followed by minor local curettage to remove remains of the developing tooth-germ at that site.

13.8.2 Delayed eruption

Delayed eruption of primary teeth may arise from either systemic or local factors. It may be associated with prematurity or low birth weight.

Delayed eruption of teeth of both dentitions may occur in association with Down syndrome and Turner's syndrome. Delayed eruption may also be associated with nutritional abnormalities or endocrine disorders such as hypothyroidism or hypopituitarism.

Cleidocranial dysplasia is an autosomal dominant condition characterized by aplasia or hypoplasia of the clavicles and widespread cranial changes. These include a brachycephalic skull (short in the antero-posterior dimension), frontal and parietal bossing, hypoplasia of the maxilla and zygomatic arches, hypertelorism as well as delayed closure of the anterior fontanelle and skull sutures. Multiple wormian bones are present in the line of the cranial sutures, particularly the lambdoid suture. With respect to the jaws, the most striking dental feature is the presence of multiple supernumerary teeth, particularly of the permanent dentition, and particularly in the anterior parts of the jaws. Permanent tooth eruption is often delayed or there is failure of eruption, partly because of the number of supernumerary teeth. The primary teeth may fail to resorb. Although it has been suggested that there may be hypoplasia of cementum on the roots of the teeth, this has not been definitively established. The proportion of cellular to acellular cementum does not seem to be significant.

Hereditary gingival fibromatosis may be associated with delayed eruption, presumably because of a local effect whereby the teeth are unable to penetrate the enlarged and thickened gingivae. Other, truly localized causes of delayed eruption include ectopic crypt position. This most often affects the maxillary or mandibular permanent canines, or may present with the impaction of the maxillary first permanent molars against the distal aspect of the adjacent primary second molar.

Local causes such as the presence of supernumeraries or odontomes may also interfere with eruption of an adjacent permanent tooth (Fig. 13.6(a) and (b)). A delay of more than 6 months between the eruption of a tooth and its antimere requires investigation, most usually radiographically.

The position of the permanent canines, particularly those in the maxilla, should be ascertained by palpation not later than the 10th birthday of the child. Any uncertainty as to their presence or position should be followed by radiographic examination. The potential for palatal impaction of these teeth may be identified by this simple measure and simple intervention in selected cases, by the prompt removal of the primary canine, may prevent the need for later surgery (Chapter 14).

Delayed eruption of permanent teeth may also be due to dilaceration of developing roots and crowns as a result of trauma to the primary dentition (Chapter 12).

Early extraction of a primary tooth may be associated with delayed eruption of the permanent successor due to thickening of the overlying mucosa.

Treatment

Any systemic condition may require treatment if this is available. Local obstructions such as supernumerary teeth or odontomes need to be removed. Surgical exposure and orthodontic traction may be necessary for late-presenting permanent canines and patients with hereditary gingival fibromatosis may require gingivectomy.

In cleidocranial dysplasia, a combined restorative and surgical and occlusal management approach to treatment planning is required. Retained primary teeth will likely need to be extracted, together with the surgical removal of unerupted supernumerary teeth. This requires careful treatment planning, as the successful eruption of the permanent dentition cannot be guaranteed. Orthodontic treatment to guide the teeth into occlusion may be one of the treatment options, with prosthetic replacement of the teeth being considered should the teeth fail to erupt.

13.9 DISTURBANCES OF EXFOLIATION

13.9.1 Premature exfoliation

Premature exfoliation is always a cause for further investigation. Its association with hypophosphatasia has been considered above (Section 13.7.4). Premature exfoliation may also be seen in cases of severe congenital neutropaenia, cyclical neutropaenia, Chediak-Higashi syndrome (where it is associated with gross periodontal destruction) and in the Langerhans cell histiocytoses

13.9.2 Delayed exfoliation

Infraocclusion

The terms infraocclusion, submerged teeth and ankylosed teeth are often used to describe teeth which have failed to come into normal occlusion or, more typically, have remained in their relative position in the arch while other teeth have continued to erupt. This is most commonly seen when one or more premolars fails to develop, hence the primary molars have no stimulus to become resorbed. As the adjacent permanent teeth erupt alveolar growth occurs, but in some cases the primary molars become ankylosed within the bone and fail to alter their position (Fig. 13.45(a)). As a result, there is an open bite in the affected area with the occlusal plane of the primary molars being lower than that of the adjacent permanent teeth. It should be recognized that the process of physiological resorption of primary teeth is not unremitting and there are phases of resorption and repair. If there is an imbalance between the two, with the latter predominating (particularly in the absence of

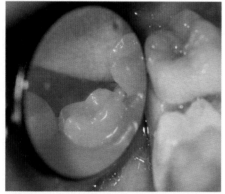

(a)

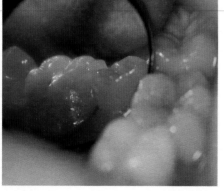

(b)

Fig. 13.45   Infra-occlusion tooth 75; before and after restoration with a laboratory made composite inlay.

normal physiological stimulus for resorption), then the net result is ankylosis. Genetic factors may be important but the aetiology has not yet been resolved.

Treatment

A substantial study has shown that removal of infraoccluded primary molars will lead to progressive space loss at that site with a potential either to give rise to or to focus crowding at that site; that all of the infraoccluded teeth in the study were shed within the expected time limits and that a more conservative approach to the management of these teeth may be indicated.

Where there is no permanent successor, the infraoccluded primary teeth may be retained and the crowns built up with acid-etch composite restorations or other restorative material. Onlays, either in metal or laboratory cured composite, may be considered. (Fig. 13.45(b)) If extraction is contemplated, then consideration needs to be given to orthodontic alignment, a denture, bridge, or implant.

Other causes of delayed exfoliation

Delayed exfoliation of primary teeth may be seen in association with a number of local causes, including fused/geminated primary teeth, ectopically developing permanent teeth and subsequent to trauma or severe infection of primary teeth.

Key points

- There is a time range in which teeth erupt—but this range will affect the dentition as a whole.
- Dentitions falling substantially outside this range, or individually affected teeth delayed by 6 months, should be investigated.
- Premature exfoliation always demands investigation.
- There is a place for a conservative approach to the management of infraoccluded primary teeth.

When seeking a diagnosis of a developmental dental condition please remember:

Common things occur commonly (rarities are rarely seen!)

Is this a chronological distribution?

Are any other members of the family affected?

Are all the teeth (more or less) equally affected?

And finally, 'When everything else has been excluded, that which remains, however improbable, must be the answer' (Sherlock Holmes—paraphrase).

13.10 SUMMARY

1. Dental anomalies may have both a functional and psycho-social impact on the child and their family.
2. The presence of one dental anomaly may be associated with others. Thorough clinical examination and radiographic investigations are essential.
3. An anomaly in the primary dentition may be associated with a similar anomaly in the permanent dentition.
4. All cases of missing teeth require treatment planning with multidisciplinary input.

5. Both developmental enamel defects and developmental dentine defects may be genetic or environmental in origin.

6. Both development enamel defects and developmental dentine defects may be seen in isolation or in association with extraoral features.

7. The distribution of an environmentally induced enamel defect will depend upon the stage of tooth development at the time of the insult.

8. Excessive fluoride ingestion can cause enamel defects.

9. Dental professionals have an important part to play in the diagnosis and care of children with these conditions.

10. Careful monitoring of dental development, together with interception when appropriate, may reduce the impact of these conditions.

13.11 FURTHER READING

Aldred, M. J., Crawford, P. J. M., Savarirayan, R. (2003). Amelogenesis imperfecta—a classification and catalogue for the 21st century. *Oral Diseases*, 9, 19–23.

Aldred, M. J., Crawford, P. J. M. (1997). Molecular biology of hereditary enamel defects. In *Dental Enamel*. pp. 200–209, Chichester: Wiley.

Aldred, M. J. (2003). Human Genetics. In *Oxford Handbook of Applied Dental Science* (ed. C. Scully), pp. 389–406. Oxford Medical Publications, Oxford.

Brook, A. H., Winter, G. B. (1970). Double teeth. A retrospective study of 'geminated' and 'fused' teeth in children. *British Dental Journal*, **4**, 129(3), 123–30.

Crawford, P. J. M., Aldred, M. J. (1989). Regional odontodysplasia: a bibliography. *Journal of Oral Pathology Medicine*, **18**, 251–63.

Crawford, P. J. M., Aldred, M. J. (1992). X-linked amelogenesis imperfecta. Presentation of two kindreds and a review of the literature. *Oral surgery, Oral Medicine, and Oral Patholgy* **73**, 449–55.

Gorlin, R. J., Cohen, M. M., Cohen, R., and Hennekam, R. (2001). *Syndromes of the Head and Neck* (Oxford Monographs on Medical Genetics). Oxford University Press, Oxford.

Hall, R. K., Bankier, A., Aldred, M. J., Kan, K., Lucas, J. O., and Perks, A. G. B. (1997). Solitary median maxillary central incisor, short stature, choanal atresia/midnasal stenosis (SMMCI) syndrome: an analysis of the clinical features of 19 consecutive cases of the syndrome, a review of the literature and consideration of its aetiology. Oral Surgery, *Oral Medicine, and Oral Pathology* **84**, 651–662.

Kurol, J. and Koch, G. (1985). The effect of extraction of infraoccluded deciduous primary molars: A longitudinal study. *American Journal of Orthodontics*, **87**(1), 46–55.

Online Mendelian Inheritance in Man, OMIM (TM). McKusick-Nathans Institute for Genetic Medicine, Johns Hopkins University (Baltimore, MD) and National Center for Biotechnology Information, National Library of Medicine (Bethesda, MD), 2000. www.ncbi.nlm.nih.gov/womim/

The paedodontic/orthodontic interface

14 The paedodontic/orthodontic interface

N. E. Carter

14.1 INTRODUCTION

The long-term management of a child's developing occlusion often benefits greatly from a good working relationship between the paediatric dentist and the orthodontist. Typical problems range from minimizing damage to the occlusion caused by enforced extraction of poor quality teeth, through the management of specific local abnormalities such as impacted teeth, to referral for comprehensive treatment of all aspects of the malocclusion. This chapter discusses the principles of when to refer to a specialist colleague, and looks at some common clinical situations where collaboration is often needed.

14.2 RECOGNITION OF MALOCCLUSION

14.2.1 Orthodontic assessment

All children from the age of 8 years should be screened for the presence of malocclusion when they attend for a routine dental examination. Although orthodontic treatment is usually carried out in the late mixed and early permanent dentition, some conditions do benefit from treatment at an earlier stage. The screening need only be a brief clinical assessment, but it should be carried out systematically to ensure that no important findings are overlooked.

An outline of a basic orthodontic assessment is given in Table 14.1. With practice this can be carried out quite quickly to give an overall impression of the nature and severity of a malocclusion. In essence, it comprises assessments of the following elements:

(1) the patient's awareness of their malocclusion (the complaint, if any);
(2) their general level of dental awareness;
(3) an extraoral examination of facial form (skeletal pattern and soft tissues);
(4) general oral condition—oral hygiene and tooth quality;
(5) the presence or absence of all teeth;
(6) the alignment and form of each arch;
(7) the teeth in occlusion.

Radiographs are not necessary routinely when screening for the presence of malocclusion, and should only be taken when there is a clinical indication. A panoramic radiograph gives a useful general scan of the dentition and indicates the presence or absence of teeth. Some authorities advise that it should be supplemented with a naso-occlusal view as the premaxillary region is often poorly shown on panoramic views and is commonly the site of dental anomalies. But, provided that the panoramic view is of reasonable quality, intraoral views of this region are only necessary if there is a specific indication for them, such as delayed eruption of an

Table 14.1 Orthodontic assessment

Complaint	Aesthetic or functional concerns about the position of the teeth
Medical history:	May affect decisions about extractions, or where appliances may compromise gingival health
Dental history:	Caries experience, previous extractions, dental awareness
Attitude to treatment:	Of patient and parents. Likely level of co-operation: with dentistry generally, with orthodontic appliances, monthly adjustment visits (time off school, travelling), etc
Extraoral examination	
General	Height, developmental stage (pre-, during, or postpubertal growth spurt)
Facial skeletal pattern	
Anteroposterior:	Facial profile—skeletal class I, II, or III. Mild, moderate, severe
Vertical:	Steepness of mandibular plane. Facial proportions—increased, normal, reduced
Transverse:	Facial asymmetry. Discrepancies in widths of upper and lower arches
Soft tissues	
Lips:	Competent or incompetent. Relationship of lower lip to upper incisors
Tongue:	Tongue thrust (rare); tongue to lower lip seal
Habits:	Digit sucking or other habit
TMJ	Pain, clicks, limitation of opening, mandibular deviation
Intra-oral examination	
Dentition:	Teeth present in the mouth. Delayed eruption of teeth. Oral hygiene. Teeth of poor prognosis: caries, extensive restorations, trauma
Lower arch:	Crowding, misplaced teeth. Angulation of incisors and canines
Upper arch:	Crowding, misplaced teeth. Palpate for unerupted canines. Angulation of incisors and canines
Incisor relationship:	Overjet (mm). Overbite—increased or reduced, complete or incomplete. Centrelines—coincident, correct within face? Anterior cross-bites. Check for premature occlusal contact and associated displacement of mandible on closure—forward and/or lateral
Posterior occlusion:	Both sides: class I, II, or III. Check first molars and canines. Posterior cross-bites—local, unilateral, bilateral. Mandibular displacement?
Radiographs	Presence of permanent teeth: absent teeth, supernumerary teeth, ectopic teeth. Pathology. (Skeletal assessment using cephalometric radiographs is not needed for routine screening for malocclusion)

incisor or a history of trauma. A radiographic assessment must always be made when considering any extractions.

Good quality study models are often helpful when planning orthodontic treatment, and full orthodontic records comprising study models, relevant radiographs, and photographs should be obtained before any active treatment is started. Full-face and profile photographs are a record of facial form, including lip morphology. Intraoral photographs are a further record of the malocclusion, give some indication of the standard of oral hygiene, and are valuable where enamel defects are present before treatment.

14.2.2 Need and demand for orthodontic treatment

The Index of Orthodontic Treatment Need (IOTN) is based upon the severity of the malocclusion, and has been developed to try to establish a consensus within the profession as to which malocclusions will gain a worthwhile benefit from orthodontic treatment. The complexity and difficulty of treatment do not necessarily depend upon the severity of the malocclusion, and mild malocclusions often need extensive and sophisticated treatment if any improvement is to be made at all. Other indices have been developed to assess the complexity and success of treatment. The IOTN has two components:

1. *The Dental Health Component* categorizes malocclusion into five grades (Table 14.2) according to severity, based upon current evidence for the detrimental effects of various occlusal features. A malocclusion is graded according to its worst feature. Patients in grades 1 and 2 have little or no indication for treatment on dental health grounds, while those in grades 4 and 5 are considered to have a definite need for treatment. The borderline cases in grade 3 require a degree

Table 14.2 Dental health component of the Index of Orthodontic Treatment Need

Grade 5 (need treatment)

5.i	Impeded eruption of teeth (except for third molars) due to crowding, displacement, the presence of supernumerary teeth, retained primary teeth and any pathological cause
5.h	Extensive hypodontia with restorative implications (more than one tooth missing in any quadrant) requiring pre-restorative orthodontics
5.a	Increased overjet greater than 9 mm
5.m	Reversed overjet greater than 3.5 mm with reported masticatory and speech difficulties
5.p	Defects of cleft lip and palate and other craniofacial anomalies
5.s	Submerged primary teeth

Grade 4 (need treatment)

4.h	Less extensive hypodontia requiring pre-restorative orthodontics or orthodontic space closure to obviate the need for a prosthesis
4.a	Increased overjet greater than 6 mm but less than or equal to 9 mm
4.b	Reverse overjet greater than 3.5 mm with no masticatory or speech difficulties
4.m	Reverse overjet greater than 1 mm but less than 3.5 mm with recorded masticatory and speech difficulties
4.c	Anterior or posterior cross-bites with greater than 2 mm discrepancy between retruded contact position and intercuspal position
4.l	Posterior lingual cross-bite with no functional occlusal contact in one or both buccal segments
4.d	Severe contact point displacements greater than 4 mm
4.e	Extreme lateral or anterior open bites greater than 4 mm
4.f	Increased and complete overbite with gingival or palatal trauma
4.t	Partially erupted teeth, tipped and impacted against adjacent teeth
4.x	Presence of supernumerary teeth

Grade 3 (borderline need)

3.a	Increased overjet greater than 3.5 mm but less than or equal to 6 mm with incompetent lips
3.b	Reverse overjet greater than 1 mm but less than or equal to 3.5 mm
3.c	Anterior or posterior cross-bites with greater than 1 mm but less than or equal to 2 mm discrepancy between retruded contact position and intercuspal position
3.d	Contact point displacements greater than 2 mm but less than or equal to 4 mm
3.e	Lateral or anterior open bites greater than 2 mm but less than or equal to 4 mm
3.f	Deep overbite complete on gingival or palatal tissues but no trauma

Grade 2 (little)

2.a	Increased overjet greater than 3.5 mm but less than or equal to 6 mm with competent lips
2.b	Reverse overjet greater than 0 mm but less than or equal to 1 mm
2.c	Anterior or posterior cross-bites with less than or equal to 1 mm discrepancy between retruded contact position and intercuspal position
2.d	Contact point displacements greater than 1 mm but less than or equal to 2 mm
2.e	Lateral or anterior open bites greater than 1 mm but less than or equal to 2 mm
2.f	Increased overbite greater than or equal to 3.5 mm without gingival contact
2.g	Pre-normal or post-normal occlusions with no other anomalies (includes up to half a unit discrepancy)

Grade 1 (none)

1	Extremely minor malocclusions including contact point displacements less than 1 mm

(P. Brook and W. Shaw 1989. Reproduced with kind permission of the Editor of the *European Journal of Orthodontics*.)

of judgement when deciding upon their need for treatment, and the appearance of the dentition can be taken into account using the Aesthetic Component of the IOTN.

2. *The Aesthetic Component* of the IOTN uses a scale of 10 photographs showing different levels of dental attractiveness (Fig. 14.1). The appearance of the dentition is rated using the photographs as a guideline. Grades 1–4 indicate little or no need, for treatment on aesthetic grounds, grades 5–7 are borderline, and patients in grades 8–10 would clearly benefit from orthodontic treatment. It is, however, difficult to be truly objective when making judgements of this kind about an individual's appearance, and the Aesthetic Component has not achieved universal use because of its subjective nature.

Demand for orthodontic treatment is affected by many factors. Patients vary enormously in how they perceive their own dental appearance, some apparently being unaware of obvious malocclusions while others express dissatisfaction about very minor irregularities. Demand for treatment thus depends upon the severity of the malocclusion as perceived by patients and parents rather than by dentists. It is also affected by patients' attitudes to wearing orthodontic appliances, which are influenced by the appearance of the appliances and how acceptable they think appliance treatment is among their peers. Demand for orthodontic treatment tends to increase as appliances become more common and accepted among a population, but it is also greatly affected by the availability of treatment (geographic accessibility, waiting lists, etc.).

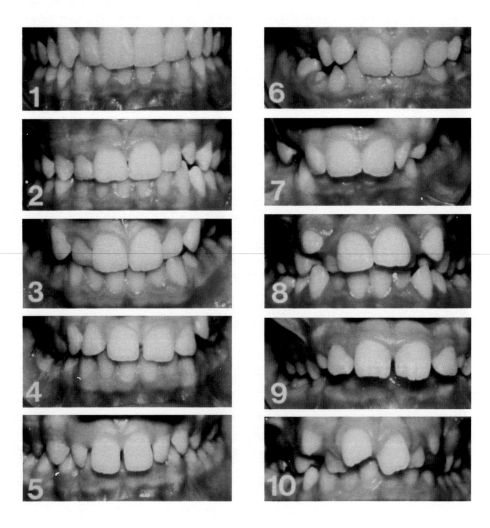

Fig. 14.1 The Aesthetic Component of the Index of Orthodontic Treatment Need. (R. Evans and W. Shaw (1987). Reproduced with kind permission of the Editor of the *European Journal of Orthodontics*.)

14.2.3 Referral for orthodontic advice

The referring dentist can give the orthodontist a lot of invaluable information.

Timing of referral

The right time for orthodontic intervention will vary according to the condition, but if specialist advice is needed it is better to refer too early rather than too late. The majority of orthodontic treatments are carried out in the late mixed and early permanent dentition, but some conditions may be treated earlier (see Section 14.4), and some treatments, such as functional appliances, depend on active facial growth and should not be delayed too long before starting.

Patient and family attitudes

In many cases the dentist will have known the family for some time, and will know their level of dental awareness, their degree of concern about the malocclusion, and their attendance record. This information can be difficult for the orthodontist to pick up during one or two short consultations, but is vital when assessing the likely compliance with orthodontic treatment.

Oral hygiene

Appliance therapy is inappropriate for patients whose oral hygiene is poor and in general this should be improved before referring for orthodontic treatment. However, this should not be at the expense of excessive delay in referring those patients with more severe malocclusions who may gain some benefit from simple interceptive measures.

Prognosis of teeth

The family dentist is in a much better position than the orthodontist to estimate the prognosis of restored or traumatized teeth.

Radiographs

Any relevant radiographs should be forwarded with the referral to avoid unnecessary repetition.

Key Points

Screening

- All children should be screened for malocclusion from 8 years of age.
- Judge the need for treatment using the Index of Treatment Need (IOTN): dental health and aesthetics.
- Check the oral hygiene and attitude to treatment.
- Refer in good time and give as much background information as possible.

14.3 EXTRACTIONS IN THE MIXED DENTITION

The extraction of teeth in children may be needed as part of orthodontic treatment, or may be necessary because of caries, trauma, or developmental anomalies. The extraction of teeth in the mixed dentition for purely orthodontic reasons, usually crowding, can sometimes be helpful, but managing the enforced extraction of carious or poor quality teeth is a matter of trying to minimize disruption of the developing dentition.

14.3.1 Extraction of primary teeth

In general, where a child has a tendency to dental crowding, the extraction of primary teeth will worsen this as it allows the adjacent teeth to drift into the resulting space. Usually, it is the teeth distal to the extraction that migrate forwards as a result of mesial drift. This drifting is generally unhelpful where the extraction is enforced, but in some situations it can be harnessed to help with the management of dental crowding.

As there is a significant increase in the size of the arches during the mixed dentition stage, decisions about the treatment of crowding should be deferred until the permanent incisors have erupted for at least a year, usually at about 8½–9 years of age. Where there is severe crowding, the extraction of primary teeth may be considered at this point as part of a programme of serial extractions, but where the crowding is mild the decision should be delayed until the permanent canines and premolars are erupting.

The term 'balancing extraction' refers to the contralateral tooth in the same arch, while a 'compensating extraction' refers to the equivalent tooth in the opposite arch.

14.3.2 Serial extraction

Serial extraction is a form of interceptive orthodontic treatment which aims to relieve crowding at an early stage so that the permanent teeth can erupt into good alignment, thus reducing or avoiding the need for later appliance therapy. It consists of a planned sequence of extractions:

1. *Primary canines*—extracted as the permanent lateral incisors erupt to allow them space to align.
2. *First primary molars*—about 1 year later, or when the roots of the first primary molars are half resorbed or more, to encourage eruption of the first premolars. In the lower arch these often tend to erupt after the canines.
3. *First premolars*—on eruption to make space for the eruption of the permanent canines into alignment.

In effect, the extraction of primary canines transfers the crowding from the incisors to the canine regions where it is more easily treated by extracting the first premolars (Fig. 14.2). It is essential to carry out a full orthodontic assessment before embarking on a course of serial extractions. The indications for serial extraction are:

(1) significant incisor crowding;
(2) patient aged about 9 years;
(3) class I occlusion without a deep overbite;
(4) all permanent teeth present;
(5) first permanent molars in good condition.

The intended advantage of serial extraction is to minimize or eliminate the need for appliances to align the arches after the permanent teeth have erupted. Sometimes this is very successful (Fig. 14.3), but the results can be disappointing. Where crowding is severe it may be necessary to fit a space maintainer following extraction of the first premolars, to ensure that mesial drift of posterior teeth does not leave the canines short of space (see Section 14.4.4).

The great disadvantage of serial extraction is the multiple episodes of extractions, starting when the child is quite young. These may well be a child's first experience of dental treatment and might cause subsequent psychological problems with their attitude to dentistry, especially as the experience is to be repeated as the programme of extractions proceeds. The likely benefit of the extractions must be considered very carefully, and in only a small minority of cases would general anaesthesia be

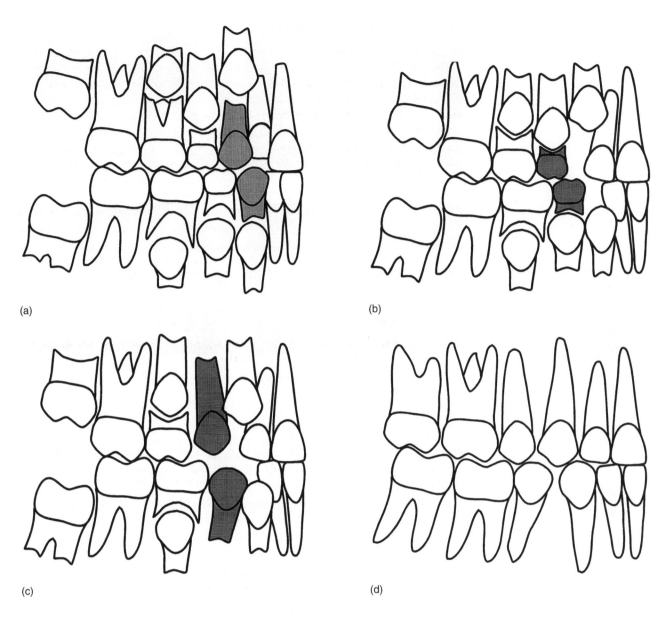

(a)

(b)

(c)

(d)

justified for this purpose. In practice, the extraction of the first primary molars is usually omitted, and the decision thus becomes whether the primary canines should be extracted. Extraction of these teeth might be indicated where it is clear that orthodontic appliances should be minimized or avoided for some reason, or where the crowding is obviously severe and is causing gross incisor displacement or cross-bite. It is also sometimes indicated to encourage the eruption of an ectopic permanent tooth (see Section 14.5.4). However, it must always be borne in mind that the extractions will allow some mesial migration of the buccal segments, so increasing the crowding. The extractions should always be balanced by removing the contralateral canine to prevent a centreline shift, but it is not necessary to compensate by extracting the canines in the opposite arch.

14.3.3 Enforced extraction of primary teeth

The main complication of the enforced extraction of poor quality primary teeth is mesial drift of the teeth distal to the extraction space, causing crowding of the permanent successors. Mesial drift is greatest where there is a tendency to crowding,

Fig. 14.2 Serial extractions. (a) Class I occlusion with incisor crowding in the mixed dentition. (b) Improved incisor alignment following extraction of primary canines. The primary first molars are extracted to encourage eruption of the first premolars. (c) First premolars are extracted on eruption to relieve crowding of the permanent canines. (d) The result following eruption of the canines.

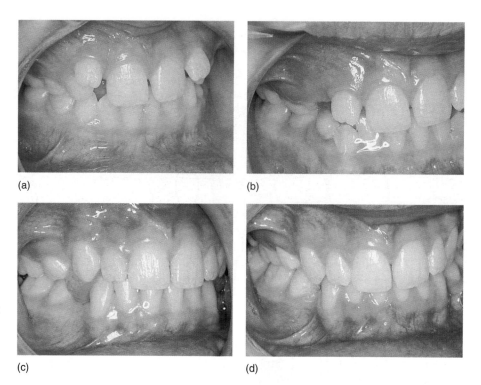

Fig. 14.3 (a) Class I occlusion with crowding of the lateral incisors in an 8½– year old patient, before extraction of primary canines.
(b) Aged 10½–, 6 months before extraction of first premolars. Upper canines palpable in buccal sulcus, lower canines crowded buccally.
(c) Aged 13—excess space in lower arch.
(d) Aged 15—upper spaces closed, lower spaces reducing. (Photos courtesy of Mr T. G. Bennett.)

and it also becomes greater the more distal the tooth to be extracted is. It is greater in the upper arch than in the lower, as the upper permanent molars are distally inclined on eruption and readily move mesially by uprighting, whereas the lower permanent molars are mesially inclined on eruption and move forward less readily, but tilt mesially as they do so.

Extraction of *primary incisors* usually causes virtually no drifting of other teeth, but if done very early may delay the eruption of the permanent incisors. (Loss of a permanent incisor is a very different matter—see Section 14.7.1.)

Extraction of a *primary canine* causes some mesial drift of the buccal segment, depending upon the degree of crowding. There is also drift of the incisors into the space, which causes a centreline shift towards the extraction site. This should be prevented by balancing the extraction with loss of the contralateral canine. In the same way the extraction of a *primary first molar* allows mesial drift of the teeth distal to it, more than with the loss of a canine, and there may also be some effect on the centreline. Where the distribution of caries indicates loss of a primary canine on one side and a primary first molar on the other, these extractions can be regarded as balancing each other reasonably well and the contralateral teeth can be retained.

Extraction of a *primary second molar* allows significant mesial migration of the first permanent molar in that quadrant, causing potentially severe local crowding with displacement or impaction of the second premolar, especially in the upper arch where mesial drift is greatest (Fig. 14.4). How severe this is depends on the degree of crowding, and in a spaced arch the extraction has little effect. In principle, however, the loss of a primary second molar should be avoided if at all possible, especially in the upper arch. A space maintainer, either removable or fixed, can be considered, unless the patient's caries rate is high or the oral hygiene is poor. Primary second molar extractions should never be balanced on the contralateral side as there is very little effect on the centreline and the potential crowding becomes complicated even further.

In general, there is no need to compensate primary tooth extractions with extractions in the opposing arch.

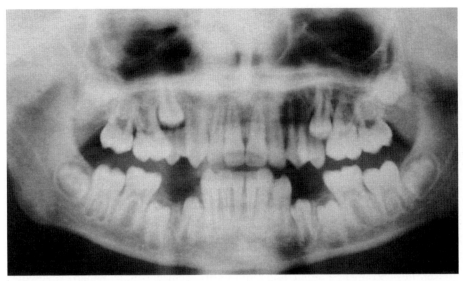

(a)

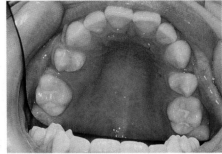

(b)

Fig. 14.4 (a) and (b) Localized crowding of upper second premolars due to the early loss of primary upper second molars. (Photos courtesy of Professor J. H. Nunn.)

Key Points

Mixed dentition extractions

- Early loss of primary teeth generally worsens crowding.
- Primary second molars should be preserved if at all possible.
- Extraction of primary canines may help incisor crowding.
- Benefit of this must be balanced against the trauma of extractions.
- Extraction of primary canines should be balanced on the contralateral side.

14.3.4 Enforced extraction of first permanent molars

First permanent molars are very rarely the teeth of choice for extraction for orthodontic reasons—in practice their removal often makes treatment more difficult.

1. The space they provide is remote from the labial segments and is poorly placed either for the relief of anterior crowding or for overjet reduction.
2. Depending on the timing of the extractions, much of the space is lost to mesial migration of the second molars, especially in the upper arch (see Section 14.3.3).
3. The behaviour of the lower second molars is fairly unpredictable following loss of lower first permanent molars and is greatly influenced by the timing of the extractions.

In general, therefore, first permanent molars are only extracted if their long-term prognosis is felt to be poor, and the orthodontic management of these extractions aims to minimize disruption of the developing dentition. Where the loss of one or more first molars is necessary in the mixed dentition, the management of the extractions depends on whether or not the patient is likely to have active treatment with orthodontic appliances in the future—often a difficult judgement to make.

A panoramic radiograph must be taken to confirm the presence of all permanent teeth (except for third molars) before finalizing the extractions. The following discussion assumes the presence of all permanent teeth—if a premolar is congenitally absent then the first molar in that quadrant should be saved if possible.

Extraction of first permanent molars where no orthodontic treatment is planned

The objective is to minimize disruption of the occlusion. Following the extraction of a first molar, the paths of eruption of adjacent unerupted teeth alter, and erupted

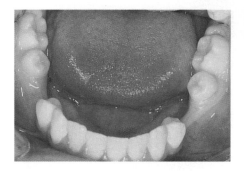

Fig. 14.5 Spaces between the lower first and second premolars resulting from very early extraction of the lower first molars.

adjacent and opposing teeth also start to drift. Many of these changes are unhelpful, but some can be used to advantage with careful planning.

In general, the most obvious change is mesial drift of the second molar, especially in the upper arch. However, in the lower arch some distal movement of premolars and canines may also be expected, especially where the arch is crowded. The extraction of first molars can be a convenient way of relieving pre-molar crowding, especially in the lower arch. In the lower arch the timing of the extraction is important. If carried out very early the unerupted lower second pre-molar migrates distally, sometimes leaving a space between the first and second premolars if the arch is uncrowded (Fig. 14.5). If carried out late, as or after the lower second molars erupts, that tooth tilts mesially under occlusal forces and can cause an occlusal interference—especially if the opposing upper first molar overerupts into the lower extraction space (Fig. 14.6(a) and (b)). There is often residual space mesial to the tilted second molar and this poor relationship with the second premolar may cause a stagnation area. These unwanted effects can be minimized in two ways:

1. Extraction of the upper first molar—this eliminates the problem of overeruption of the opposing first molar, and removes the occlusal contact which exaggerates mesial tilting of the lower second molar (Fig. 14.7(a) and (b)).

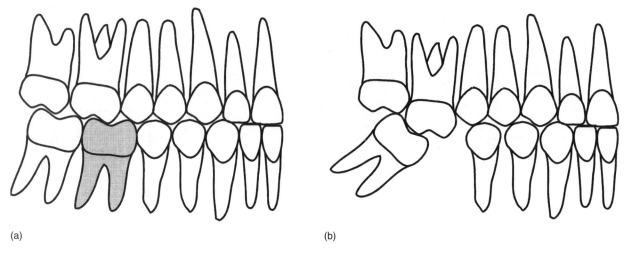

(a)

(b)

Fig. 14.6 (a) and (b) Loss of the lower first molar after eruption of the second molars causes severe tipping of the lower second molar and overeruption of the upper first molar.

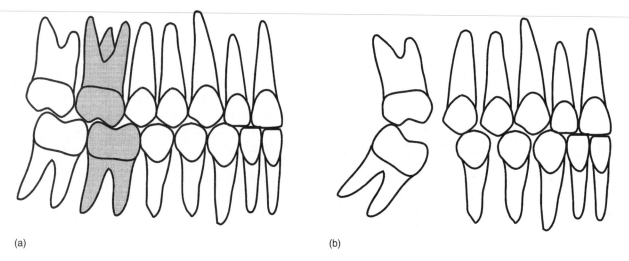

(a)

(b)

Fig. 14.7 (a) and (b) Extraction of the upper first molar as well as the lower prevents overeruption of the opposing first molar and reduces the mesial tilting of the lower second molar.

2. Careful timing of the extractions—ideally when the bifurcation of the roots of the lower second molar is starting to calcify, usually at about 8½–9½ years of age (Fig. 14.8(a) and (b)).

In the *upper arch* the behaviour of the second molar is more predictable, although timing is still important. The tendency to mesial drift is much greater than in the lower arch, and there is almost no distal drift of the upper premolars. If the upper first molar is extracted early, the unerupted second molar migrates mesially so that it erupts into the position of the first molar. If the second molar has erupted before the extraction it still migrates forward, taking up most or all of the space depending on the degree of crowding, and it usually tilts mesially and rotates mesiopalatally about the palatal root. However, compensating extraction of the lower first molar is not indicated (Fig. 14.9(a) and (b)).

Balancing extractions of the contralateral first permanent molars are not routinely necessary unless they also are in poor condition. Where the arch is crowded an extraction on the opposite side is usually needed to relieve crowding and prevent any

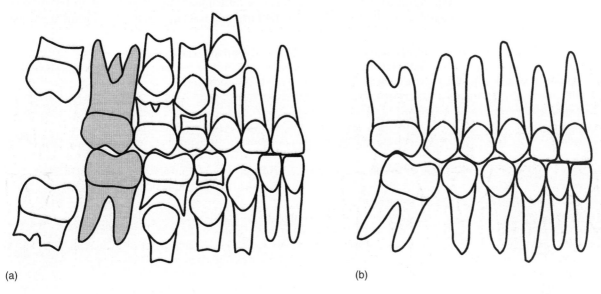

(a)   (b)

Fig. 14.8 (a) and (b) Extraction of the first molars when the bifurcation of the roots of the lower second molar is starting to calcify, usually 8½–9½ years of age, gives the best chance of a good result.

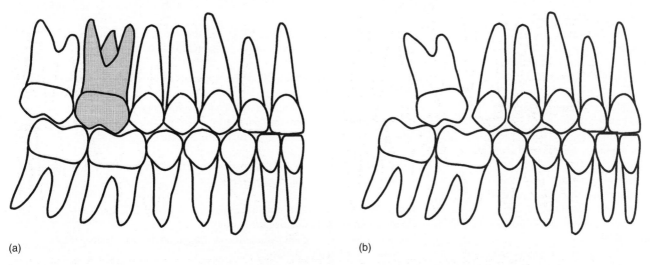

(a)   (b)

Fig. 14.9 (a) and (b) Extraction of the upper first molar does not need to be compensated with extraction of the lower first molar.

shift of the centreline, but if the first permanent molars are in good condition the extraction of first premolars may well be more appropriate.

Key Points

First permanent molar extractions

- These are never the teeth of choice for orthodontic extraction.
- The best age for loss is 8½–9½ years.
- Extraction of the upper first molar may reduce occlusal disturbance where the lower first molar has to be extracted.
- There is no need to extract the lower first molar if the upper first molar has to be extracted.
- Contralateral extractions depend on the degree of crowding.

Extraction of first permanent molars where orthodontic treatment is planned

Where future appliance treatment is anticipated, the objective is to try to avoid complicating it. It is difficult to give hard and fast rules as the management strategy

Table 14.3 Management of enforced extraction of first permanent molars in the mixed dentition. These guidelines are very broad and their application will vary greatly between individual patients. They assume that only one first molar is of poor prognosis, and with crowding their application should be modified where more than one first molar is of poor prognosis

Extraction of lower first molar

1. Class I malocclusion Little or no crowding No appliance treatment planned	Extract at 'ideal' age—8½–9½ years. Usually compensate with extraction of opposing upper 6. Do not balance with contralateral extractions
2. Class I malocclusion Significant crowding No appliance treatment planned	If possible delay until after eruption of second molars. Compensate with loss of opposing upper 6. Contralateral extractions usually required: 4s often better if 6's sound
3. Class I with crowding Later appliance treatment planned	If possible delay extraction until after eruption of second molars. Do not compensate or balance with loss of opposing upper 6 or contralateral 6s
4. Class II Little or no crowding Later appliance treatment planned	Extract at 'ideal' age—8½–9½ years. Do not compensate with extraction of opposing upper 6. Do not balance with contralateral extractions
5. Class II with crowding Later appliance treatment planned	If possible delay extraction until after eruption of second molars. Do not compensate or balance with loss of opposing upper 6 or contralateral 6s
6. Class III Both where appliance treatment is and is not planned	Extract at 'ideal' age—8½–9½ years. Do not compensate or balance with extraction of further 6's

Extraction of upper first molar

7. Class I malocclusion Little or no crowding No appliance treatment planned	Extract at 'ideal' age—8½–9½ years. Do not compensate or balance with extraction of opposing lower 6 or contralateral extractions
8. Class I malocclusion Significant crowding No appliance treatment planned	If possible delay extraction until after eruption of second molars. Plan lower arch extractions on their own merits. Balancing contralateral upper arch extraction required, but 4 may be more suitable if 6 is in good condition.
9. Class I malocclusion Significant crowding Later appliance treatment planned	If possible delay extraction until after eruption of upper second molars. Leave other extractions until ready for orthodontic treatment
10. Class II Little or no crowding Later appliance treatment planned	Usually extract carious 6 and plan orthodontic treatment on its own merits. Do not compensate or balance the extraction
11. Class II with crowding Later appliance treatment planned	If possible delay extraction until after eruption of upper second molars. Do not compensate or balance the extraction
12. Class III Both where appliance treatment is and is not planned	Extract carious 6 and plan orthodontic treatment on its own merits. Do not compensate or balance the extraction

will differ for each patient, but the main factor to consider is the amount of space that will be needed. Where the extraction space is to be used to relieve crowding or reduce an increased overjet, unwanted mesial drift of the second permanent molars must be minimized. On the other hand, where there will be excess space, mesial drift of the second permanent molars should be encouraged.

In the *lower arch* the extractions are managed according to severity of crowding. Where there is little or no crowding the extraction should, if possible, be carried out at the 'ideal' age of about 8½–9½ years, so as to encourage mesial migration of the second molar. Where there is significant crowding it is better to delay the extraction, if possible, until after the lower second molar has erupted, so that the space is available for alignment of the arch.

The *upper arch* is also managed according to space requirements, but these are determined not only by the amount of crowding but also by the class of malocclusion. Where there is significant crowding the upper first molars should be preserved if possible until after the upper second molars have erupted and can be included in an appliance. Similarly, in a class II malocclusion space will be useful to reduce an increased overjet and, again, where possible the extractions should be delayed. If the upper first molar has to be removed earlier it is sometimes possible to start treatment with appliances before the upper second molars have erupted, but the treatment tends to be more complex, with headgear to move the upper premolars distally.

Conversely, excess upper arch space in a class III malocclusion complicates treatment, as proclining the upper incisors is a form of expansion which itself creates more space.

Clearly, where active orthodontic treatment is planned the loss of a lower first molar is not automatically compensated by the extraction of the opposing upper first molar.

The broad principles of the management of enforced extraction of first molars are summarized in Table 14.3.

14.4 APPLIANCE TREATMENT IN THE MIXED DENTITION

The great majority of orthodontic treatments are carried out during the late mixed and early permanent dentitions, to avoid prolonged appliance wear while permanent teeth erupt. However, a few conditions can benefit from earlier intervention.

14.4.1 Anterior cross-bite

Although it may be a sign of a developing class III problem, a local anterior cross-bite involving one or two incisors is often simply due to the positions of the developing tooth-germs causing the teeth to erupt into cross-bite. Possible complications of a localized anterior cross-bite include a premature contact with the tooth in cross-bite, which causes the mandible to displace forwards as the teeth come into maximum intercuspal position, or one lower incisor in cross-bite may be driven labially through the supporting tissues, causing localized gingival recession (Fig. 14.10). Early correction encourages development of a class I occlusion, and treatment in the mixed dentition is often straightforward provided that these criteria are met:

1. *Normal skeletal pattern.* Treatment of obvious class III problems should be delayed until the nature of the patient's growth pattern becomes clearer. However, it is essential to check for the presence of a forward displacement of the mandible, as this can make a normal facial pattern appear to be slightly prognathic.

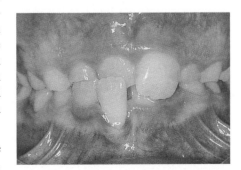

Fig. 14.10 Localized gingival recession associated with incisor cross-bite.

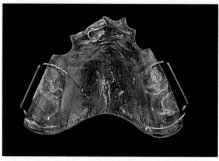

(a)

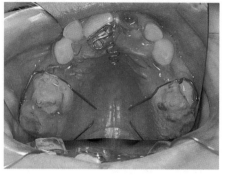

(b)

Fig. 14.11 (a) and (b) Appliance to procline upper incisor. Note posterior capping to disengage occlusion and retention anterior to 6|6 to resist the displacing force generated by the Z-spring.

2. *Adequate space in the arch.* There must be enough space to accommodate the tooth in alignment. In a crowded upper arch, space may be made for alignment of upper lateral incisors by extracting the primary upper canines (see serial extraction, Section 14.3.2). This treatment must be started fairly early while the permanent canine is still high, because labial movement of the lateral incisor will be prevented if the canine crown is labial to the root of the lateral. It is therefore essential to palpate the position of the permanent canine crown, and, if it has come down too far, treatment must be delayed until the first premolars have erupted.

3. *Adequate overbite.* Stable correction of the cross-bite depends on there being positive overbite after treatment. Labial tipping of upper incisors with a removable appliance tends to reduce overbite, and specialist advice should be sought where lack of overbite is a problem.

There are many designs of removable appliance to correct anterior cross-bites and a typical example is shown in Fig. 14.11(a) and (b). Its essential features are:

1. *An active component* such as a Z-spring or a screw palatal to the tooth to be moved.

2. *Retention* as far anteriorly as possible to resist the tendency of the spring to displace the front of the appliance.

3. *Posterior capping* to open the occlusion while the upper incisor moves labially over the lowers.

14.4.2 Posterior cross-bite with displacement

Bilateral posterior cross-bites are often accepted as they usually reflect a transverse skeletal discrepancy and cause no functional problem. Where the upper arch is slightly narrow, the buccal teeth may initially occlude cusp to cusp and only achieve full intercuspation when the mandible displaces laterally (Fig. 14.12(a) and (b)), causing a unilateral posterior cross-bite. This can be difficult to detect if the patient cannot relax the jaw muscles fully during examination, but it is important to determine whether or not there is a lateral displacement. A unilateral posterior cross-bite with a displacement is easily corrected during the mixed dentition, but one without an associated displacement is probably skeletal in origin and correction should not be attempted.

A unilateral posterior cross-bite with a displacement is treated by expansion of the upper arch to remove the initial cusp-to-cusp contact, using an appliance such as that shown in Fig. 14.12(c). It has a mid-line expansion screw which is turned by the parent once or twice a week, and double Adams clasps on 6e|e6. The d|d are usually unsuitable for clasping as they have little or no undercut. The appliance should contact c|c as these usually need to be expanded, but need not contact the incisors unless a bite plane is required.

14.4.3 Increased overjet

The incidence of trauma to the upper incisors is greater where the overjet is increased, to the extent that among 13 year olds twice as many children with overjets of 10 mm or more have traumatized upper incisors compared with children with overjets of less than 5 mm. Boys are at greater risk than girls. Reducing the risk of trauma is a good reason for early reduction of a large overjet, even without cosmetic considerations.

In the mixed dentition this is usually done with a functional appliance. Details of the management and effects of these appliances can be found in orthodontic texts, but they induce correction of the incisor and molar relationships by a combination

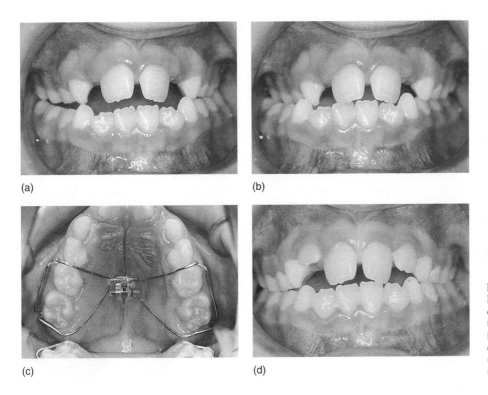

(a)

(b)

(c)

(d)

Fig. 14.12 Unilateral posterior cross-bite with lateral mandibular displacement. (a) Initial contact on closure. (b) Lateral displacement of the mandible on closure into maximum intercuspal position causing unilateral posterior cross-bite. (c) Upper expansion appliance. (d) Displacement has been eliminated after upper arch displacement.

of dentoalveolar and skeletal changes. This is not done by active components such as springs, but instead the appliances harness forces generated by the masticatory and facial musculature. They achieve this by holding the mandible in a forward postured position, and all designs of functional appliance are similar in that they engage both dental arches and cause mandibular posturing and displacement of the condyles within the glenoid fossae (Fig. 14.13(a)–(f)).

Functional appliances have two main limitations: they only work in growing children, most effectively during periods of rapid growth; and, while they change the occlusion between the arches, they cannot treat irregularities of arch alignment such as crowding.

In practice, these limitations mean that functional appliance treatment can become very lengthy when started early. Progress can be slow in prepubertal children because of their relatively slow growth rate, and dwindling co-operation with these demanding appliances can become a real problem during prolonged treatments. The appliance should be worn as a retainer until after the pubertal growth spurt, which in boys may be 15 or 16 years of age—a long time if treatment started at the age of 9. Treatment for crowding can usually only begin after the premolars start to erupt, and the patient effectively has two courses of treatment—one to reduce the overjet and one to align the arches. A potential difficulty of this approach is that the overjet reduction must be retained while the crowding is being treated, which can make management complex.

Early treatment is often justifiable for patients with severe overjets, but the possible disadvantages must be balanced carefully against the potential benefits.

14.4.4 Space maintenance

It is often important that drifting of teeth into an extraction space is prevented, such as: following loss of a primary molar (Section 14.3.3); following loss of an upper incisor (Section 14.7.2); where the crowding is severe enough that extractions give only just enough space.

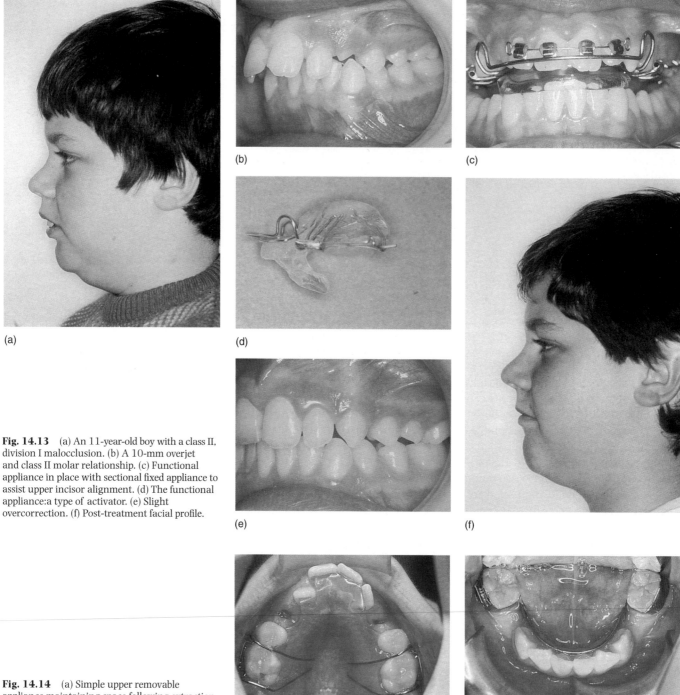

Fig. 14.13 (a) An 11-year-old boy with a class II, division I malocclusion. (b) A 10-mm overjet and class II molar relationship. (c) Functional appliance in place with sectional fixed appliance to assist upper incisor alignment. (d) The functional appliance: a type of activator. (e) Slight overcorrection. (f) Post-treatment facial profile.

Fig. 14.14 (a) Simple upper removable appliance maintaining space following extraction of 4|4 while 3|3 erupt. (b) Lower lingual arch serving as a space maintainer.

In these situations a space maintainer is indicated. In the upper arch this can be a simple acrylic appliance with clasps, but in the lower a lingual arch is better tolerated (Fig. 14.14(a) and (b)).

14.4.5 Digit-sucking habits

Thumb- and finger-sucking habits which persist into the mixed dentition may cause: anterior open bite; increased overjet; unilateral posterior cross-bite with displacement.

A unilateral posterior cross-bite can occur because during digit sucking the tongue position is low, allowing activity of the buccal musculature to narrow the upper arch slightly (see Section 14.4.2).

Although a few children continue the habit into their teenage years, nearly all grow out of it by about 10 years of age. An anterior open bite caused by a sucking habit (Fig. 14.15(a)) will usually then resolve, but it may persist and require treatment if the tongue has adapted to the open bite by contacting the lower lip to make an anterior seal during swallowing. Correction of an increased overjet or a posterior cross-bite will need active treatment, and in most cases the presence of an appliance in the mouth finally breaks the habit. For these reasons a sucking habit in a young child is rarely a cause for concern, and parents can be reassured that drastic measures to stop the habit are unnecessary.

'Habit-breaking' appliances are thus rarely indicated and do not always work, but they may be considered if the effect on the occlusion is severe or if the habit is unusually persistent (Fig. 14.15(b)). There are many designs of habit-breakers, some quite barbaric, but a common one is an upper removable appliance with a steeply inclined anterior bite plane (Fig. 14.16(a)–(c)). The mid-line split in the acrylic of an expansion appliance may also help by breaking the suction.

14.4.6 Incisor spacing—mid-line diastema

This is mentioned only to point out that treatment just for spacing is rarely indicated in the mixed dentition stage. Parents are often concerned about spacing of the upper incisors, and they can be reassured that it will often reduce as the permanent upper canines erupt. It is, however, important to ensure that an upper mid-line diastema is not due to a supernumerary tooth (see Section 14.6.1). A diastema may also be due to generalized spacing, diminutive teeth, congenital absence of upper lateral incisors, or to a fleshy upper labial frenum. There is some disagreement about the role of frenectomy in the treatment of diastemata, but it is very rarely indicated in the mixed dentition stage and is probably best carried out during active orthodontic treatment.

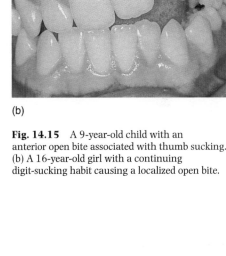

(a)

(b)

Fig. 14.15 A 9-year-old child with an anterior open bite associated with thumb sucking. (b) A 16-year-old girl with a continuing digit-sucking habit causing a localized open bite.

Key Points

Mixed dentition

- Cross-bites with displacement may be treated in the mixed dentition.
- Treatment of increased overjet can become lengthy if started early.
- Persistent digit-sucking habits usually resolve when appliance treatment is started.
- Upper incisor spacing usually reduces as the permanent canines erupt.
- An upper mid-line diastema may be a sign of an anomaly of tooth size or number.

Fig. 14.16 (a) A 12-year-old girl whose digit-sucking habit has caused an anterior open bite and increased overjet. (b) and (c) Split plate with a steep anterior bite plane to break the habit while the overjet is being reduced.

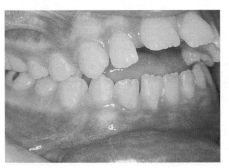

(a)

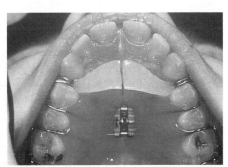

(b)

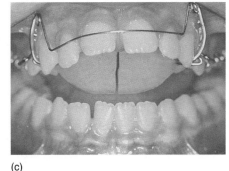

(c)

14.5 ANOMALIES OF ERUPTION—THE ECTOPIC MAXILLARY CANINE

The path of eruption of any tooth can become disturbed. Sometimes the reason is obvious, such as a supernumerary tooth impeding an upper incisor (see Section 14.6.1), but often it is obscure. In clinical orthodontics, the most common problem of aberrant eruption is the impacted maxillary canine, which is second only to the third molar in the frequency of impaction.

14.5.1 Prevalence of impacted maxillary canines

Ectopic maxillary canines occur in about 2% of the population, of which about 85% of canines are palatal and 15% buccal to the line of the upper arch. The risk of impaction of the upper canine is greater where the lateral incisor is diminutive or absent—the lateral incisor root is known to guide the erupting canine. An impacted canine can sometimes resorb adjacent incisor roots, and this risk may be as high as 12%. Incisor resorption is sometimes quite dramatic (Fig. 14.17).

14.5.2 Clinical assessment

During the mixed dentition stage the normal path of eruption of the maxillary canines is slightly buccal to the line of the arch, and from about 10 years of age the crowns should be palpable as bulges on the buccal aspect of the alveolus.

If not, an abnormal path of eruption should be suspected, particularly where eruption of one canine is very delayed compared with the other side. Unerupted maxillary canines should be palpated routinely on all children from the age of 10 years until eruption.

14.5.3 Radiographic assessment

Where the canine is not palpable it should be assessed radiographically. A periapical radiograph shows whether the primary canine root is resorbing normally and whether the canine follicle is enlarged. If the apex of the primary canine is not resorbing, with either no root resorption or only lateral resorption, the path of eruption of the permanent canine may be abnormal. However, a single radiograph cannot fully determine the unerupted canine's position relative to the other teeth—two views are needed for this, either at right angles to each other or for the parallax technique.

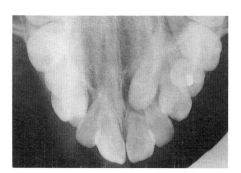

Fig. 14.17   An ⌊3 causing root resorption of ⌊12.

Parallax technique

This method, also known as the tube-shift method, compares two views of the area taken with the X-ray tube in two different positions. Figure 14.18(a) shows a palatal canine on a periapical film being taken with the tube positioned forward or mesially. A second film taken with the tube positioned further distally gives an image which apparently shows the canine crown in a different position relative to the adjacent roots (Fig. 14.18(b)). In this case the image of the canine appears to have shifted distally when compared with the first film, that is in the same direction that the tube was moved, which indicates that the canine is palatal to the other teeth. An apparent shift in the opposite direction to the tube shift would indicate that the tooth is lying buccally to the other teeth.

The parallax technique works best using two periapical views, but with care it can also be applied to a panoramic tomogram with a standard occlusal view, using vertical shift (Fig. 14.19(a) and (b)). The tube position is low down for the panoramic tomogram and much higher for the occlusal view, and so in this example the palatal

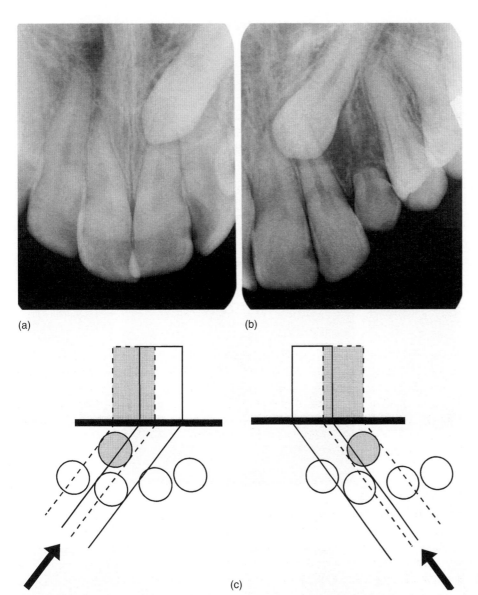

Fig. 14.18 Parallax location of $\underline{|3}$.
(a) Radiograph taken with the tube positioned forward shows that the image of the canine crown is slightly mesial to the image of $\underline{|1}$.
(b) Radiograph taken with the tube positioned further distally shows that the image of $\underline{|3}$ is further distally. The image of $\underline{|3}$ has shifted in the same direction as the tube shift: $\underline{|3}$ is therefore nearer to the film than $\underline{|1}$, i.e. it is palatal to the line of the arch. (c) Diagrammatic representation of how a palatally positioned tooth moves 'with' the tube from left to right.

canine appears to be nearer the incisor apices in the occlusal view, i.e. its apparent movement is upwards with the tube. The size of the image of a displaced tooth on a panoramic radiograph is another indicator, being enlarged if it is palatal and reduced if it is labial or buccal. However, a periapical view is still necessary to check for associated pathology, and this can be used with the occlusal view to make another parallax pair. The combination of panoramic, standard occlusal, and periapical views, such as that in Fig. 14.19, allows comprehensive assessment of a maxillary canine.

Two films at right angles

This method is more applicable to the specialist as it involves a taking lateral skull view and a posteroanterior (p-a) view: possibly a p-a skull, but more commonly using a panoramic radiograph for the same purpose (Fig. 14.20(a) and (b)). The lateral skull view shows whether the canine crown is buccal or palatal to the incisor roots, and the p-a or panoramic view shows how close it is to the mid-line. The angulation of the tooth and its vertical position are assessed using both views. An intraoral view must also be taken to check for any associated pathology.

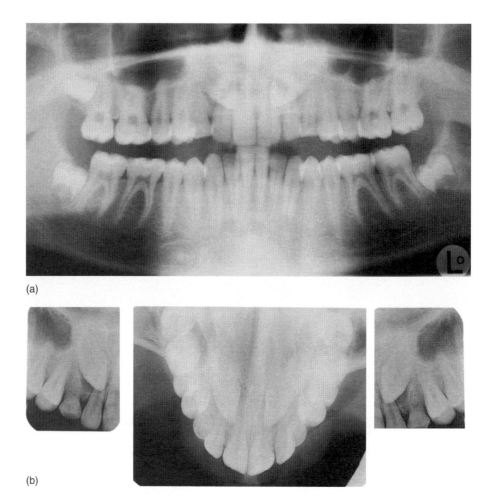

Fig. 14.19 (a) and (b) This combination of views allows the use of vertical and horizontal parallax to assess ectopic canines.

(a)

(b)

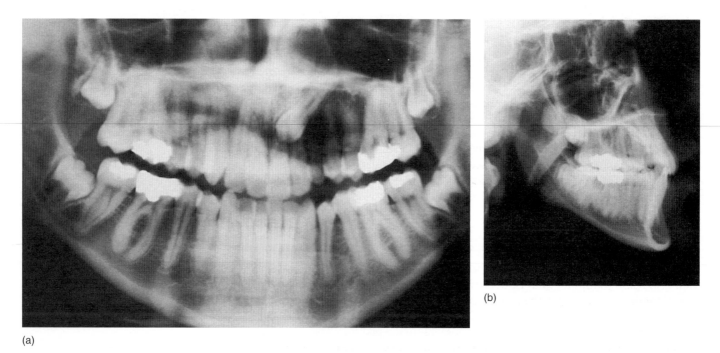

(a)

(b)

Fig. 14.20 (a) The panoramic view shows that the crown of the ⌐3 is close to the mid-line. (b) The lateral view shows that it is palatal to the roots of the incisors.

The position of the impacted canine's crown should be determined as being buccal, palatal, or in the line of the arch. The degree of displacement should be assessed horizontally, that is how close it is to the mid-line, in terms of how far it overlaps the roots of the incisors. The canine crown's vertical position is assessed relative to the incisor apices. An estimate should also be made of the tooth's angulation and the position of its apex relative to the line of the arch.

Other radiographic signs that may suggest an abnormal path of eruption are: obvious asymmetry between the positions of the two upper canines; lack of resorption of the root of the primary canine on the affected side (Fig. 14.19); and resorption of permanent incisor roots (Fig. 14.17). If there are signs of incisor resorption, urgent advice and treatment should be sought.

14.5.4 Early treatment

During the later mixed dentition, if an upper canine is not palpable normally and is found to be ectopic, extraction of the primary canine has a good chance of correcting or improving the path of eruption of the permanent canine, provided it is not too severely displaced. Extraction of the primary canine is only appropriate under these conditions:

(1) early detection—mixed dentition;
(2) canine crown overlap of no more than half the width of the adjacent incisor root as seen on a panoramic view;
(3) canine crown no higher than the apex of the adjacent incisor root;
(4) angle of 30° or less between the canine's long axis and the mid-sagittal plane;
(5) reasonable space available in the arch—no more than moderate crowding.

Unless the upper arch is spaced, the contralateral primary canine should also be removed to prevent the upper centreline shifting. Eruption of the permanent canine should be monitored clinically and if necessary radiographically, and specialist advice sought if it fails to show reasonable improvement after a year.

The main disadvantage of extracting the primary canine is losing the option of retaining it if the permanent canine fails to erupt. It may also allow forward drift of the upper buccal teeth where there is a tendency to crowding, and if space is critical a space maintainer should be fitted.

14.5.5 Later treatment

The treatment options in the permanent dentition are to:

(1) expose the canine and align it orthodontically;
(2) transplant the canine;
(3) extract the canine;
(4) leave the impacted canine *in situ*.

Exposure and orthodontic alignment

This is the treatment of choice for a well-motivated patient, provided the impaction is not too severe. The canine should lie within these limits:

(1) canine crown overlapping no more than half the width of the central incisor root;
(2) canine crown no higher than the apex of the adjacent incisor root;
(3) canine apex in the line of the arch.

The tooth can either be exposed into the mouth and the wound packed open, or a bracket attached to a gold chain can be bonded to it and the wound closed. An orthodontic appliance, usually fixed, then applies traction to bring the tooth into alignment. This treatment can take up to 2 years, depending on the severity of the canine's displacement. Exposure works well for palatally impacted canines, but buccally impacted canines usually have a poor gingival contour following exposure, even when an apically repositioned flap procedure has been used. For this reason some operators prefer to attach a chain to buccally impacted canines and to close the wound, so that the unerupted canine is brought down to erupt through attached, rather than free, gingiva.

Transplantation

The attraction of transplantation is that orthodontic treatment is avoided and yet the canine is brought into function. Two criteria must be met: the canine can be removed intact with a minimum of root handling; and there must be adequate space for the canine in the arch.

The major cause of failure is root resorption, but the incidence of this is reduced if the surgical technique is atraumatic and the transplanted tooth is root- filled with calcium hydroxide shortly after surgery. The success rate for canine transplantation is about 70% survival at 5 years, but many clinicians regard it as being appropriate in only a few cases.

Extraction of the permanent canine

This is appropriate if the position of the canine puts it beyond orthodontic correction, or if the patient does not want appliance treatment. If present, the primary canine can be left *in situ*, and although the prognosis is unpredictable, a canine with a good root may last for many years. When it is eventually lost a prosthesis will be needed, and provision of this can be difficult if the overbite is deep—another factor to be taken into account when considering treatment options.

Extraction of the permanent canine may also be considered where the lateral incisor and premolar are in contact, giving a good appearance. In this case it is often expedient to accept the erupted teeth and extract the canine.

Leaving the unerupted canine *in situ*

During the early teenage years there is a risk of resorption of adjacent incisor roots so that annual radiographic review is necessary, although the risk of root resorption reduces with increasing age. The onset of root resorption can be quite rapid, and for this reason many impacted canines are removed. There may be a case for retaining the canine in the short term in a younger patient, in case they have a change of heart about orthodontic treatment to align the tooth.

Key Points

Ectopic canines

- About 2% of children have ectopic upper canines, of which 85% are palatal.
- Always palpate for upper canines from the age of 10 years until eruption.
- Non-palpable upper canines should be located radiographically or referred for investigation.
- Consider extraction of a primary canine if a permanent canine is *mildly* displaced.
- Untreated, unerupted permanent canines may resorb incisor roots and should be radiographed annually during the teenage years.

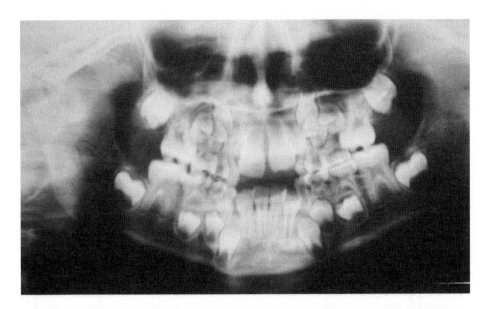

Fig. 14.21 Impaction of ⌊6 causing distal resorption of ⌊e.

14.5.6 Other anomalies of eruption

In the mixed dentition, three other anomalies of eruption are fairly common:

1. *Infraoccluded primary teeth* (Chapter 13) usually exfoliate provided that the permanent successors are present, but they should be kept under review. If they are not shed and eruption of the permanent tooth is seriously delayed, or if the infraocclusion becomes very marked, then they should be extracted and a space maintainer fitted if appropriate.

2. *Impaction of the upper first permanent molar* into the distal of the upper second primary molar causing resorption (Fig. 14.21). It is possible to disimpact the tooth with an appliance, but the problem usually resolves spontaneously when the primary molar is shed. The resorption may cause pain if it involves the pulp, in which case the primary molar should be removed. This allows the permanent molar to move rapidly mesially, and a space maintainer or an active appliance to move it distally should be considered (see Section 14.3.3).

3. *Second premolars* in unfavourable positions are sometimes seen as incidental findings on panoramic radiographs, but fortunately they usually correct spontaneously and eventually erupt satisfactorily. Very occasionally this does not happen, and a few cases have been reported of a lower second premolar migrating towards the mandibular ramus. Upper or lower second premolars that are blocked out of the arch because of crowding usually erupt, but are displaced lingually.

14.6 ANOMALIES OF TOOTH SIZE AND NUMBER

These anomalies are discussed in Chapter 13, but their clinical management often has orthodontic implications.

14.6.1 Supernumerary teeth

Supernumerary teeth are very common in the premaxilla, and can interfere with the eruption of normal teeth, or cause localized crowding if they erupt. In terms of clinical

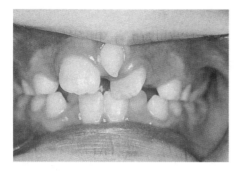

Fig. 14.22 An erupted conical mid-line supernumerary which has not prevented eruption of 1|1, but has displaced |1.

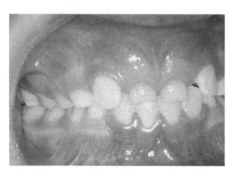

(a)

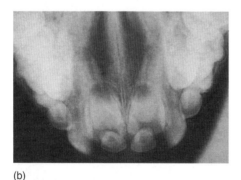

(b)

Fig. 14.23 (a) and (b) Failure of eruption of 1|1 due to the presence of two tuberculate supernumerary teeth. (Photos courtesy of Mr T. G. Bennett.)

management, supernumeraries in the upper labial segment fall into three groups:

1. *Conical supernumeraries* are usually close to the mid-line between the central incisors (mesiodens), and are usually one or two in number. They are sometimes inverted, and their positions can range from having erupted to lying above the incisor apices. The majority do not prevent eruption of incisors, but may cause some displacement or a median diastema, in which case they should be extracted (Fig. 14.22). They should also be extracted if they erupt or if the adjacent incisors are to be moved orthodontically. However, they can otherwise be left *in situ* if high and symptom-free.

2. *Tuberculate supernumeraries* are the main cause of failure of eruption of upper permanent incisors (Fig. 14.23(a) and (b)). Early detection improves the prognosis for treatment. A central incisor which fails to erupt before the adjacent lateral incisor should be radiographed, and any supernumerary teeth localized (see Section 14.5.3). These should be removed surgically as soon as possible, and it is essential that the space is maintained or, if already lost, re-opened with an appliance. About 75% of unerupted incisors erupt spontaneously within 2 years of removal of supernumeraries, so it is worth waiting for at least 18 months before considering surgical exposure. Even if the incisor has not erupted it has usually come down such that the crown is just submucosal and only requires minimal exposure of the incisal edge, aiming to minimize loss of attached gingiva (Fig. 14.24(a)–(c)).

3. *Supplemental teeth* of normal morphology cause localized crowding unless there is generalized spacing in the arch. Figure 14.25 shows a supplemental upper lateral incisor, and treatment consists of extracting one of the two lateral incisors in that quadrant. One is often smaller than the other and, if possible, the tooth that matches the contralateral incisor should be retained, but the severity of displacement and difficulty of orthodontic alignment must also be taken into account.

14.6.2 Hypodontia

Any tooth in the arch can be congenitally absent but, aside from third molars, the teeth most commonly affected are lower second premolars and upper lateral incisors (Chapter 13). Where one or two teeth are absent the orthodontic options are to open, maintain, or close the space. Where multiple teeth are absent orthodontic treatment may be able to give a more favourable basis for restorative replacement.

Second premolars

Where the arch is aligned or spaced the primary second molar should be left *in situ*, but where there is crowding the space can be used for arch alignment. In the upper arch, and in a significantly crowded lower arch, the primary second molar should be

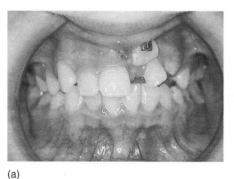

(a)

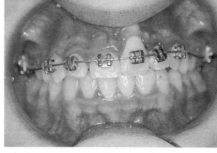

(b)

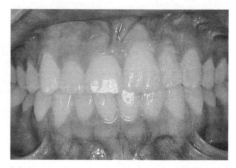

(c)

Fig. 14.24 (a) Surgical exposure of unerupted |1. (b) Orthodontic alignment of |1. (note the poor gingival contour as a result of exposure). (c) Poor gingival contour persists for several years after treatment.

retained until the start of orthodontic treatment. Where there is mild lower arch crowding which is to be treated, the primary second molar can be extracted earlier to allow some of the space to be lost to mesial drifting of the first molar.

Upper lateral incisors

Where one or both upper lateral incisors are absent in an uncrowded arch the excess space is often distributed as generalized anterior spacing (Fig. 14.26(a)–(e)). An upper fixed appliance can be used to localize the space in the lateral incisor area prior to provision of bridgework. Some overbite reduction is often needed to create enough interocclusal space for the retaining wings of the bridge. The bridge should not be made for at least 6 months after removal of the fixed appliance, during which time a removable retainer should be worn which has wire spurs to prevent any drifting into the reopened space. The bridge itself often acts as a permanent orthodontic retainer, and careful thought should be given to this aspect of its design. For example, if an upper canine has been moved distally, a fixed–fixed design ensures that the canine cannot relapse mesially. A cantilever design might allow relapse, causing the lateral incisor pontic to overlap the central incisor.

Where the upper arch is inherently crowded, the lateral incisor space could be closed. There is some debate as to the merits or otherwise of the resulting aesthetics, but, in general, it seems unfortunate to extract a sound premolar to open space for a prosthesis, and in the long term the appearance following space closure is usually acceptable (Fig. 14.27(a) and (b)). The quality of the appearance depends on the shape of the canine, but pointed canines can be made to look more like lateral incisors by reducing the cusp tip and adding composite mesio-incisally.

More severe hypodontia with multiple missing teeth

This often needs complex treatment. Preliminary orthodontic treatment can often help restoration by making the space distribution more favourable, uprighting tilted teeth, and reducing the overbite. Fixed appliances are usually needed and orthodontic retention requires careful management (Fig. 14.28(a)–(f)).

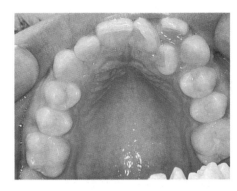

Fig. 14.25 Supplemental lateral incisor causing localized crowding.

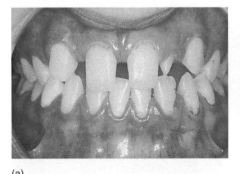

(a)

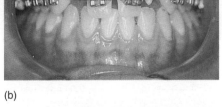

(b)

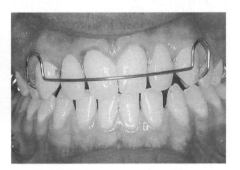

(c)

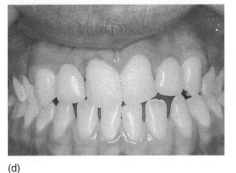

(d)

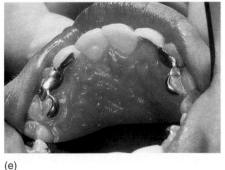

(e)

Fig. 14.26 (a) Spaced arch complicated by the absence of 2| and a very diminutive |2. (b) |2 to be extracted and fixed appliance opening space for replacement 2|2. (c) Removable retainer—note wire spurs to ensure space is maintained. (d) Adhesive bridges in place, and composite additions to enlarge 1|1. (e) Bridge design.

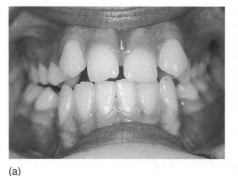

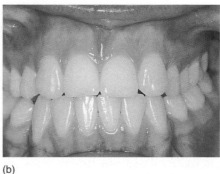

Fig. 14.27 (a) Congenital absence of 2|2, where crowding tendency indicates space closure. (b) After alignment, with 31|13 in contact.

(a)   (b)

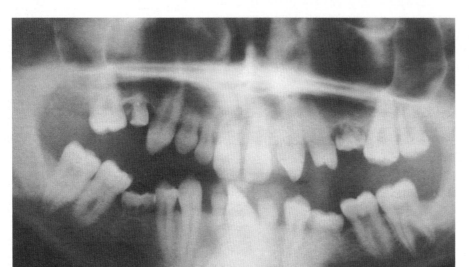

a)

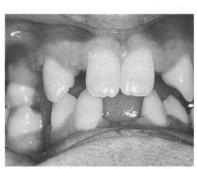

(d)

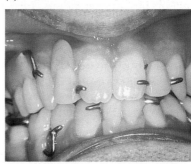

(e)

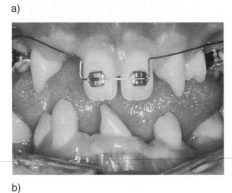

b)

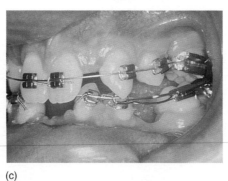

(c)

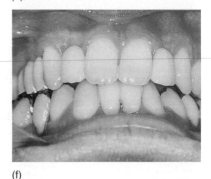

(f)

Fig. 14.28 (a) Severe hypodontia. (b) Note tilted teeth and unfavourable space distribution. (c) Fixed appliances to upright the teeth and redistribute space. (d) Result of orthodontic treatment. (e) Initial retention with partial dentures incorporating spurs to prevent any orthodontic relapse. (f) Definitive fixed restorations.

14.6.3 Anomalies of tooth size

Anomalies of tooth size are discussed in Chapter 13. Any tooth may be affected, but the upper lateral incisor is most commonly involved.

Megadontia

If the upper and lower teeth do not match for size it is impossible for them to be both aligned and in normal occlusion. An abnormally large upper incisor is associated with

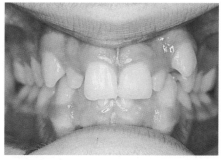

crowding or increased overjet, or both. A grossly oversized tooth may have to be extracted and replaced with a pontic after completion of any orthodontic treatment. In milder cases it is possible to narrow the tooth by reducing the enamel interdentally. Up to 1 mm may be removed after the teeth have been aligned but before appliances are removed, so that the resulting spaces can be closed.

Microdontia

Upper lateral incisors are most commonly affected. Any orthodontic treatment should precede the restoration of a diminutive tooth, and should leave adequate space for it to be enlarged (Fig. 14.29(a)–(c)). The retainer should carry interdental spurs to prevent adjacent teeth from drifting into the space, and it should be worn for at least 3 months before the tooth is built up. Where the upper arch is inherently crowded but the lateral incisors are diminutive on one side and congenitally absent on the other, it may be appropriate to extract the diminutive tooth and close the spaces. This relieves the crowding and gives a symmetrical appearance.

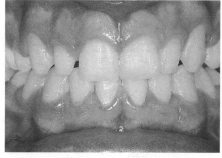

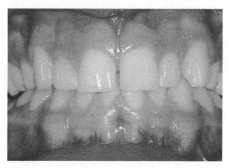

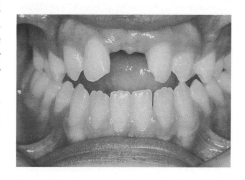

Fig. 14.29 (a) Patient with crowding and diminutive 2|2. (b) Following orthodontic treatment to align the arches. (c) Dimutive 2|2 enlarged with composite.

14.7 ORTHODONTICS AND DENTAL TRAUMA

Orthodontic brackets are often used as an immediate measure after trauma to stabilize loosened or reimplanted teeth, to realign displaced teeth, or to extrude teeth that have been intruded (Chapter 12). Teeth that have been fractured at the gingival level may require extrusion later, to facilitate restoration.

14.7.1 Orthodontic considerations for the missing upper incisor

Upper central incisor

The space starts to close very quickly, within days of losing the tooth, and it should be maintained by inserting a partial denture immediately (Fig. 14.30). In a crowded arch it is often possible to move the lateral incisor into the central space, but the resulting appearance is usually very poor. Building up or crowning the lateral incisor to mimic the central tooth is rarely satisfactory as it gives the tooth a very triangular shape, and it is difficult to maintain periodontal health around the enlarged crown.

Where a premolar is to be extracted for orthodontic reasons it can sometimes be transplanted into the central incisor site, and then restored to mimic the missing incisor.

Upper lateral incisor

Lateral incisor spaces can be either maintained or closed, depending on the amount of crowding in the arch (see Section 14.6.2).

Fig. 14.30 Space loss following avulsion of 1|1.

14.7.2 Orthodontic movement of traumatized teeth

In general, root-filled teeth can be moved orthodontically quite normally, with no increased risk of external root resorption compared with normal teeth. The risk factors associated with root resorption during orthodontic treatment are discussed in Section 14.8.3. Traumatized teeth, however, are already at an increased risk of root resorption, especially those which have been displaced or reimplanted—orthodontic treatment increases the risk further. In these cases the need for orthodontics should be assessed very carefully, but where it is needed the risk of resorption during tooth movement should be minimized by: (1) maintaining a calcium hydroxide dressing in the root canal during orthodontic treatment, and (2) ensuring that orthodontic forces are as light as possible.

Fixed appliances should be used with great care as they can easily generate high forces, and treatment with them should be kept to a minimum. Functional appliances are useful for reducing an overjet as they do not apply high forces to individual teeth.

A tooth that has become ankylosed cannot be moved orthodontically and will eventually be lost, but in the shorter term it will serve as a space maintainer unless the ankylosis causes excessive infraocclusion.

> **Key Points**
> Trauma
> - A space maintainer should be fitted *immediately* if an upper incisor is lost.
> - Traumatized teeth may resorb during orthodontic treatment. This is minimized by putting calcium hydroxide in the root canal and keeping orthodontic forces light.
> - Teeth with a poor prognosis serve as useful space maintainers in the short term.

14.8 COMPLICATIONS OF ORTHODONTIC TREATMENT

The most common problem with orthodontic treatment is lack of co-operation by the patient, which in some cases can lead to the treatment conferring no benefit or even making the malocclusion worse (see Section 14.2.2). Discussed below are four issues which may concern the paediatric dentist.

14.8.1 Postorthodontic decalcification

White spots of enamel decalcification are sometimes left after orthodontic treatment if the patient's compliance with oral hygiene and preventive advice has been poor (Fig. 14.31(a) and (b)). The problem is greatest with fixed appliances, with decalcification being mostly related to areas of plaque accumulation around the brackets, and commonly involving the labial surfaces of anterior teeth. The lesions can develop very quickly, within a few weeks, and consist of some softening of the enamel surface with progressive mineral loss of the subsurface layer to a depth of up to 100 μm.

Prevention of the problem starts with careful patient selection, but if oral hygiene during treatment is poor, and especially if there are signs of decalcification, preventive measures should be implemented immediately, These include:

(1) regular reinforcement of oral hygiene (see Section 14.8.2);

(2) dietary advice;

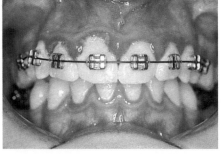

(a)

(b)

Fig. 14.31 (a) Neglected fixed appliance with associated gingival inflammation and decalcification. (b) The decalcification is obvious following bracket removal.

(3)   prescription of daily sodium fluoride mouthwashes.

If the patient does not respond then the orthodontic treatment should be stopped as quickly as possible, and it is often better to leave some residual malocclusion than to continue and risk severe damage.

If white enamel lesions are present when the appliance is removed, a daily sodium fluoride mouthwash should be started (if not already in use). This encourages remineralization, and the chalky appearance and degree of opacity of the lesions usually reduce during the 3 months following appliance removal. The majority of lesions that remain unsightly respond to the hydrochloric acid–pumice microabrasion technique (Chapter 10), but severe lesions and those with surface breakdown may require localized composite restorations or even veneers.

14.8.2 Orthodontics and periodontal health

Fixed appliances

Gingival inflammation is a frequent complication of fixed appliances (Fig. 14.31), and the patient must be encouraged to maintain good oral hygiene. They must recognize that it takes longer to clean the teeth with fixed appliances than without. A standard toothbrush with a fairly small two- or three-row head is suitable in most cases, or special orthodontic brushes are available with a groove which is intended to facilitate cleaning behind the archwire. Some patients find interspace brushes helpful, especially for local problem areas.

Marginal gingival inflammation resolves when the brackets and bands are removed, and there is no evidence that orthodontic treatment causes clinically significant long-term damage to the periodontium (Chapter 11). However, excessive arch expansion or proclination of teeth, especially the lower incisors, should be avoided as there is a risk of fenestration of the buccal alveolar bone or even gingival clefting.

Removable appliances

Mild palatal marginal gingivitis is quite common under removable appliances, but resolves at the end of treatment. Good oral and appliance hygiene is very important. The patient should take the appliance out to brush it and to clean the teeth at least twice a day, and to rinse it after meals. More widespread candidal infection occasionally occurs under the acrylic, but usually resolves if the patient wears the appliance part-time for a few days. Severe inflammation palatal to the upper incisors can occur during overjet reduction, due to compression of the tissues between the acrylic and the teeth (Fig. 14.32(a) and (b)). This should be avoided by keeping the appliance under frequent review, and ensuring at each visit that enough palatal acrylic has been trimmed away to allow tooth movement.

14.8.3 Root resorption

Most orthodontic treatments probably cause some resorption of root apices. In most cases it is slight, but significant apical resorption does occur in a few patients (Fig. 14.33 and Fig. 11.11). Any tooth can be affected, although studies have focused on the maxillary incisors. The aetiology is multifactorial and individual susceptibility to resorption is very variable, but factors associated with increased risk include:

(1)   history of trauma to maxillary incisors;

(2)   signs of pre-existing resorption: short roots or blunted apices;

(3)   thin, pipette-shaped root apices;

(4)   prolonged use of fixed appliances, especially intermaxillary elastics;

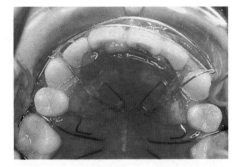
(a)

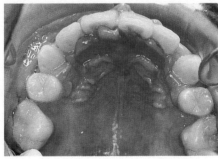
(b)

Fig. 14.32   (a) Upper removable appliance for retraction of the upper incisors. (b) Severe gingival inflammation resulting from compression of the gingival tissues under the appliance during incisor retraction.

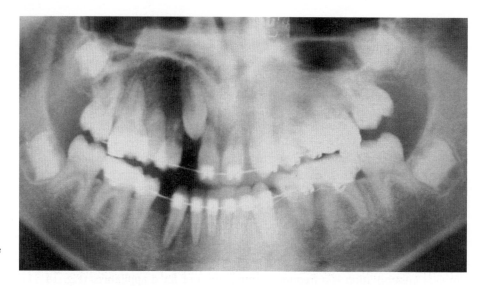

Fig. 14.33 Panoramic radiograph showing widespread root resorption during fixed appliance orthodontic treatment.

(5)   intrusive forces and torquing of apices;

(6)   reduction of large overjets, other than with functional appliances;

(7)   treatment to align impacted maxillary canines.

Orthodontic treatment for patients in the first three categories should be as short and simple as possible, keeping fixed appliances to a minimum and ensuring that forces are very light. Functional appliances avoid applying high forces to incisors during overjet reduction. Mild malocclusions are better left untreated in these circumstances.

14.8.4 Orthodontics and temporomandibular joint (TMJ) disorders

In general, the presence of malocclusion is not associated with an increased prevalence of TMJ disorders. There is a slightly greater prevalence in subjects with malocclusions of the type that often have associated occlusal interferences, including class III cases, cross-bites, and open bites, but the correlation is weak. Even so, simple orthodontic treatment, often in the mixed dentition, to correct a cross-bite with an associated mandibular displacement is well worthwhile. In older patients, orthodontic treatment to remove the interference can be complex and an alternative approach may be better, such as occlusal adjustment, unless treatment is needed anyway for other aspects of the malocclusion. Orthodontic treatment should always aim to leave the occlusion with no interferences.

It has been claimed that many forms of orthodontic treatment cause TMJ disorders, with premolar extractions coming under the greatest attack. However, extensive studies have found no evidence of an increased prevalence of TMJ disorders in subjects who have had orthodontic treatment, including extractions, compared with untreated controls.

14.9 TEMPOROMANDIBULAR JOINT (TMJ) DISORDERS

Although several studies include children aged 5–7 years, most observations have been made on the young adolescent. A small number of temporomandibular problems are associated with functional malocclusion (occlusal interferences) and morphological malocclusion such as cross-bite and anterior open bites, but bruxism and muscular hyperactivity probably play an important part in the development of TMJ disorders in childhood.

> **Key Points**
>
> Orthodontic injury
>
> - Teeth with blunted or thin roots have a greater risk of resorption during orthodontic treatment.
> - Prolonged treatment with high forces increases the risk or root resorption.
> - There is little evidence that malocclusion or orthodontic treatment are associated with temporomandibular joint disorders.
> - There is no evidence of significant long-term periodontal disease associated with orthodontic treatment.
> - Good oral hygiene and diet control are especially important during orthodontic treatment.
> - Daily fluoride mouthwashes reduce enamel decalcification.

The commonest clinical symptoms in children and adolescents are clicking (10–30%) and muscle tenderness on palpation (20–60%). Clinical signs such as reduced opening, pain and movement, and tenderness of the joints on palpation are less frequent than in adults. There seems to be no consistent pattern in the development of either subjective symptoms or clinical signs during growth. Headache is common in children (girls more than boys) and its prevalence increases with age. The connection between headache, bruxism, hyperactivity of jaw muscles, and mandibular dysfunction is well recognized and should not be missed.

Children with TMJ symptoms and those starting orthodontic treatment should have a full examination for occlusion, tooth wear, mandibular mobility, TMJ function and palpation, and jaw musculature function and palpation. One clinical symptom that has consistently disclosed the presence of a TMJ dysfunction is reduced opening.

Treatment principles used in adults can be broadly applied to children and adolescents, after taking into account the dynamic changes in occlusion in connection with tooth eruption and facial growth. The majority of treatment is by activators and/or splints. Occlusal adjustment is not generally undertaken in the young permanent dentition as most occlusal displacement in growing individuals will change with time. However, selective grinding may be necessary when a direct causal connection is suspected. It may be difficult to motivate children and adolescents to do jaw exercises, compared with adults. Training in one or two movements against resistance is usually accepted.

The TMJ can also be affected by diseases or conditions which might influence mandibular growth. The most frequent are juvenile idiopathic arthritis (JIA), traumatic injuries, unilateral hyperplasia, and congenital aplasia. JIA affects the TMJ in over 50% of those with the disease. This causes destruction of the condyles and glenoid fossa leading to mandibular micrognathia, mandibular asymmetry, open bite, abnormal bite, reduced opening, and loss of muscle strength. Traumatic injuries involving the condyles can lead to abnormal growth and development and should be followed closely.

Unilateral hyperplasia of the condyle, although rare, may occur around puberty. This can lead to cross-bite and mid-line deviation, as well as asymmetrical jaw movements and tenderness and pain from muscles and joints. Congenital aplasia of the TMJ may occur in syndromes such as hemifacial microsomia and Treacher–Collins syndrome, and results in abnormal growth and function. Such cases require a combined interdisciplinary approach.

14.10 CLEFT LIP AND PALATE

Patients with clefts of the lip and palate commonly need extensive and specialized treatment, provided by a multidisciplinary team of specialists including plastic surgeon, orthodontist, paediatric dentist, speech therapist, maxillofacial surgeon, ENT surgeon, and others. Approaches to management vary greatly. It is not the purpose of this section to discuss the details of the condition or its treatment, for which the reader is referred to specialist texts, but rather to highlight the crucial part the dentist plays in maintaining dental health throughout the prolonged period over which the treatment usually extends.

Management begins at birth with counselling of the parents to reassure them, explain the likely course of events, and to give practical advice on feeding. Sometimes presurgical intraoral appliances are fitted to try to reduce the size of the defect and facilitate surgical repair. The lip is repaired within the first few weeks or months, followed later by closure of the palate. The primary repairs are followed by a period of observation, usually in multidisciplinary clinics attended by the various specialists. As well as observing facial development, speech is monitored and corrective measures, such as speech therapy or palatopharyngeal surgery, instituted where necessary. These children often suffer middle ear infections for which ENT advice will be needed. As with all children, advice on preventive dental care should be given to the family and reinforced regularly.

A complication of surgical repair is that scar contraction in the palate causes narrowing of the upper arch. Sometimes this is quite dramatic, although modern techniques are reducing the severity of this problem. Orthodontic treatment often begins during the mixed dentition stage, at about 8 or 9 years, with expansion of the upper arch in preparation for a bone graft into the alveolar defect at about the age of 10 years. Grafting at this age provides bone into which teeth can erupt, particularly the adjacent canine, and greatly aids occlusal development. Clefts are often associated with other dental anomalies such as supernumerary, microdont, or impacted teeth.

Further orthodontic treatment, normally with fixed appliances, is needed when the permanent dentition has erupted—if this includes significant arch expansion, the patient will have to wear an appliance permanently to prevent relapse of the expansion. Secondary surgery to the lip and palate repairs may be needed. If scarring has restricted forward growth of the maxilla, surgical correction of a class III facial deformity may be considered in the late teenage years after growth is complete. This usually requires orthodontic preparation to give a satisfactory postoperative occlusion. Finally, restorative treatment may be needed because of missing teeth or other defects, and often to provide permanent retention of the orthodontic tooth movement.

It is obvious that the success of all this treatment depends on the maintenance of a sound dentition over many years, and that the loss of teeth due to caries greatly complicates and hinders treatment. The dentist thus has a vitally important part in maintaining continuity of routine preventive and restorative care. It is well recognized that patient compliance with long and complex treatments dwindles, and unfortunately many patients with clefts, and their families, do not give routine dentistry a high enough priority compared with other aspects of their treatment such as surgery. An enthusiastic and supportive dental team must therefore play a central part in the multidisciplinary management of clefts of the lip and palate.

14.11 SUMMARY

1. All children from the age of 8 years should be screened for malocclusion.
2. Unerupted maxillary canines should be palpated routinely on all children from the age of 10 years until eruption.
3. A maxillary canine which is not palpable should be investigated.
4. Significant variation from the normal sequence of eruption should be investigated, e.g. upper lateral incisor erupting before upper central incisor.

5. Refer for orthodontic advice in good time and give as much background information as possible.

6. Good oral hygiene and co-operation are essential for successful orthodontic appliance treatment.

7. Consider orthodontic aspects when extractions in the mixed dentition are necessary.

8. A space maintainer should be fitted immediately if a traumatized upper incisor is lost.

9. Cross-bites with displacement may be treated in the mixed dentition.

10. Treatment of increased overjet in the mixed dentition can become lengthy.

11. Persistent digit-sucking habits usually resolve when appliance treatment is started.

14.12 FURTHER READING

Andreason, J. O. and Andreason, F. M. (1994). *Textbook and color atlas of traumatic injuries to the teeth*, (3rd edn). Munksgaard, Copenhagen. (*Comprehensive coverage of the management of dental trauma, including the role of orthodontics.*)

Houston, W. J. B., Stephens, C. D., and Tulley, W. J. (1992). *A textbook of orthodontics*, (2nd edn). Wright, Oxford. (*An excellent introductory textbook*).

Isaacson, K. G., Reed, R. T., and Stephens, C. D. (1990). *Functional orthodontic appliances*. Blackwell Scientific, Oxford. (*A clear and thorough review of the role, management and effects of functional appliances.*)

Okeson, J. P. (1989). Temporomandibular disorders in children. *Pediatric Dentistry*, **11**, 325–9. (*A useful short summary on the subject.*)

Proffitt, W. R. (1993). *Contemporary orthodontics* (2nd edn). Mosby, St Louis. (*A superb, comprehensive orthodontic textbook.*)

Richardson, A. (1989). *Interceptive orthodontics* (2nd edn). *British Dental Journal* Publications, London. (*A concise handbook of the role of orthodontics in the mixed dentition.*)

Shaw, W. C. (ed.) (1993). *Orthodontics and occlusal management*. Butterworth–Heinemann, London. (*An authoritative orthodontic textbook, including cleft lip and palate, and risk/benefit of treatment.*)

14.13 REFERENCES

Brook, P. and Shaw, W. (1989). The development of an index of orthodontic treatment priority. *European Journal of Orthodontics*, **11**, 309–20.

Evans, R. and Shaw, W. (1987). Preliminary evaluation of an illustrated scale for raising dental attractiveness. *European Journal of Orthodontics*, **9**, 314–18.

15

Oral pathology and oral surgery

15 Oral pathology and oral surgery

J. G. Meechan

15.1 INTRODUCTION

The incidence of pathological conditions of the mouth and perioral structures differs between children and adults. For example, mucoceles are more common in the young, whereas squamous cell carcinomas occur more frequently in older individuals. The management of pathology in the child differs from that in the adult. Growth and development may be affected by the disease, or its treatment. On a more practical basis, anaesthetic considerations for surgical treatment of simple pathological conditions can make management more complex. This chapter deals with those conditions that occur exclusively, or more commonly in children. It is not an exhaustive guide to paediatric oral pathology, for which readers should refer to oral pathology textbooks. Surgical treatment of the simpler conditions is discussed in the oral surgery section of this chapter (Section 15.5).

15.2 LESIONS OF THE ORAL SOFT TISSUES

Conditions affecting the oral mucosa and associated soft tissues can be classified as: infections, ulcers, vesiculobullous lesions, white lesions, cysts, and tumours.

15.2.1 Infections

Viruses, bacteria, fungi, or protozoa may cause infections of the oral mucosa. Odontogenic infections will be discussed under 'oral surgery' later in this chapter.

Viral infections

HERPETIC INFECTIONS

PRIMARY HERPES SIMPLEX INFECTION

This condition usually occurs in children between the ages of 6 months and 5 years. Circulating maternal antibodies usually protects young babies. The symptoms, signs, and treatment are covered in Chapter 11.

SECONDARY HERPES SIMPLEX INFECTION

Secondary infection with herpes simplex usually occurs at the labial mucocutaneous junction and presents as a vesicular lesion which ruptures and produces crusting (Chapter 11).

Herpes varicella-zoster

Shingles, which is caused by the varicella zoster virus, is much commoner in adults than children. The vesicular lesion develops within the peripheral distribution of a branch of the trigeminal nerve. Chickenpox, a more common presentation of varicella-zoster in children, produces a vesicular rash on the skin. The intraoral lesions of chickenpox resemble those of primary herpetic infection. The condition is highly contagious.

MUMPS

Mumps produces a painful enlargement of the parotid glands. It is usually bilateral. The causative agent is a myxovirus. Associated complaints include headache, vomiting, and fever. Symptoms last for about a week and the condition is contagious.

MEASLES

The intraoral manifestation of measles occurs on the buccal mucosa. The lesions appear as white speckling surrounded by a red margin and are known as Koplick's spots. The oral signs usually precede the skin lesions and disappear early in the course of the disease. The skin rash of measles normally appears as a red maculopapular lesion. Fever is present and the disease is contagious.

RUBELLA

German measles does not usually produce signs in the oral mucosa; however, the tonsils may be affected. Protection against the diseases of mumps, measles, and rubella can be achieved by vaccinating children in their early years with MMR vaccine.

HERPANGINA

This is a coxsackievirus A infection. It can be differentiated from primary herpetic infection by the different location of the vesicles, which are found in the tonsillar or pharyngeal region. Herpangina lesions do not coalesce to form large areas of ulceration. The condition is short-lived.

HAND, FOOT, AND MOUTH DISEASE

This coxsackievirus A infection produces a maculopapular rash on the hands and feet. The Intraoral vesicles rupture to produce painful ulceration. The condition lasts for 10–14 days.

INFECTIOUS MONONUCLEOSIS

The Epstein–Barr virus, causes this condition. It is not uncommon among teenagers. The usual form of transmission is by kissing. Oral ulceration and petechial haemorrhage at the hard/soft palate junction may occur. There is lymph node enlargement and associated fever. There is no specific treatment. It should be noted that the prescription of ampicillin and amoxicillin (amoxycillin) can cause a rash in those suffering from infectious mononucleosis. These antibiotics should be avoided during the course of the disease. Treatment of the viral illnesses is symptomatic and relies on analgesia and maintenance of fluid intake. It must be remembered that aspirin should be avoided in children under 12 years of age (see later).

HUMAN PAPILLOMAVIRUS

This is associated with a number of tumour-like lesions of the oral mucosa, which are discussed below.

Bacterial infection

STAPHYLOCOCCAL INFECTIONS

Staphylococci and streptococci may be cause impetigo. This can affect the angles of the mouth and the lips (Fig. 15.1). It presents as crusting vesiculobullous lesions. The vesicles coalesce to produce ulceration over a wide area. Pigmentation may occur during healing. The condition is self-limiting, although antibiotics may be prescribed in some cases. Staphylococcal organisms can cause osteomyelitis of the

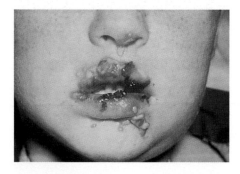

Fig. 15.1 Bacterial infection on the lip of an immunocompromised child. (By kind permission of *Dental Update*.)

jaws in children. Although the introduction of antibiotics has reduced the incidence of severe forms of the condition, it can still be devastating. In addition to aggressive antibiotic therapy, surgical intervention is required to remove bony sequestrae.

STREPTOCOCCAL INFECTION

Streptococcal infections in childhood vary from a mucopurulent nasal discharge to tonsillitis, pharyngitis, and gingivitis. Scarlet fever is a β-haemolytic streptococcal infection consisting of a skin rash with maculopapular lesions of the oral mucosa. It is associated with tonsillitis and pharyngitis. The tongue shows characteristic changes from a strawberry appearance in the early stages to a raspberry-like form in the later stages.

CONGENITAL SYPHILIS

Congenital syphilis is transmitted from an infected mother to the fetus. Oral mucosal changes such as rhagades, which is a pattern of scarring at the angle of the mouth, may occur. In addition, this disease may cause characteristic dental changes in the permanent dentition. These include Hutchinson's incisors (the teeth taper towards the incisal edge rather than the cervical margin) and mulberry molars (globular masses of enamel over the occlusal surface).

TUBERCULOSIS

Tuberculous lesions of the oral cavity are rare; however, tuberculous lymphadenitis affecting submandibular and cervical lymph nodes is occasionally seen. These present as tender enlarged nodes, which may progress to abscess formation with discharge through the skin. Surgical removal of infected glands produces a much neater scar than that caused by spontaneous rupture through the skin if the disease is allowed to progress.

CAT-SCRATCH DISEASE

This is a self-limiting disease which presents as an enlargement of regional lymph nodes. The nodes are painful and enlargement occurs up to 3 weeks following a cat scratch. The nodes become suppurative and may perforate the skin. Treatment often involves incision and drainage.

Fungal infections

CANDIDA

Neonatal acute candidiasis (thrush) contracted during birth is not uncommon. Likewise young children may develop the condition when resistance is lowered or after antibiotic therapy (Fig. 15.2). Easily removed white patches on an erythematous or bleeding base are found. Treatment with nystatin or miconazole is effective (those under 2 years of age should receive 2.5 ml of a miconazole gel (25 mg/ml) twice daily; 5 ml twice daily is prescribed for those under 6 years of age, and 5 ml four times a day for those over 6 years of age).

Actinomycosis

Actinomycosis can occur in children. It may follow intraoral trauma including dental extractions. The organisms spread through the tissues and can cause dysphagia if the submandibular region is involved. Abscesses may rupture on to the skin and long-term antibiotic therapy is required. Penicillin should be prescribed and maintained for at least 2 weeks following clinical cure.

Protozoal infections

Infection by *Toxoplasma gondii* may occasionally occur in children. The principal reservoir of infection being cats. Glandular toxoplasmosis is similar in presentation

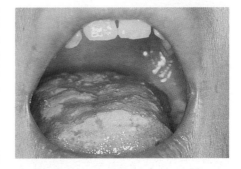

Fig. 15.2 Oral candidiasis in an immunocompromised child undergoing chemotherapy for acute lymphoblastic leukaemia. (By kind permission of *Dental Update*.)

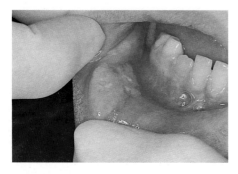

Fig. 15.3 Ulceration of the lower lip produced by biting while still anaesthetized from an inferior block.

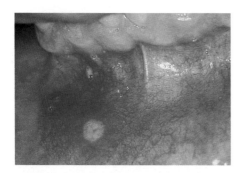

Fig. 15.4 Minor aphthous ulceration. (By kind permission of Wolfe Publishing.)

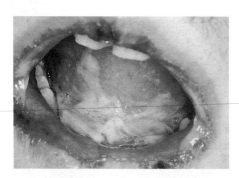

Fig. 15.5 Erythema multiforme in a teenager.

to infectious mononucleosis and is found mainly in children and young adults. There may be a granulomatous reaction in the oral mucosa and there can be parotid gland enlargement. The disease is self-limiting, although an anti-protozoal such as pyrimethamine may be used in cases of severe infection.

15.2.2 Ulcers

Traumatic ulceration of the tongue, lips, and cheek may occur in children, especially after local anaesthesia has been administered (Fig. 15.3). Recurrent aphthous oral ulceration not associated with systemic disease is often found in children (Fig. 15.4). One or more small ulcers in the non-attached gingiva may occur at frequent intervals. In the young child the symptoms may be mistaken for toothache by a parent. The majority of aphthous ulcers in children are of the minor variety (less than 5 mm in diameter). These usually heal within 10–14 days. Treatment other than reassurance is often unnecessary; however, topical steroids (Adcortyl in Orabase or Corlan pellets) may be prescribed in severe cases. Older children may benefit from the use of antiseptic rinses to prevent secondary infection. In the absence of a history of major aphthous ulceration any ulcer lasting for longer than 2 weeks should be regarded with suspicion and biopsied.

15.2.3 Vesiculobullous lesions

Vesiculobullous lesions cause ulcers in the later stages of such conditions. Viral causes have been mentioned above. Similarly, conditions such as epidermolysis bullosa and erythema multiforme can produce oral ulceration in children. The major vesiculobullous conditions such as pemphigus and pemphigoid are rare in young patients.

Epidermolysis bullosa is a term that covers a number of syndromes, some of which are incompatible with life. The skin is extremely fragile and mucosal involvement may occur. The act of suckling may induce bullae formation in babies. In older children effective oral hygiene may be difficult as even mild trauma can produce painful lesions.

The oral lesions of erythema multiforme usually affect the lips and anterior oral mucosa (Fig. 15.5). There is initial erythema followed by bullae formation and ulceration. The pathogenesis of the condition is still unclear, however, precipitating factors include drug therapy and infection. Treatment includes the use of steroids and oral antiseptic and analgesic rinses to ease the pain.

15.2.4 White lesions

Trauma of either a chemical or physical nature, for example, burns and occlusal trauma, can cause white patches intraorally.

WHITE SPONGY NAEVUS

The white spongy naevus (also known as the oral epithelial naevus) is a rough folded lesion that can affect any part of the oral mucosa. It often appears in infancy. It is benign.

LEUCOEDEMA

This is a folded, white translucent appearance found in children of races who exhibit pigmentation of the oral mucosa. It is considered a variation of normal.

CANDIDIASIS

The white patches of acute fungal candidiasis mentioned above are readily removed, in contrast to the white lesions discussed here.

GEOGRAPHIC TONGUE

This condition may be seen in children. It is normally symptomless, although some patients complain of discomfort with spicy foods. Areas of the tongue appear shiny and red due to loss of filiform papillae (Fig. 15.6). These red patches are surrounded by white margins. These areas disappear before reappearing in other regions of the tongue. The condition is benign and requires no treatment apart from reassurance to the child and parent.

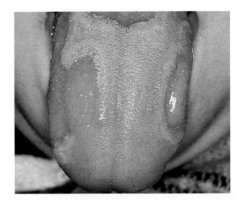

Fig. 15.6 Geographic tongue. (By kind permission of Wolfe Publishing.)

15.2.5 Cysts

MUCOCELES

The peak incidence of mucoceles is in the second decade of life; however, they are not uncommon in younger children (Fig. 15.7) including neonates. Mucoceles are caused by trauma to minor salivary glands or ducts and are often located on the lower lip. They are the commonest non-infective cause of salivary gland swelling in children. Salivary tumours are rare in this age group.

RANULA

This appears as a bluish swelling of the floor of the mouth (Fig. 15.8). It is essentially a large mucocele. It may arise from part of the sublingual salivary gland.

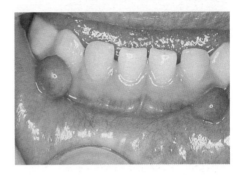

Fig. 15.7 Bilateral mucoceles in a 3-year-old girl. (By kind permission of the *Journal of Dentistry for Children*.)

BOHN'S NODULES

These gingival cysts arise from remnants of the dental lamina. They are found in Neonates. They usually disappear spontaneously in the early months of life.

EPSTEIN'S PEARLS

These small cystic lesions are located along the palatal mid-line. They are thought to arise from trapped epithelium in the palatal raphe. They are present in about 80% of neonates and disappear within a few weeks of birth.

DERMOID CYSTS

These are rare lesions of the floor of the mouth. They appear as intraoral and submental swellings (Fig. 15.9). They are derived from epithelial remnants remaining from fusion of the mandibular processes.

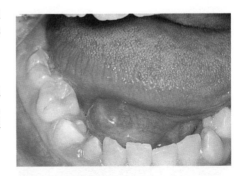

Fig. 15.8 A ranula in a 14-year-old girl.

LYMPHOEPITHELIAL CYST

In the past this was termed branchial arch cyst as it was thought to arise from epithelial remnants of a branchial arch. They are normally found in the sternomastoid region, although they can present in the floor of the mouth. Histologically the cyst wall contains lymph tissue. The tissue of origin is thought to be salivary epithelium.

THYROGLOSSAL CYST

This cyst, which arises from the thyroglossal duct epithelium, may present intraorally. The mouth however, is a rare site. Most arise in the region of the hyoid bone.

15.2.6 Tumours

CONGENITAL EPULIS

This is a rare lesion that occurs in neonates. It normally presents in the anterior maxilla. It consists of granular cells covered by epithelium and is thought to be reactive in nature. This is a benign lesion and simple excision is curative.

MELANOTIC NEUROECTODERMAL TUMOUR

This rare tumour occurs in the early months of life, usually in the maxilla. The lesion consists of epithelial cells containing melanin with a fibrous stroma. Some localized bone expansion may occur. The condition is benign and simple excision is curative.

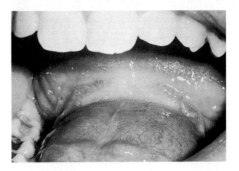

Fig. 15.9 A dermoid cyst.

SQUAMOUS-CELL PAPILLOMA

This is a benign condition that occurs in children. The small cauliflower-like growths, which vary in colour from pink to white (Fig. 15.10), are usually solitary lesions. They may be due to the human papillomavirus.

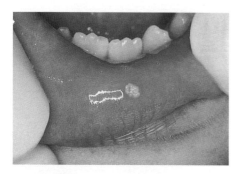

Fig. 15.10   Squamous-cell papilloma in a 9-year-old girl. (By kind permission of *Dental Update*.)

VERRUCA VULGARIS

This condition also known as the common wart may present as solitary or multiple intraoral lesions. These may be associated with skin warts. They are probably caused by the human papillomavirus.

FOCAL EPITHELIAL HYPERPLASIA

This is a rare condition also known as Heck's disease. It is associated with human papillomavirus. It presents as multiple small elevations of the oral mucosa especially in the lower lip.

FIBROEPITHELIAL POLYP

This is a fairly common lesion that presents as a firm pink lump. It normally affects the buccal mucosa at the occlusal level. They are caused by trauma. They are usually symptomless unless further traumatized and are easily removed.

FIBROUS EPULIS

This presents as a mass on the gingiva. Colour varies from pink to red depending upon the degree of vascularity of the lesion. (Fig. 15.11). It consists of an inflammatory cell infiltrate and mature fibrous tissue, occasionally a calcified variant is found. Surgical excision is curative.

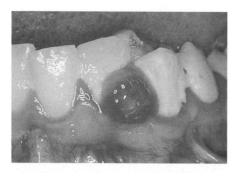

Fig. 15.11   A fibrous epulis in a 10-year-old girl (a pyogenic granuloma appears similar).

PYOGENIC GRANULOMA

These commonly occur on the gingiva usually in the anterior maxilla. They are probably a reaction to chronic trauma, especially from a sub-gingival calculus. Due to their aetiology they have a tendency to recur after removal.

PERIPHERAL GIANT-CELL GRANULOMA

This dark-red swelling of the gingiva can occur in children. It often arises interdentally. Radiographs may reveal some loss of the interdental crest. The central giant-cell granuloma (see below) shows much greater bone destruction. This condition is thought to be a reactive hyperplasia. Unless excision is complete it will recur.

HAEMANGIOMAS

Haemangiomas are relatively common in children. They are malformations of blood vessels. They are divided into cavernous and capillary variants, although some lesions contain elements of both. Capillary haemangiomas may present as facial birthmarks. The cavernous haemangioma is a hazard during surgery if involved within the surgical site. It is a large blood-filled sinus that will bleed profusely if damaged (Fig 15.12). The extent of a cavernous haemangioma can be established prior to surgery using either angiography or magnetic resonance imaging (MRI) scanning. Small haemangiomas are readily treated by excision or cryotherapy. Larger lesions are amenable to laser therapy.

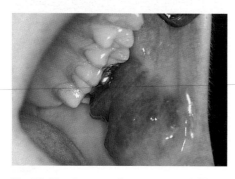

Fig. 15.12   Cavernous haemangioma of the right buccal mucosa. (By kind permission of Wolfe Publishing.)

STURGE–WEBER SYNDROME

Sturge–Weber angiomatosis is a syndrome consisting of a haemangioma of the leptomeninges with an epithelial facial haemangioma closely related to the distribution of branches of the trigeminal nerve. Mental deficiency, hemiplegia, and ocular defects can occur. Intraoral involvement may interfere with the timing of eruption of the teeth (both early and delayed eruption have been reported).

LYMPHANGIOMAS

Lymphangiomas are benign tumours of the lymphatics. The vast majority are found in children. The head and neck region is a common site (Fig 15.13). The cystic hygroma is a variant that appears as a large neck swelling, which may extend intraorally to involve the floor of the mouth and tongue.

NEUROFIBROMAS

These may present as solitary or multiple lesions. They are considered hamartomas (a haphazard arrangement of tissue). They present intraorally as mucosal swellings on the tongue or gingivae. Multiple oral neuromas are a feature of the multiple endocrine neoplasia syndrome. As the oral signs may precede the development of more serious aspects of this condition (such as carcinoma of the thyroid), children presenting with multiple lesions should be referred to an endocrinologist.

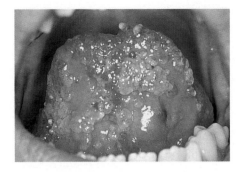

Fig. 15.13 Lymphangioma of the tongue and floor of the mouth. (By kind permission of Professor C. Scully.)

Orofacial granulomatosis

Orofacial granulomatosis (OFG) is not a tumour in the true sense nor a distinct disease entity, but describes a clinical appearance. Typically there is diffuse swelling of one or both lips and cheeks, folding of the buccal reflected mucosa and occasionally gingival swelling and oral ulceration (Fig. 15.14(a) and (b)). This may represent a localized disturbance due to an allergic reaction to foodstuffs, toothpaste, or even dental materials. Alternatively, the appearance may be due to an underlying systemic condition such as sarcoidosis or Crohn's disease.

MELKERSSON–ROSSENTHAL SYNDROME

This is a condition that generally begins during childhood. It consists of chronic facial swelling (usually the lips), facial nerve paralysis, and fissured (scrotal) tongue.

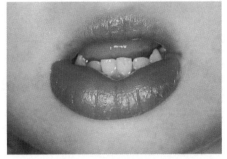

(a)

Malignant tumours of the oral soft tissues

EPITHELIAL TUMOURS

Malignant tumours of the oral epithelium, such as squamous-cell carcinoma, are rare in children. Malignant salivary neoplasms are also uncommon, although mucoepidermoid carcinomas have been reported in young patients.

LYMPHOMAS

Hodgkin's and non-Hodgkin's lymphomas have been reported in children; however, they are relatively rare in the paediatric age group. An exception is Burkitt's lymphoma, which is endemic in parts of Africa and occurs in those under 14 years of age. Indeed, in these areas the condition accounts for almost half of all malignancy in children. Burkitt's lymphoma is multifocal, but a jaw tumour (more often in the maxilla) is often the presenting symptom. Burkitt's lymphoma is strongly linked to the Epstein–Barr virus as a causal agent.

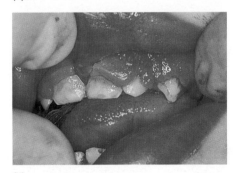

(b)

Fig. 15.14 (a) and (b) Swelling of the lower lip and attached mucosa and gingiva in a 3-year-old girl with orofacial granulomatosis.

RHABDOMYOSARCOMAS

These malignant tumours of skeletal muscle present in patients around 9 to 12 years of age. The usual site is the tongue. Metastases are common and the prognosis is poor.

15.3 LESIONS OF THE JAWS

These can be divided into: cysts, developmental conditions, osteodystrophies, and tumours.

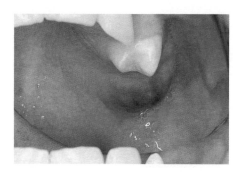

Fig. 15.15 Eruption cyst prior to the appearance of the upper permanent first molar.

15.3.1 Cysts

ERUPTION

Eruption cysts are really dentigerous cysts (see below) that present as swellings of the alveolar mucosa. They may precede the eruption of both primary and permanent teeth (Fig. 15.15). When filled with blood they are often called eruption haematomas. The treatment of eruption cysts is discussed in Section 15.5.5.

DENTIGEROUS

This is the commonest jaw cyst in children (Fig. 15.16). Its origin is the reduced enamel epithelium, and attachment to the tooth occurs at the amelocemental junction. There are often no symptoms but eruption of the affected tooth will be prevented. The treatment of dentigerous cysts is discussed in Section 15.5.5.

RADICULAR

These cysts related to the apex of a non-vital tooth do occur in children, although they are rare in the primary dentition. They are often symptomless and are discovered radiographically. Extraction, apicectomy, or conventional endodontics will effect a cure.

Lateral periodontal cysts are very rare in children.

ODONTOGENIC KERATOCYSTS

The odontogenic keratocyst is the most aggressive of the jaw cysts. It has a high rate of recurrence due to the fact that remnants left after subtotal removal will regenerate. These cysts may be found in children and may be associated with the Gorlin–Goltz syndrome. Keratocysts associated with this syndrome appear in the first decade of life, whereas the syndromic basal-cell carcinomas are rare before puberty. Other signs and symptoms include: multiple basal-cell carcinomas, bifid ribs, calcification of the falx cerebri, hypertelorism, and frontal and temporal bossing.

NON-ODONTOGENIC

These include the nasopalatine duct cyst which may occur clinically as a swelling in the anterior mid-line of the hard palate. The radiographic appearance is a radiolucency of greater than 6 mm in diameter in the position of the nasopalatine duct. The anterior teeth have vital pulps. Surgical excision is curative. The so-called globulomaxillary cyst, which occurs between the lateral incisor and canine teeth, is now thought to be odontogenic in origin. It is either a radicular cyst or an odontogenic keratocyst.

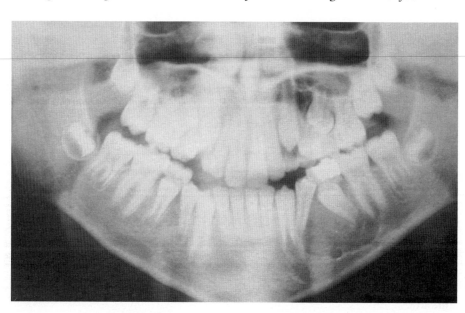

Fig. 15.16 Radiographic appearance of a dentigerous cyst associated with a lower second premolar. (By kind permission of *Dental Update*.)

The haemorrhagic bone cyst is a condition that may be found in children and adolescents. It occurs most commonly in the mandible in the premolar/molar region. It is often a chance radiographic finding and normally asymptomatic. Radiographically it appears as a scalloped radiolucency between the roots of the teeth. It regresses spontaneously or after surgical investigation.

15.3.2 Developmental conditions

Numerous developmental conditions may affect the oral and perioral structures. These range from minor problems (e.g. tongue-tie) that are readily treated under local anaesthesia, to severe craniofacial disorders (e.g. Crouzon's syndrome) requiring a combined interdisciplinary approach between maxillofacial and neurosurgery. Readers should refer to specialized texts for a full description of congenital jaw abnormalities. It is important to remember that patients with developmental orofacial abnormalities may have other congenital disorders, such as cardiac defects, which may influence routine dental treatment.

15.3.3 Osteodystrophies

FIBROUS DYSPLASIA

This can occur as one of three variants, namely: monostotic, polyostotic, or as part of Allbright's syndrome (where associated conditions include skin pigmentation and precocious puberty in females). The monostotic type is the most common to affect the jaws, especially the maxilla. The disease presents as a slow-growing bony expansion that produces facial asymmetry and malalignment of teeth. Radiographically there is a fine granular radiopacity (Fig. 15.17). Surgery can correct the asymmetry.

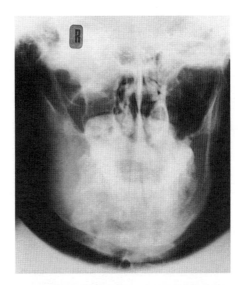

Fig. 15.17 Monostotic fibrous dysplasia of right mandibular angle and ascending ramus in a 15-year-old boy.

CHERUBIM

In this rare condition there is a characteristic fullness of the cheeks and jaws. Initial presentation is commonly between 2 and 4 years of age. Size increases during growth. It is self-limiting and regression occurs in adulthood. Cosmetic surgery may be employed after active growth has finished. Multilocular radiographic radiolucencies occur at the angles of the mandible (Fig. 15.18) and the maxillary tuberosities. Histologically the lesion is similar to the giant-cell granuloma.

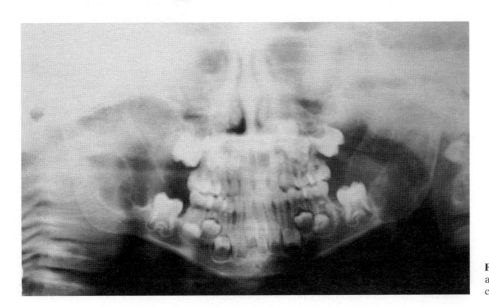

Fig. 15.18 Bilateral multilocular radiolucencies affecting the angles of the mandible in a 5-year-old child with cherubism.

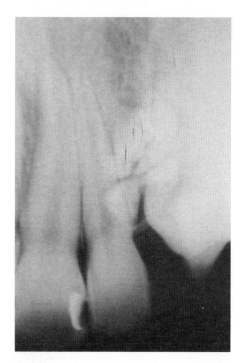

Fig. 15.19 Compound odontome in the upper left canine region.

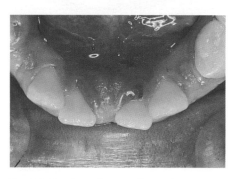

Fig. 15.20 Central giant-cell granuloma in a 9-year-old girl.

15.3.4 Tumours of the jaws

ODONTOMES

Odontomes are hamartomas that contain dental calcified tissue. They are classified as compound (a collection of discrete tooth-like structures) and complex (a haphazard arrangement of dental tissue). Compound odontomes are most commonly found in the anterior maxilla (Fig. 15.19). The complex type are usually located in the premolar/molar regions of both jaws. Odontomes are usually symptomless and are diagnosed radiographically. The mean age of patients at diagnosis is 15 years. Occasionally an odontome will become infected when partially erupted and surgical excision is required. Similarly, removal is indicated if an odontome is interfering with the eruption of a neighbouring tooth or is needed as part of an orthodontic treatment plan.

JUVENILE OSSIFYING FIBROMA

This benign lesion differs from the adult ossifying (or cemento-ossifying) fibroma in that growth is rapid. It consists of fibrous tissue with a varying amount of mineralized material. It usually affects the mandible. Radiographs show a well-circumscribed radiolucency with 'speckling'. Surgical excision is required.

CENTRAL GIANT-CELL GRANULOMA

This swelling of bone usually affects the mandible (Fig. 15.20). Radiographically there is a well-defined radiolucency with occasional resorption of associated teeth. Histologically there are large numbers of osteoclast-like cells in a vascular stroma. Surgical curettage is curative.

HISTIOCYTOSES

Langerhans' cell histiocytosis, formerly known as histiocytosis X is a condition that predominantly affects children (Chapter 11). Bone is replaced by Langerhans' cells, so producing sharply defined radiographic radiolucencies.

AMELOBLASTOMA

Although more commonly found in adults, this locally invasive neoplasm can occur in children. It is usually found in the mandible. It is slow growing, and is often symptomless in the early stages. As it progresses it causes a bony swelling, which appears as a multi-locular radiolucency in the jaw. Surgical resection to sound bone is necessary for a cure.

AMELOBLASTIC FIBROMA

This rare lesion usually affects a younger age group than the ameloblastoma. The average age of patients at diagnosis is 14 years. It is a benign tumour. A related lesion is the ameloblastic fibro-odontoma. This lesion contains dentine and enamel and occurs in children under 10 years of age.

PRIMARY INTRAOSSEOUS CARCINOMA

This is a very rare tumour but when it occurs it is usually in children. It is thought to arise from odontogenic epithelium and shows rapid growth.

SARCOMAS

Sarcomas of the jaws are rare; however, the highly malignant Ewing's sarcoma occurs in children between the ages of 5 and 15 years of age. The mandible is usually the bone affected and the prognosis is poor.

15.4 ORAL MANIFESTATIONS OF SYSTEMIC DISEASE

In addition to specific pathological oral conditions, diseases that affect other systems of the body can produce oral manifestations, for example, Crohn's disease. In addition, disorders such as chronic renal failure and diabetes can predispose to periodontal disease and there may be poor resistance to the spread of odontogenic infection.

It is not only the oral soft tissues that are affected by systemic conditions. The temporomandibular joint can be involved in juvenile rheumatoid arthritis and the jaws can be affected in hyperparathyroidism (giant-cell tumours). In some cases an oral condition may be the presenting feature of a systemic disease and dental practitioners should not hesitate to refer children with abnormal oral signs for further investigation.

15.5 ORAL SURGERY

This section deals with dental extractions and minor oral surgical procedures for children. The procedures described are those that can be performed under local anaesthesia with or without sedation (normally inhalational) or day-stay general anaesthesia in healthy children. Oral surgery procedures that require in-patient facilities, other than the treatment of severe infection, will not be considered in this text.

15.5.1 Exodontia

Differences between primary and permanent teeth

1. *Size*. Primary teeth are smaller in every dimension compared with their permanent counterparts. Although the roots of primary teeth are smaller than those of the permanent dentition they do form a proportionately greater part of the tooth.
2. *Shape*. The crowns of primary teeth are more bulbous than the crowns of permanent teeth. The roots of primary molars are more splayed than the roots of permanent molar teeth. The furcation of primary molar roots is positioned more cervically than in the corresponding permanent teeth.
3. *Physiology*. The roots of primary teeth resorb naturally, whereas in the permanent dentition resorption is normally a sign of pathology.
4. *Support*. The bone of the alveolus is much more elastic in the younger patient. These differences mean that there are some modifications to extraction techniques in children. The types of forceps employed for the removal of primary teeth differ from that used for the removal of permanent teeth. The beaks and handles are smaller. In addition, to accommodate the more bulbous crown, the beaks are more curved in forceps designed for the removal of primary teeth.

The wide splaying of primary molar roots means that more expansion of the socket is required for the extraction of primary teeth. The more elastic alveolus of the younger patient allows this to be achieved.

Due to the relatively cervical position of the bifurcation in primary molars it is injudicious to use forceps with deeply plunging beaks (such as the adult cowhorn design) as these could damage the underlying permanent successors. This is especially so with the lower primary molars.

As primary roots are resorbed it is often preferable to leave small fragments *in situ* if the root fractures. When part of a fractured root is visible then it should be removed. Blind investigation of primary sockets should not be performed as there is a danger of damaging the underlying permanent successor. Similarly, blind investigation of the distal root socket of first permanent molar teeth must not be carried out in children with unerupted second molars, as unintentional elevation of the second molar can occur.

Problems peculiar to the child patient

A number of problems peculiar to the child patient will affect the way in which extractions are carried out. The following should be considered:

(1) natal and neonatal teeth;
(2) infraocclusion of teeth;
(3) fusion/gemination of two teeth;
(4) damage to the permanent successor;
(5) dislocation of the mandible.

NATAL AND NEONATAL TEETH

Most neonatal teeth (85%) are found in the mandible. About 5% of these are supernumeraries. Their management is discussed in Chapter 13.

INFRAOCCLUSION

Surgical division is sometimes necessary to remove these teeth (Chapter 13).

FUSION/GEMINATION (CONNATION)

Such teeth may not lend themselves to forceps extraction due to their unusual coronal shape. Elevators are usually employed, with or without tooth division and bone removal, to effect extraction.

DAMAGE TO PERMANENT SUCCESSOR

This may occur if forceps with large beaks are used or during root elevation.

DISLOCATION OF THE MANDIBLE

It is very easy to dislocate a child's mandible during extractions under general anaesthesia (when the muscles are relaxed) unless adequate support is provided by the 'non-working' hand. This is because the articular eminence is not as pronounced in young patients as in adults. It is essential to verify that dislocation has not occurred before the patient is allowed to regain consciousness.

15.5.2 Extraction techniques

PATIENT POSITION

The child should be seated in a dental chair reclined about 30° to the vertical for extractions under local anaesthesia. Under general anaesthesia the patient is usually supine. When removing upper teeth under local anaesthesia the operator stands in front of the patient, with a straight back and the patient's mouth at a level just below the operator's shoulder. A right-handed operator removes lower left teeth from a similar position in front of the patient, except that the patient's mouth is at a height just below the operator's elbow. When removing teeth from the lower right the right-handed operator stands behind the patient with the chair as low as possible to allow good vision. When performing extractions in the supine patient under general anaesthesia the patient's mouth is usually at a level just below the operator's elbow. Once again, lower right teeth are removed from behind, with all others being extracted by the operator standing in front of the patient. It does save time during general anaesthesia if teeth can be removed ambidextrously as all teeth can be extracted with the operator standing in front of the patient. The removal of primary teeth with the non-dominant hand is not difficult to master and is a useful skill to acquire.

The non-working hand

The sections below describe the instruments and technique used by the operator's working hand. The 'non-working' hand also has important roles to play (Fig. 15.21):

1. It retracts soft tissues to allow visibility and access.
2. It protects the tissues if the instrument slips.

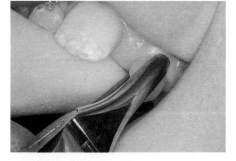

Fig. 15.21 The non-working hand supports the tooth for extraction and reflects the soft tissues.

3. It provides resistance to the extraction force on the mandible to prevent dislocation.
4. It provides 'feel' to the operator during the extraction and gives information about resistance to removal.

Order of extraction

When performing multiple extractions in all quadrants of the mouth (especially if under general anaesthesia) the order of extraction is as follows:

1. Symptomatic teeth are extracted before 'balancing extractions' on the opposite side.
2. Lower teeth are extracted before upper teeth (to eliminate bleeding interfering with the surgical field).
3. If there are symptomatic teeth in all quadrants right-handed operators should begin with lower right extractions. This minimizes the number of changes of position of the surgeon, which will reduce general anaesthetic time.

UPPER PRIMARY AND PERMANENT ANTERIORS

When these teeth are in a normal position in the dental arch they should be removed by applying the forceps beaks to the root and then using clockwise and anticlockwise rotations about the long axis (the action one would employ when using a screwdriver). In older children some additional buccal expansion may be required for the removal of the permanent upper canine. When removing primary upper anteriors, upper primary anterior or upper primary root forceps are used; for the permanent maxillary anteriors upper straight forceps are employed.

Malpositioned permanent upper anteriors are frequently encountered and modifications to technique must be employed. Labially placed upper lateral incisors and canines have very little buccal support and are easily removed, either by using straight forceps applied mesially and distally and using a slight rotatory movement as described earlier or by the use of elevators. The most useful elevators under these circumstances are the straight and curved Warwick James and Couplands. The straight elevators are applied along the length of the mesial and distal surfaces of the root and directed in a rotatory manner towards the apex (Fig. 15.22). The mesiobuccal and distobuccal surfaces are used alternately, although in many instances the tooth will be elevated after application to only one of these surfaces. When the curved Warwick James elevators are used, the right-sided Warwick James is positioned on the mesiobuccal surface of upper right teeth and the distobuccal surface of upper left teeth, and then rotated towards the mid-line of the tooth. The left-sided instrument is used on the opposite root surface in a similar fashion.

Palatally positioned lateral incisors and canines are usually not accessible with forceps and thus elevators are used as described above, with the exception that they are applied on the palatomesial and palatodistal surfaces. When the curved elevators are used the right-sided instrument is applied distally on the right side and mesially on the left side.

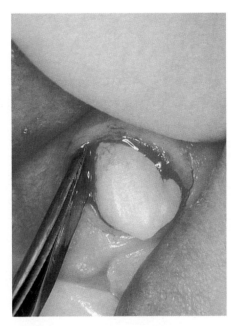

Fig. 15.22 Use of a Coupland elevator to deliver a buccally placed upper canine.

UPPER PRIMARY MOLARS

These teeth display the most widely splayed roots found in either dentition and thus considerable expansion of the socket is required. Upper primary molar forceps are used and applied to the roots. The initial movement after application of the forceps is palatal, to expand the socket in this direction. The tooth is then subjected to a continuous bucally directed force, which results in delivery. Occasionally, buccal movement is not adequately obtained due to gross caries on the palatal aspect causing slippage of the forceps beak on the palatal side during buccal expansion. This may be overcome by completing the extraction by continued palatal expansion, the elastic bone of younger patients allowing this to be performed.

UPPER PREMOLARS

The two-rooted, upper first premolar is best removed by buccal expansion using upper premolar forceps. The upper second premolar is often single rooted and, although buccal expansion with premolar forceps should be attempted in the first instance, this tooth can also be subjected to a rotation about its long axis to effect delivery. Palatally displaced upper premolars are difficult to remove with forceps. The use of elevators in a manner similar to that described for palatally placed canines is preferred.

UPPER PERMANENT MOLARS

These teeth are removed using left and right upper molar forceps. Following application of the forceps to the roots of the tooth (the pointed beak being driven towards the buccal root bifurcation) the tooth is delivered by expanding the socket in a buccal direction. The use of palatal expansion is not as successful in the removal of permanent molars, but it may be worth attempting if buccal expansion fails to deliver the tooth. The problem with palatal expansion when extracting permanent molars is that it can cause fracture of the palatal root, which is usually the most closely associated with the maxillary antrum.

LOWER PRIMARY ANTERIORS

These teeth are extracted in the same manner as their upper counterparts, in that, rotation about the long axis using lower primary anterior or root forceps is employed.

LOWER PERMANENT ANTERIORS

Permanent lower incisors are not readily removed by rotation as their roots are thin mesiodistally and rotation is likely to cause root fracture. The most effective method of removal is to apply lower root forceps and expand the socket labially. Permanent lower canines may be delivered by a rotatory movement about the long axis or by buccal expansion. Labially displaced lower canines are removed in a manner similar to that described for buccally placed upper anteriors. Mesial and distal application of forceps or straight elevators are used. Straight elevators are used on lower incisors that are labially placed. The position of lingually placed lower anteriors normally precludes the use of forceps and straight elevators applied mesially and distally should be employed.

LOWER PRIMARY MOLARS

These teeth are removed by buccolingual expansion of the socket. They can be extracted using either lower primary molar or lower primary root forceps. Lower primary molar forceps are similar in design to the permanent molar forceps. They have two pointed beaks which engage the bifurcation. Lower primary root forceps are used by applying the beaks to the mesial root of the primary molar. Lower first primary molars are usually more easily removed with lower primary root forceps. After application of the forceps a small lingual movement is followed by a continuous buccal force, which delivers the tooth.

LOWER PREMOLARS

When these teeth are fully erupted in the arch of the young patient they are usually simply removed by a rotatory movement around the long axis of the root using lower premolar forceps. Malpositioned lower second premolars are normally lingually positioned and can be difficult to remove with lower forceps. When lingually placed, lower premolars may be extracted using straight elevators applied mesially, lingually, and distally. Alternatively, it is often possible to apply the beaks of upper fine root forceps mesially and distally to the crown of the lingually placed tooth when the forceps are directed from the opposite side of the jaw. Gentle rotation of the tooth with the forceps may then effect removal.

LOWER PERMANENT MOLARS

Two designs of forceps are used to extract lower molar teeth. The lower molar forceps have two pointed beaks that are applied in the region of the bifurcation buccally and lingually. Once applied the forceps are used to move the tooth in a buccal direction to expand the buccal cortical plate. When buccal expansion is not sufficient to deliver the tooth then the forceps should be moved in a figure-of-eight fashion to expand the socket lingually as well as buccally, and this is generally successful.

A different technique is used with forceps of the cowhorn design. These forceps have two beaks that taper to a point. The points are applied to the bifurcation of the lower molar in a manner identical to that described above. The next movement is to squeeze the forceps handles together, which results in the beaks approaching one another at the base of the bifurcation. The only way the beaks can approach each other is by displacing the tooth in an occlusal direction resulting in extraction of the tooth. Both the methods are successful in removing permanent molar teeth in children and the choice of technique depends mainly on the preference of the operator.

Management of buried teeth

Buried teeth (including supernumeraries) are treated in children for several reasons:

(1) symptomatic (e.g. pain);
(2) radiographic signs of pathology (e.g. dentigerous cyst formation);
(3) part of an orthodontic treatment plan.

If buried teeth are symptomless, have no associated pathology, and are not causing orthodontic problems (either by their absence or in preventing the orthodontic movement of erupted teeth) they should be left alone. Such teeth should be kept under clinical and radiographic review so that any developing pathology may be detected and treated. In cases where unerupted teeth are to be removed the first step in management is to localize the buried tooth by clinical examination and radiographic techniques. A number of radiographic views may be used:

(1) parallax periapicals;
(2) orthopantomogram;
(3) occlusal views;
(4) true lateral facial bones.

In practice, parallax periapicals and an orthopantomogram are usually sufficient. The periapical films will help to establish the buccolingual position of the buried tooth in relation to the erupted dentition. The orthopantomogram will supply information concerning the overall shape of the tooth, its relationship to neighbouring structures (such as the antrum, inferior alveolar nerve canal, other unerupted teeth), and the extent of any associated pathology. Once the tooth has been located and the difficulty of removal and patient co-operation assessed then the method of anaesthesia should be determined.

Extraction of buried teeth

When removing buried dental tissue in children it is imperative to have an excellent view of the operative field. This is especially important when removing unerupted teeth or supernumeraries closely associated with other unerupted teeth that are to be retained. In these circumstances the tooth of interest and its unerupted neighbours must be clearly identified.

FLAP DESIGN

Flaps should:

- be mucoperiosteal;
- be cut at 90° to bone;

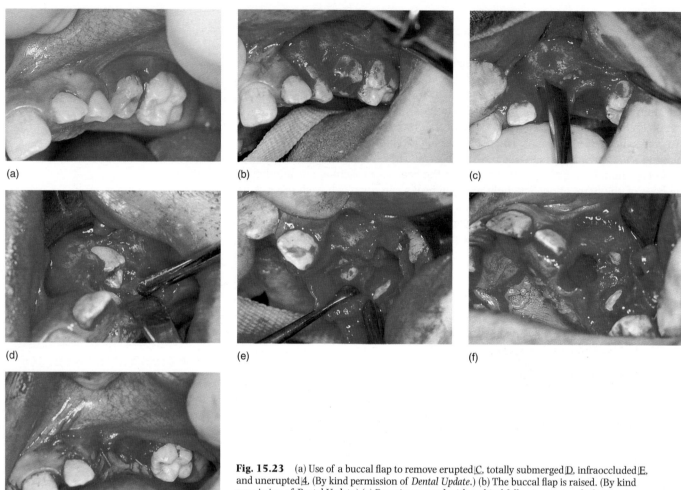

Fig. 15.23   (a) Use of a buccal flap to remove erupted |C, totally submerged |D, infraoccluded |E, and unerupted |4. (By kind permission of *Dental Update*.) (b) The buccal flap is raised. (By kind permission of *Dental Update*.) (c) Bone is removed with a chisel following removal of |CE. (By kind permission of *Dental Update*.) (d) Totally submerged |D is identified by occlusal amalgam. (By kind permission of *Dental Update*.) (e) |D Removed and |4 located. (By kind permission of *Dental Update*.) (f) |4 removed. (By kind permission of *Dental Update*.) (g) Wound Closure. (By kind permission of *Dental Update*.)

- have a good blood supply;
- avoid damage to important structures;
- allow atraumatic reflection;
- provide adequate access and visibility; and
- permit reapposition of the wound margins over sound bone.

FLAPS FOR BUCCALLY PLACED TEETH

Two designs of flap may be used for the removal of buccally placed teeth. The first of these includes the gingival margin as the horizontal component and a vertical relief incision into the depth of the buccal sulcus (Fig. 15.23(a)–(g)). It allows good exposure, easy orientation, can be readily extended and, for the most part the wound edge will be replaced over sound bone at the end of the procedure. If this design is used in the mandible in the region of the mental foramen care must be taken to ensure that the vertical relief is at least one tooth in front of the foramen (which will have been localized from the orthopantomogram). The only problem with this type of flap is that it may disrupt the gingival contour, but this is not a major long-term problem in the child. The second design of flap for buccally placed teeth is a semilunar incision. At least 5 mm of attached gingiva should be maintained at the narrowest point to ensure a good blood supply to the marginal gingivae. This flap does not provide such good exposure or orientation as the previous design, and it is

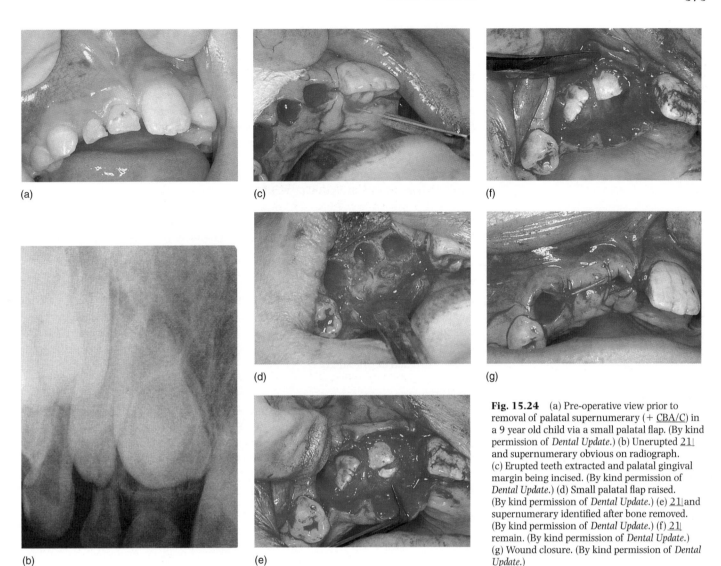

Fig. 15.24 (a) Pre-operative view prior to removal of palatal supernumerary (+ <u>CBA/C</u>) in a 9 year old child via a small palatal flap. (By kind permission of *Dental Update*.) (b) Unerupted <u>21|</u> and supernumerary obvious on radiograph. (c) Erupted teeth extracted and palatal gingival margin being incised. (By kind permission of *Dental Update*.) (d) Small palatal flap raised. (By kind permission of *Dental Update*.) (e) <u>21|</u> and supernumerary identified after bone removed. (By kind permission of *Dental Update*.) (f) <u>21|</u> remain. (By kind permission of *Dental Update*.) (g) Wound closure. (By kind permission of *Dental Update*.)

easy at the end of surgery to be left with a large part of the wound margin over a bony defect. This can lead to wound breakdown.

FLAPS FOR PALATALLY/LINGUALLY PLACED TEETH

Palatally positioned teeth are best removed via an incision that follows the palatal gingival margin (Fig. 15.24(a)–(g)). Such an incision maintains the integrity of the greater palatine nerves and blood vessels. It is often possible to raise this flap without sacrificing the neurovascular bundle that leaves the incisive foramen. This bundle will stretch to a certain degree; however, if access demands it should be cut. This rarely results in any postoperative complications. The extent of the palatal gingival incision depends upon the surgery involved. A flap extending between the mesial aspect of both first permanent molars is not unusual for the removal of bilateral impacted maxillary canines. Smaller flaps may be sufficient to remove palatally placed teeth or supernumeraries near the mid-line. In the lower jaw adequate access to the lingual side is obtained by raising the lingual gingiva and reflected mucosa via an incision run around the lingual gingival margin.

BONE REMOVAL

When working close to buried teeth that are to be retained it is essential that bone is removed with care. This may be carried out using a handpiece and bur very slowly. The use of chisels with hand pressure (mallets are not used unless working under general anaesthesia and are seldom required in children) is much safer because this is unlikely to damage coronal tissue.

TOOTH REMOVAL

Once sufficient bone has been removed to allow identification of the tooth to be extracted and exposure of the greatest diameter of its crown, the tooth should be elevated. If this is likely to produce undue pressure on neighbouring erupted or buried teeth then the tooth should be divided using a handpiece and bur and removed in parts. Mandibular teeth that are impacted within the line of the arch are best removed by the so-called 'broken instrument technique', in which pressure is applied from one side of the tooth (e.g. using a straight Warwick James elevator) to force it out of the other side.

SUTURING

Resorbable sutures should be used in children whenever possible: 3/0 or 4/0 softgut is ideal.

DISCHARGE

Any bleeding should be arrested before the patient is allowed to leave the surgery. The patient and parent should receive instructions on simple methods of haemorrhage control. The patient is encouraged to maintain good oral hygiene and may be given an antiseptic mouthwash. The problem of self-inflicted trauma in anaesthetized areas is stressed at this stage.

PAIN RELIEF

Simple analgesics are usually required, but aspirin must be avoided in those under 12 years of age due to its association with Reye's syndrome. Paracetamol elixir (120 mg/5 ml four times daily for those under 6 years of age; 250 mg/5 ml four times daily for children aged 6–12 years) is ideal. The patient is given a review appointment but should return sooner if there are any problems with bleeding, excessive pain, or swelling. A telephone number for contact in an emergency must be provided.

REVIEW

The patient should be reviewed 1 week after surgery, at which stage resorbable sutures may have disappeared. The surgical site should be examined for undue swelling, the area of local anaesthesia examined for evidence of self-inflicted trauma, and the patient questioned about any residual altered sensation.

It is often necessary to reinforce good oral hygiene at this stage.

POSTEXTRACTION PROBLEMS

Fortunately, postextraction problems are rare in children. Dry socket does not seem to occur after the removal of primary teeth but it can affect older children following permanent molar extractions, although the incidence is not as great as in adults. Local measures such as irrigation and dressing with a sedative pack, plus the prescription of an analgesic are sufficient. Postoperative haemorrhage is an occasional problem with children and can be impressive following multiple extractions under general anaesthesia. Usually pressure applied with gauze or a handkerchief is effective. If not, sutures with or without haemostatic gauze must be used. Severe blood loss is very rare, but if this occurs it is important to exclude a systemic cause to ensure subsequent treatment can be performed safely.

15.5.3 Surgical aids to orthodontics

Surgical exposure of teeth

The exposure of buried teeth may involve either the extraction of erupted teeth or the removal of buried dental elements, but in some cases all that is required is excision of overlying soft tissue. If the tooth can be exposed adequately through a collar of attached gingiva then the procedure is quite simple:

1. Erupted primary predecessors may be extracted.

2. A flap is raised in the manner described above.

3. Any unerupted supernumeraries or buried teeth are extracted.

4. The bony impaction is relieved and the widest diameter of the crown exposed. At this stage it may be possible to place an orthodontic bracket to aid eruption, although this is by no means essential.

5. A pack, for example, Whitehead's varnish on ½-inch (about 1.25 cm) or ¼-inch (about 0.63 cm) ribbon gauze or a periodontal dressing, is then placed around the tooth and the flap replaced around the pack. It is not always necessary to sacrifice soft tissue if the tooth is exposed, and the pack can be placed via primary tooth sockets. Alternatively it is possible in some cases (such as the exposure of a palatally placed canine) to incorporate a periodontal pack on to the acrylic of an upper removable orthodontic appliance to maintain exposure during healing.

6. The use of non-resorbable sutures to maintain the pack is recommended, although other parts of the incision can be closed with resorbable sutures.

7. In cases in which the removal of soft tissue from the palate or crest of the ridge is all that is required to expose a tooth then it is unnecessary to raise a full flap. All that is needed is to sacrifice the overlying tissue and pack the wound (Fig. 15.25(a) and (b)). Occasionally this can cause excessive bleeding in the palate. This is controlled by passing a non-resorbable suture across the full thickness of the palatal mucoperiosteum just posterior to the wound edge to ligate the greater palatine artery.

8. When an unerupted tooth, classically a canine, is palpable high in the buccal sulcus under reflected mucosa it should not be exposed by sacrificing the overlying soft tissue. This would result in the cervical collar of the tooth being surrounded by non-keratinized mucosa. To overcome this problem a flap containing keratinized gingiva must be raised coronal to the impacted tooth, bone removed if necessary, and the flap replaced in a more apical position to allow a collar of attached gingiva around the tooth at eruption.

9. The pack and any remaining non-resorbable sutures should be removed after 7–10 days.

Bonding of orthodontic appliances to unerupted teeth

When it is impossible to reposition a flap apically around an unerupted tooth an alternative is to bond either a gold chain or a magnet to the buried tooth (Fig. 15.26(a) and (b)). When performing this technique the tooth is localized as described above and the gold chain or magnet attached to the tooth using composite resin and a bonding agent. When a gold chain has been attached (Fig. 15.26(a)) the chain is brought through the edges of the wound in the area of natural eruption of the tooth. The free end of the chain is then either bonded to an erupted tooth or sutured to the mucosa during the healing period before orthodontic activation. When a magnet is used (Fig. 15.26(b)) the soft tissues are relocated in their original position and sutured. A magnet with the opposite polarity is incorporated within a removable appliance and this is placed over the wound to apply the magnetic force.

Surgical anchorage

Occasionally there is insufficient erupted dentition to allow orthodontic anchorage. This is especially the case for the patient with hypodontia (Chapter 13). Extraoral anchorage may be employed in such cases. Another technique is to provide

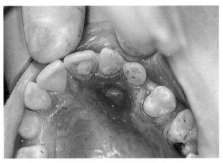

(a)

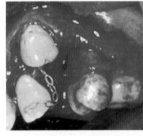

(b)

Fig. 15.25 (a) Exposure of palatal canine by tissue sacrifice. (By kind permission of *Dental Update*.) (b) Ribbon gauze pack sutured in defect. (By kind permission of *Dental Update*.)

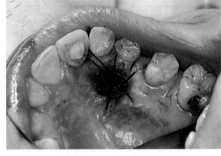

(a)

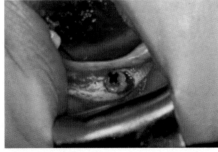

(b)

Fig. 15.26 (a) Gold chain bonded to unerupted maxillary permanent canine. The free end of the chain will be bonded to the erupted maxillary permanent incisor following flap replacement. (b) Magnet bonded to unerupted lower second premolar tooth following bone removal. Following flap replacement an acrylic splint containing the magnet with the opposite pole will be positioned over the mucosa.

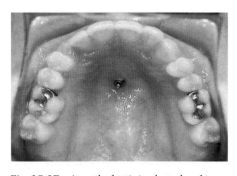

Fig. 15.27 An orthodontic implant placed in the mid-line of the palate and used to provide anchorage. (Image kindly supplied by Straumann Ltd.)

anchorage by the provision of implants. Standard dental implants are not normally used in children as they act as ankylosed teeth and may disturb the growth of the jaws (see below). Orthodontic implants, however, may be placed, for example, in the midline of the palate (Fig 15.27). Orthodontic appliances can then be attached to these implants, which are removed at the end of treatment.

15.5.4 Apical surgery

Apicectomy is rarely performed in children. As with adult patients the best treatment for pulpal pathology is normally conventional endodontic therapy. However, there are some indications for the technique, most commonly teeth with intransigent open apices. A number of different flap designs may be used. The best is the triangular flap involving the gingival margin and vertical relief incision described above for the removal of buccally placed buried teeth. Principally this is because the extent of apical pathology is often more extensive in children than is suggested radiographically, and use of the semilunar flap can lead to parts of the incision being left over a bony defect at the end of surgery.

Technique

The surgical technique is identical to that used in adults but there are a number of points of difference when placing the apical seal. In teeth with immature open apices through-and-through root fillings are unsatisfactory as the apex may be wider than the bulk of the canal, thus some form of retrograde restoration is required. It is often difficult to secure undercuts at the apex when dealing with a tooth that has an open apex, but this can be overcome by placing a large retrograde filling and relying on multiple microscopic undercuts to secure it.

15.5.5 Cysts interfering with eruption

Eruption and dentigerous cysts can interfere with the eruption of teeth. Eruption cysts in the young child are simply incised (when occluding teeth are present this can be achieved by the patient themselves on biting). Dentigerous cysts may be marsupialized to the oral mucosal lining following the removal of any overlying primary predecessor and the permanent tooth allowed to erupt. Some authorities advocate more aggressive treatment involving enucleation of the cyst (with or without removal of the tooth) to ensure that epithelial remnants are not left behind. Fissural cysts (such as the nasopalatine cyst) are rare in children; when found they should be enucleated.

15.5.6 Treatment of acute orofacial infection

At this point it is relevant to discuss the treatment of orofacial infection. The major cause of this condition is dental in origin. The minor oral surgical treatments discussed above may all be employed to definitively treat the source of an orofacial infection. Alternatively, conservative treatments such as endodontic therapy may be appropriate. A rapidly spreading extraoral infection, however, is a surgical emergency. This merits immediate treatment and may require admission for in-patient management. Two areas of extraoral spread are of special importance. These are the submandibular region and the angle between the eye and nose. Swelling in the submandibular region arising from posterior mandibular teeth can result in the floor of the mouth being raised. This can cause a physical obstruction to breathing and spread from this region to the parapharyngeal spaces may further obstruct the airway. The advance from dysphagia to dyspnoea can be rapid. A sub-mandibular swelling should be decompressed as a matter of urgency in children. A child with raising of the floor of the mouth requires immediate admission to hospital. The fact that trismus is invariably an associated feature makes expert anaesthetic help essential for safe management. Infection involving the angle between eye and nose (Fig. 15.28) has the potential to spread intracranially and produce a cavernous sinus thrombosis. This is a potentially life-threatening complication. The angular veins of the orbit (which have no valves) connect the cavernous sinus to the face, and if the normal extracranial flow is obstructed due to pressure from the extraoral infection then infected material can enter the sinus by reverse flow. To prevent this complication, infection in this area (which arises from upper anterior teeth, especially the canines) must be treated expeditiously.

The principles of the treatment of acute infection are to:

(1) remove the cause;
(2) institute drainage;
(3) prevent spread; and
(4) restore function.

In addition, analgesia and adequate hydration must be maintained. Removal of the cause is essential to cure an orofacial infection arising from a dental source. This usually means extraction or endodontic therapy.

Institution of drainage and prevention of spread are supportive treatments—they are not definitive cures. Drainage may be obtained during the removal of the cause, for example, a dental extraction, or may precede definitive treatment if this makes management easier, for example, incision and drainage of a submandibular abscess. Drainage may be intra or extraoral. When an extraoral incision is made it is made in a skin crease parallel to the direction of the facial nerve. In the submandibular region the incision is made more than one finger's breadth below the angle of the mandible to avoid the mandibular branch. Once skin has been incised the dissection is carried out bluntly until the infection has been located. Locules of infection are then ruptured using blunt dissection and a drain secured to the external surface. Depending on the amount of drainage the drain is secured for 24–48 hs. Any pus should be sent for culture and sensitivity testing to the microbiology laboratory. Prevention of spread may be achieved surgically or by the use of antibiotics. In severe cases intravenous antibiotics will be used. The antibiotic of choice in children is a penicillin.

It is important to remember that acute infections are painful and that analgesics, as well as antibiotics, should be prescribed. The use of paracetamol elixir is usually sufficient. Similarly, it is important that a child suffering from an acute infection is adequately hydrated. If the infection has restricted the intake of oral fluids due to dysphagia then admission to hospital for intravenous fluid replacement is required.

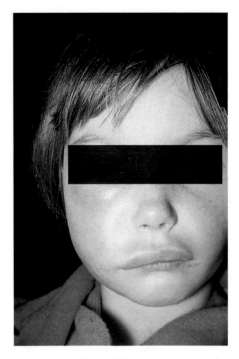

Fig. 15.28 Infection in this region can spread intracranially. (By kind permission of *Dental Update.*)

15.5.7 Autotransplantation of teeth

Replantation of an avulsed tooth due to trauma has been discussed in Chapter 12. In this section autotransplantation of teeth is discussed. Autotransplantation of teeth in children may be considered as a treatment for the following:

(1) repositioning of an ectopic tooth;
(2) replacement of an unrestorable tooth with a redundant member of the dentition.

The ectopic tooth most commonly repositioned by surgical means is the unerupted, palatally placed, upper permanent canine. An example of using autotransplantation as a means of tooth replacement is the substitution of an upper incisor that is undergoing resorption by a premolar tooth scheduled for extraction as part of an orthodontic treatment plan (Fig. 15.29 (a)–(j)). The management regimen for both treatments is similar and is as follows:

(1) assessment of donor tooth and recipient site;
(2) atraumatic extraction of donor tooth;

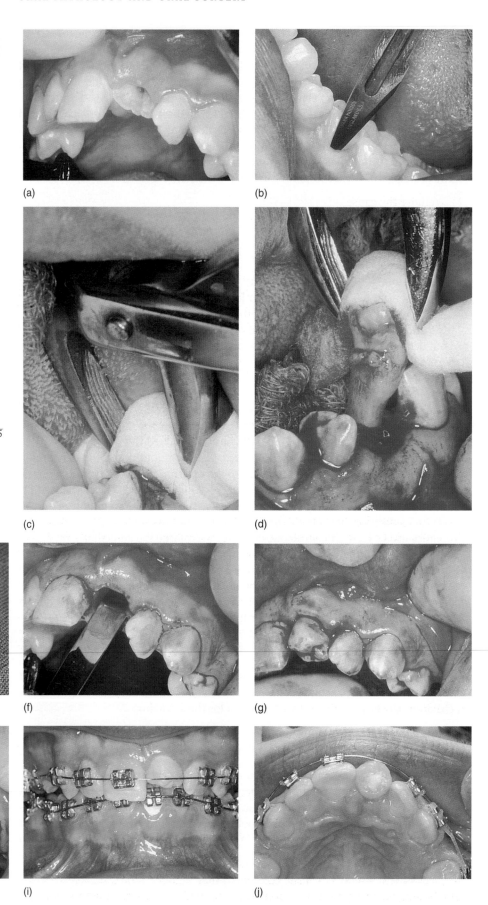

Fig. 15.29 (a) /1 for extraction to be replaced by |5 which is to be removed as part of an orthodontic treatment plan. (b) Incision of |5 gingival attachment. (c) and (d) Extraction of |5 using cotton roll to protect root. (e) Extracted |5. (f) Widening of /1 socket with chisel. (g) Transplantation of |5 to /1 socket. (h) Suturing and splinting of |5. (i) and (j) Labial and occlusal views of |5 at 3 months.

(3)   preparation of recipient site;
(4)   transplantation;
(5)   splinting of transplanted tooth;
(6)   root treatment of transplanted tooth.

In addition, when autotransplantation is used to replace a tooth in the arch some coronal preparation and orthodontic movement of the donor tooth may be required. Transplantation surgery is usually performed under antibiotic prophylaxis (either oral or intravenous amoxicillin (amoxycillin)), as the use of systemic antibiotics has been shown to decrease the incidence of root resorption.

Assessment of donor tooth and recipient site

The tooth to be transplanted has to be appraised clinically and radiographically prior to surgery. The crown of an erupted tooth can be assessed for caries and its dimensions measured. Root status and shape will be determined using periapical radiographs. Donor teeth should have an open apex with at least three-quarters of the root formed. The morphology of unerupted teeth for transplantation can only be determined radiographically. Teeth with severe root curvature are unsuitable for transplantation as it is unlikely they can be removed intact without trauma. In addition, the production of a donor site suitable for a dilacerated tooth may be difficult to produce without damaging neighbouring vital teeth.

It is important to evaluate the recipient site both clinically and radiographically. The space available for the transplanted tooth must be assessed in both the horizontal and vertical dimensions. It may be necessary to create sufficient space using preoperative orthodontics. Periapical radiographs will alert the clinician to the presence of any bony pathology or retained dental remnants at the recipient site.

Atraumatic extraction of donor tooth

It is essential to remove the donor tooth using minimal trauma and avoiding contact with the root surface. Damage to the root surface will lead to resorption or ankylosis. Thus when removing an erupted tooth for transplantation the usual rules concerning the application of forceps beaks to the root surface do not apply. The beaks are positioned on the crown. Prior to the application of the forceps a scalpel should be run around the gingival margin to the crest of the ridge to sever gingival attachments.

When an unerupted tooth is being used as a donor great care must be exercised during its removal. The entire crown must be exposed. As mentioned earlier, bone removal with hand chisels is less likely to damage the donor than the use of a bur. Once the crown has been exposed elevators or forceps (again confined to the crown) are used to extract the tooth as gently as possible. When the tooth has been extracted it should be gently replaced into its socket and maintained there until the recipient site is prepared. This is to ensure that a satisfactory tooth is obtained before recipient site surgery is performed.

Preparation of the recipient site

The recipient site may or may not contain a tooth. Following extraction of the tooth at the recipient site the socket is enlarged, if necessary, using either a chisel or a bur (an implant bur is ideal). Some operators recommend that the socket is enlarged following flap raising by removing the buccal plate of bone, which is stored in saline prior to being replaced with the cortical surface against the root. It is thought that this might decrease the incidence of ankylosis.

Transplantation

Once the socket has been prepared the donor tooth is gently placed in its new position. The occlusion is assessed to ensure that it is not traumatic to the transplanted tooth, and the gingival margin is held around the tooth with a horizontal mattress suture.

Splinting the transplanted tooth

The donor tooth should be splinted at the time of transplantation. It is important to stress that rigid splinting should not be employed as this may lead to ankylosis. A simple splint using orthodontic wire bonded to the tooth and its neighbours with composite resin is sufficient. It is essential that splinting is not maintained for too long a period as this may also lead to ankylosis—3 weeks is the maximum length of time, indeed in some cases the splint can be removed in 1 week.

Root treatment of transplanted tooth

The pulp of the transplanted tooth is extirpated after 2–3 weeks and the root canal filled with non-setting calcium hydroxide. The calcium hydroxide is replaced with gutta percha at around 6–12 months' post-transplant as long as there is no evidence of root resorption.

Follow-up of transplanted teeth

At the time of discharge the patient should be given an antiseptic mouthwash to maintain good hygiene in the surgical site. The first review is in 1 week, at which stage sutures are removed. It may be possible to remove the splint at this stage. The next review is at 2–3 weeks for splint removal and endodontic treatment. A periapical film should be taken at this stage. Further reviews should be undertaken at 3 and 6 months and then annually. Coronal reshaping can be performed at any stage.

Orthodontic movement of transplanted teeth

Transplanted teeth can be moved orthodontically. This should begin 3 months following transplantation and be completed within 9 months of the transplant.

15.6 IMPLANTOLOGY

The use of implants for orthodontic anchorage was mentioned above. The use of dental implants as prostheses in children is contraindicated except under circumstances where severe psychological stress merits such treatment. There are three reasons for avoiding implants in young patients:

1. The implant does not move with the growing alveolus—it acts as an ankylosed tooth. Thus implants should not be placed until vertical growth of the jaws is virtually complete (around 18 years of age). The exception to this rule is the lower intercanine region which can receive implants earlier in exceptional cases of hypodontia, for example, X-linked ectodermal dysplasia.
2. Implants can interfere with normal growth of the jaws.
3. Young bone does not behave in the same way as mature bone. Due to squashing and crushing, the axis of an inserted implant may deviate widely from the axis of tap.

In addition, the use of teeth for autotransplantation is often a viable alternative in young patients.

15.7 SOFT TISSUE SURGERY

The following short synopsis covers the important functional and orthodontic problems in the child and adolescent.

15.7.1 Labial frena

A prominent mid-line frenum in the maxilla may be present in association with a diastema. Whether or not the frenum is the cause of the diastema is open to question as a fleshy frenum does not always produce an aesthetic defect. Nevertheless, the excision of a mid-line maxillary frenum is often requested as part of an orthodontic treatment plan. This procedure is very simply performed under local anaesthesia (Fig. 15.30(a)–(d)). Before surgery a radiograph of the upper incisor area should be taken to eliminate other possible causes of a mid-line diastema (such as a mesiodens). A mid-line maxillary frenum should not be removed before the permanent canines have erupted, as the space may close spontaneously when these teeth appear.

Surgical removal is achieved by dissecting the mid-line tissue via incisions parallel to the frenum from the labial mucosa, at a point beyond the prominent fibrous tissue, through the interdental space to palatal mucosa. The part of the incision in attached gingiva is mucoperiosteal. The surface of the exposed bone in the interdental space should be curetted or gently burred to remove residual fibrous attachments. Primary closure of the labial part of the incision is achieved by suturing, and the defect in attached gingiva is covered by either a periodontal dressing (Coe-Pack) or ribbon gauze soaked in Whitehead's varnish, which is held in place by sutures. The pack is removed 7–10 days after surgery.

15.7.2 Lingual frena

A prominent lingual frenum should be excised if it is interfering with speech or oral hygiene. This is simply performed under local anaesthesia. The frenum is held by a pair of haemostatic forceps, a triangular section of tissue is removed, and the wound ends sutured.

15.7.3 Mucoceles

Mucoceles are common in the second decade of life, although they occasionally occur in younger children including the newborn. If these lesions cause functional or emotional problems they should be excised, but if there is no disturbance removal may be delayed until the child is older. An incision is made next to the lesion, which is removed by a blunt dissection under the epithelium. Invariably a number of minor salivary glands are obvious during surgery (they often appear like a bunch of grapes around the mucocele). These should be removed in view of the fact that mucoceles are produced as a result of trauma. Any obvious dental cause of trauma, for example, a sharp tooth, should be remedied. One type of mucocele that is best referred for specialist treatment is that found in the floor of the mouth, the so-called 'ranula' (Fig. 15.8). This lesion is often more extensive than is at first apparent and complete cure occasionally involves removing the sublingual gland.

15.7.4 Incisional biopsy

Incisional biopsies are performed to confirm a diagnosis by removing part of a lesion. It is preferable that the surgeon who is going to treat the lesion performs the incisional biopsy and therefore this procedure is best performed by an oral surgeon.

15.7.5 Excision biopsies of non–attached mucosa

Small lesions of the oral mucosa are removed by excisional biopsy, which involves the removal of an ellipse of tissue including the lesion. The long axis of the

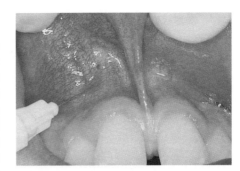

(a)

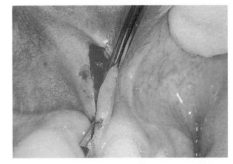

(b)

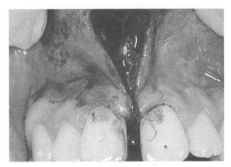

(c)

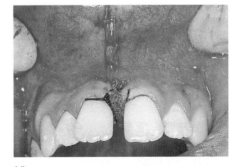

(d)

Fig. 15.30 (a) Patient for upper mid-line labial fraenectomy. (b) Incisions parallel to fraenum. (c) Defect at end of removal. (d) Wound closure with resorbable sutures in reflected mucosa and silk suture holding pack interdentally.

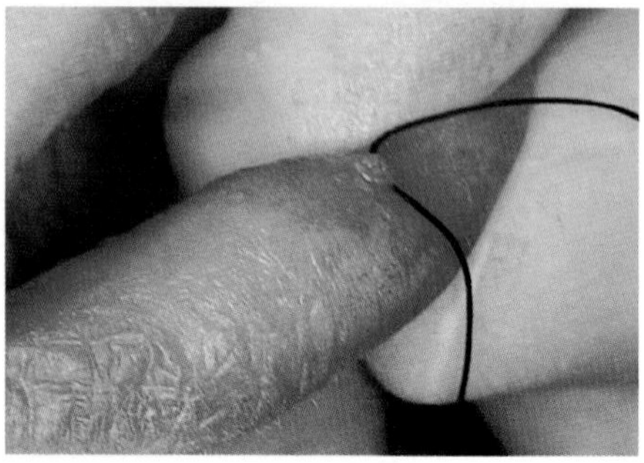

Fig. 15.31 Lip lesion held by suture. (By kind permission of *Dental Update*.)

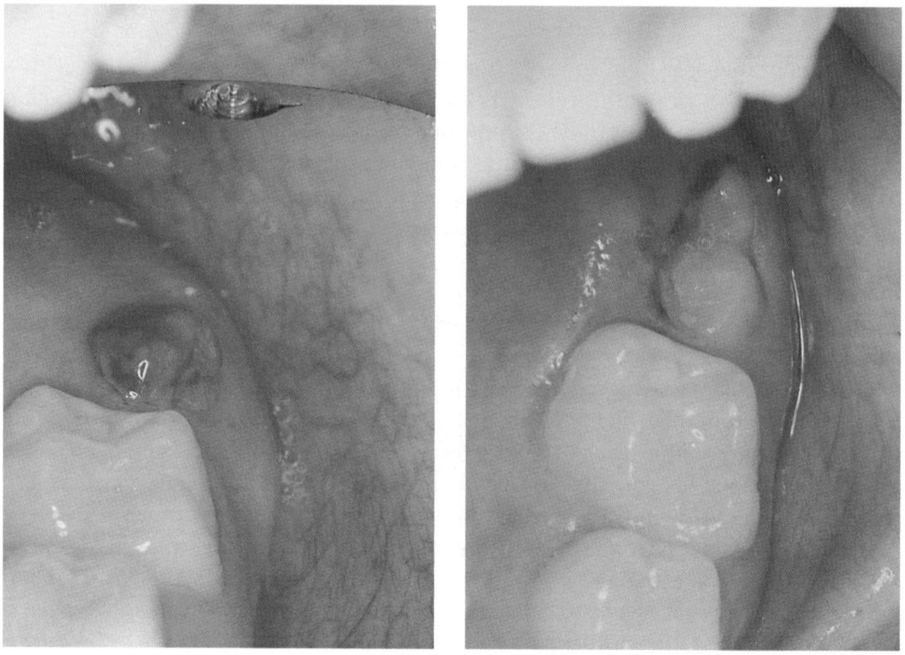

(a) (b)

Fig. 15.32 (a) and (b) Lump related to erupting |7, and view 1 week later—the lump has disappeared and the |7 has erupted—no treatment was given. (By kind permission of *Dental Update*.)

ellipse is made parallel to the direction of muscle pull, and it is best to hold the specimen with a suture passed under it to avoid crushing, which could render the specimen useless for histological examination (Fig. 15.31). All tissue surgically removed should be placed in a solution of 10% formal saline (not in water) and transported to the laboratory for histological examination. Lesions that are obviously benign and are not interfering with function or causing emotional distress can be left in the young child and removed, if necessary, at a later date (Fig. 15.32(a) and (b)).

15.7.6 Excision biopsy of attached gingiva/palate

These procedures leave a defect that is not readily treated by primary closure. Following the biopsy it is useful to lay a haemostatic material over the defect to arrest bleeding and then to cover the area either by a periodontal dressing or by securing a Whitehead's varnish, ribbon-gauze pack in the defect with non-resorbable sutures.

15.7.7 Suturing

Resorbable sutures should be used to close soft tissue wounds in children whenever possible; however, in mobile structures such as the tongue and lip these may be lost shortly after surgery as their knots may be less secure than those obtained with black silk. To overcome this problem it is useful to bury knots by taking the first bite of tissue from within the wound rather than from the mucosal surface. The second bite begins on the mucosal surface of the opposite wound edge. This ensures that the knot disappears into the wound when it is tied (Fig. 15.33).

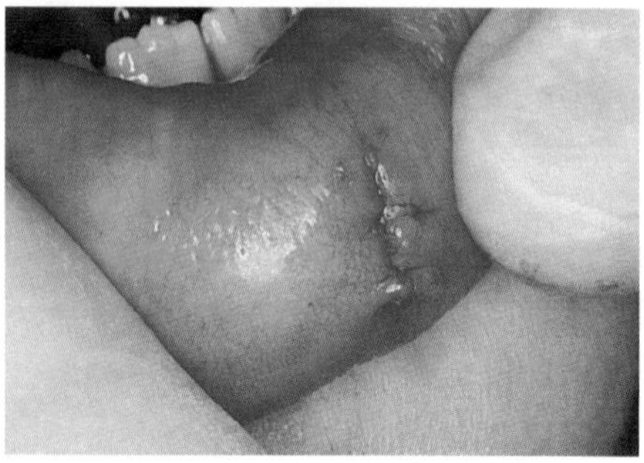

Fig. 15.33 Same patient as in Fig. 15.30 showing buried knots with soft-gut sutures. (By kind permission of *Dental Update*.)

15.8 SUMMARY

This chapter has considered:

(1) pathological conditions of the oral and perioral structures in children;
(2) dental extractions in children;
(3) minor oral surgical procedures that can be performed without in-patient anaesthetic facilities in healthy children;
(4) the management of acute spreading infection from a dental focus in children.

15.9 FURTHER READING

Andreasen, J. O. (1992). *Atlas of replantation and transplantation of teeth*. Mediglobe, Fribourg, Switzerland. (*A beautifully illustrated guide to tooth transplantation.*)

Gorlin, R. J., Cohen, M. M., and Hennekam, R. C. M. (2001). *Syndromes of the head and neck* (4th edn). Oxford University Press, Oxford. (*A valuable reference text.*)

Soames J. V. and Southam J. C. (2005). *Oral pathology* (4th edn). Oxford University Press, Oxford. (*A comprehensive oral pathology text.*)

15.10 REFERENCES

Cole, B. O. I., Shaw, A. J., Hobson, R. S., Nunn, J. H., Welbury, R. R., Meechan, J. G., and Jepson, N. J. A. (2003). The role of magnets in the management of unerupted teeth in children and adolescents. *International Journal of Paediatric Dentistry*, **13**, 204–7.

Meechan, J. G., Carter, N. E., Gilgrass, T., Hobson, R. S., Jepson, N. J. A., Nohl, F. S., Nunn, J. H. (2003). Interdisciplinary management of hypodontia: oral surgery management. *British Dentist Journal*, **194**, 423–7.

Scully, C. M., Welbury, R. R., Flaitz, C., de Almeira, O. C. (2002). *Orofacial health and disease in children and adolescents*. Martin Dunitz, London.

Medical disability

16 Medical disability

M. T. Hosey and R. R. Welbury

There are many general medical conditions that can directly affect the provision of dental care and some where the consequences of dental disease, or even dental treatment, can be life-threatening. An increasing number of children who now survive with complex medical problems due to improvements in medical care present difficulties in oral management. Dental disease can have grave consequences and so rigorous prevention is paramount. The decline in childhood mortality has led to increasing emphasis on maintaining and enhancing the quality of the child's life and ensuring that children reach adult life as physically, intellectually, and emotionally healthy as possible. Dental care can play an important part in enhancing this quality of life. Indeed, management within the primary dental services helps to 'normalize' life for these children who appreciate attending along with their family even though sometimes they might still require specialist expertise.

Even though the infant mortality rates (deaths under 1 year of age) have declined dramatically in the United Kingdom, the death rates are still higher in the first year of life than in any other single year below the age of 55 in males and 60 in females. The rates are highest for the very young. The main causes of death in the neonatal period (the first 4 weeks of life) are associated with prematurity (over 40%) and by congenital malformations (30%). In the remainder of the first year, however, the main causes of death occur at home and often nothing abnormal or suspicious is found (SUDI—sudden unexpected death in infancy and SIDS—sudden infant death syndrome). Although the unexpected death of a child over 1 year of age is rare, a few infants still succumb to respiratory and other infective diseases (e.g. meningitis), congenital malformations, and accidents.

16.1.1 The medical history

All patients should have an accurate medical history taken before any dental treatment is undertaken. This is important for several reasons:

1. To identify any medical problems that might require modification of dental treatment.
2. To prioritize children who require intensive preventive dental care.
3. To identify those requiring prophylactic antibiotic cover for potentially septic dental procedures.
4. To check whether the child is receiving any medication that could result in adverse interaction(s) with drugs or treatment administered by the dentist. This would include past medication that could have had an effect on dental development.
5. To identify systemic disease that could affect other patients or dental personnel; this is usually related to cross-infection potential.
6. To establish good rapport and effective communication with the child and their parents.

7. To determine the family and social circumstances, whether other siblings are affected by the same or similar condition and the ability of the parents to cope with attendance for dental appointments given the added burden of medical appointments and their wish to ensure adequate continued schooling.

8. To facilitate communication with medical colleagues.

9. To satisfy medico-legal requirements.

Many dental practitioners use standard questionnaires to obtain a medical history; it has been found that one of the most effective methods is to use a questionnaire followed by a pertinent personal interview with the child and their parent or guardian.

Key Points

Key medical questions—ask about:

- cardiovascular disorders;
- bleeding disorders;
- respiratory/chest problems;
- epilepsy;
- hepatitis/jaundice;
- diabetes;
- hospitalization or hospital investigation for any reason;
- previous general anaesthetic experience/any further general anaesthetic procedures planned?
- allergies;
- illness in other family members;
- medication.

16.1.2 The general examination

General observation of the child is invaluable and can provide vital information.

The child's demeanour is important in assessing their potential co-operation for dental treatment, but assessment of general outward appearance can also be helpful in determining their state of health. An impression of height (are they as tall as their peers?) and weight (undernourished or obese?) can give clues not only about nutrition but also somatic growth and dental development. Visually accessible areas, such as skin and nails, can reveal cyanosis, jaundice, and petechiae from bleeding disorders. The hands particularly are worthy of inspection and can also show alterations in the fingernails such as finger-clubbing from chronic cardiopulmonary disorders, as well as infections and splinter haemorrhages. Overall shape and symmetry of the face may be significant and there may be characteristic facies that are diagnostic of some congenital abnormalities and syndromes.

16.2 CARDIOVASCULAR DISORDERS

These can be divided into two main groups: congenital heart disease (existing before or at birth); and those disorders that are acquired after birth. Congenital heart disease occurs in approximately 8 children in every 1000 live births. There is a wide spectrum of severity, but 2–3 of these children will be symptomatic in the first year of life.

16.2.1 Congenital heart defects

The cause is rarely known in individual cases but multifactorial inheritance patterns are mainly responsible. Several chromosomal abnormalities, such as Down syndrome, are associated with severe congenital heart disease but these represent fewer than 5% of the total. The main types of congenital conditions are shown in Table 16.1. In

Table 16.1 Prevalence of congenital cardiac disease

Defect	%
Ventricular septal defect	28
Atrial septal defect	10
Pulmonary stenosis	10
Patent ductus arteriosus	10
Tetralogy of Fallot	10
Aortic stenosis	7
Coarctation of the aorta	5
Transposition of great arteries	5
Rare/diverse	15

most instances there is a combination of genetic and environmental influences, including infections, during the second month of pregnancy.

Many defects are slight and cause little disability, but a child with more severe defects may present with breathlessness on exertion, tiring easily, and suffer from recurrent respiratory infections. Those children with severe defects such as tetralogy of Fallot and valvular defects, including pulmonary atresia and tricuspid atresia, will have cyanosis, finger-clubbing, and may have delayed growth and development (Figs 16.1–16.3). Characteristically, these children will assume a squatting position to relieve their dyspnoea (breathlessness) on exertion.

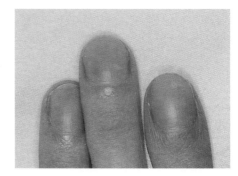

Fig. 16.1 This shows the hand of a boy with Down syndrome and Fallot's tetralogy. The cyanosis and finger-clubbing associated with his severe cardiac disease are obvious.

Heart murmurs

The incidence of congenital heart disease is falling, affecting 7–8 infants per 1000. Many parents will report that their child either has, or had, a 'heart murmur'. These may only be discovered at a routine examination, although they occur in over 30% of all children. Most of these murmurs are functional or innocent and not associated with significant abnormalities, but are the result of normal blood turbulence within the heart. Innocent murmurs are heard most frequently from 3–7 years of age. In a small minority of cases a heart murmur indicates the presence of a cardiac abnormality causing the turbulence. If the dentist is in any doubt about the significance of a murmur, then a cardiological opinion should be sought. Normally contact with the child's medical practitioner will clarify the situation. Innocent murmurs do not require any special precautions or treatment.

Ventricular septal defects (VSD)

These are the most common of the cardiac malformations. Small defects are asymptomatic and may be found during a routine physical examination. Large defects with excessive pulmonary blood flow are responsible for symptoms of breathlessness, feeding difficulties, and poor growth. Between 30% and 50% of the small defects close spontaneously, usually within the first year of life. Larger defects are usually closed surgically in the second year of life, but defects involving other cardiac structures may require complex surgery or even transplantation.

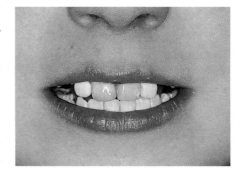

Fig. 16.2 Cyanosis affecting the lips in a boy with Fallot's tetralogy. The mucous membranes appear bluish.

Atrial septal defects (ASD)

These are not as common as the VSD in children, but are proportionately more significant in adults and more frequent in females. An isolated patent foramen ovale is of no clinical significance and not considered to be an ASD. Even an extremely large ASD rarely produces heart failure in children, but symptoms usually appear in the third decade. Surgery is usually carried out before school age.

Pulmonary stenosis

With mild to moderate stenosis of the pulmonary valve there are usually no symptoms, but exercise intolerance and cyanosis may occur if this is severe. Treatment is required for the moderate to severe forms; relief of this obstruction is now carried out in majority of children by balloon dilatation rather than surgery.

Patent ductus arteriosus

During fetal life most of the pulmonary arterial blood is shunted through the ductus arteriosus into the aorta, thus bypassing the lungs. Functional closure of the ductus arteriosus usually occurs at birth. Virtually all preterm babies weighing less than 1.75 kg have a patent ductus arteriosus in the first 24 h of life but this usually closes spontaneously. Ductus arteriosus patency is mediated by prostaglandins, and the administration of inhibitors of prostaglandin synthesis, such as indomethacin, is effective in closing the ductus in a significant number of babies. Surgical ligation,

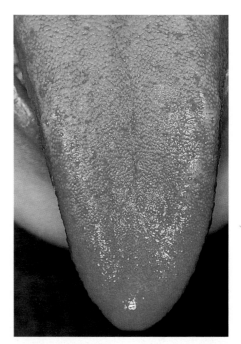

Fig. 16.3 Central cyanosis affecting the tongue of the boy shown in Fig. 16.2.

however, is a safe and effective back-up if indomethacin is contraindicated or has not been successful.

Tetralogy of Fallot

This classically consists of the combination of:

(1)   an obstruction to right ventricular outflow (pulmonary stenosis);
(2)   VSD;
(3)   dextroposition of the aorta;
(4)   right ventricular hypertrophy.

Cyanosis is one of the most obvious signs of this condition but it may not be present at birth. As the child grows, however, the obstruction to blood flow is further exaggerated. The oral mucous membranes and nail-beds are often the first places to show signs of cyanosis. Growth and development may be markedly delayed in severe untreated tetralogy of Fallot and puberty is delayed. Early medical management involves the use of prostaglandins so that adequate pulmonary blood flow can occur until surgical intervention can be carried out. Initially, a shunt procedure (usually the Blalock–Taussig shunt) is performed to anastomose the subclavian artery to the homolateral branch of the pulmonary artery. Later in childhood, total surgical correction is undertaken but the mortality rate from this procedure is 5–10%.

16.2.2 Acquired cardiovascular disease

Rheumatic fever

Rheumatic fever follows a group A streptococcal infection of the upper respiratory tract, especially in developing countries, and may occur at all ages but usually between 5 and 15 years. Environmental factors, such as overcrowding, promote the transmission of streptococcal infections and the incidence of rheumatic fever is higher among lower socio-economic groups. The clinical onset is usually acute and occurs 2–3 weeks after a sore throat. Joint pains are common and of a characteristic migratory polyarthralgia or polyarthritis. Carditis is the most serious manifestation, occurring in 40–50% of initial attacks, especially in young children. Fever is usually present, but in an insidious onset of the condition it may be low grade. Most of the carditis resolves except the lesions on the cusps of the heart valves which become fibrosed and stenotic. Rheumatic heart disease is the most important manifestation of rheumatic fever and may affect mitral, aortic, tricuspid, and pulmonary valves.

Diseases of the myocardium and pericardium

Major diseases involving the myocardium and pericardium include bacterial infections such as: diphtheria and typhoid; tuberculous, fungal, and parasitic infections; rheumatoid arthritis; systemic lupus erythematosus; uraemia; thalassaemia; hyperthyroidism; neuromuscular diseases, such as, muscular dystrophy; and glycogen storage diseases. They are relatively rare in children in developed countries.

Other cardiovascular problems

There are several other important conditions that are common in adults but not in children. These include coronary artery disease (ischaemic heart disease), cardiac arrhythmias, and hypertension. In children, secondary hypertension is more common than essential hypertension and is associated with renal abnormalities in 75–80% of those affected.

16.2.3 Dental care for children with cardiovascular disorders

The most important consideration in planning dental care for children with cardio-vascular disorders is the prevention of dental disease. As soon as a child is diagnosed as having a significant cardiac problem they should be referred for dental evaluation and an aggressive preventive regimen commenced to include dietary counselling, fluoride therapy, fissure sealants, and oral hygiene instruction. Regular monitoring, both clinically and radiographically, with reinforcement of the preventive advice is essential. Active dental disease should be treated before cardiac surgery is undertaken.

Treatment planning

If the child and parent(s) are seen in infancy and effective preventive dental procedures are instituted, then, theoretically, operative dentistry should be unnecessary. In practice, the situation may be very different. If invasive operative procedures are required then antibiotic prophylaxis will be necessary, which influences treatment planning. Ideally, treatment in children should be carried out during short appointments so that co-operation is maximized. However, if prophylactic antibiotics are required it is important to carry out as much treatment as possible under each cover but this has to be balanced against the stress of longer appointments. If multiple appointments with prophylaxis are required, then 4 weeks should be allowed between appointments when penicillin is used to allow penicillin-resistant organisms to disappear from the oral flora though alternating with non-penicillin antibiotics can circumvent this. Other problems may include prolonged bleeding following scaling or surgical procedures due to thrombocytopenia and anticoagulant medication. It is essential to check the platelet count and prothrombin time if dental extractions are planned. The patient's prothrombin time is compared with normal and called the international normalized ratio (INR). No child with symptomatic cardiac problems should have any routine dental procedures until details of the condition have been obtained and the patient's physician consulted.

Antibiotic prophylaxis

Antibiotic prophylaxis is necessary for most congenital cardiac malformations. The cardiac conditions that require antibiotic prophylaxis for dental procedures are listed in Table 16.2. Dento gingival manipulative procedures that are likely to induce an increase in the level of bacteria in the blood require antibiotic prophylaxis to prevent the development of endocarditis. The procedures are shown in Table 16.3. These include extractions, scaling, surgery involving gingival tissues, and restorative procedures where the gingival margins are likely to be traumatized either during cavity preparation or during matrix band, wedge, or rubber dam placement. Endodontic treatment should only be carried out on teeth where there is a very high probability of success. This is usually confined to permanent incisor teeth with straight canals and closed apices and is carried out as a single-visit procedure under appropriate antibiotic cover.

Antibacterial prophylaxis recommendations are constantly updated (Tables 16.4 and 16.5) and revised as new scientific evidence and drugs become available. The latest British Cardiac Society guidelines and the *British National Formulary* should be checked. The medication should be taken under supervision. There is still some controversy over which conditions do or do not require prophylactic antibiotic therapy. If any doubt exists then the paediatrician or cardiologist should be consulted before invasive dental procedures are undertaken.

At the time of writing this new edition, the British Cardiac Society have published new guidelines. These have not yet been widely adopted within the dental profession

Table 16.2   Summary of the cardiac disorders that require antibiotic prophylaxis when the dental procedure will cause intraoral bleeding

High risk
- Prosthetic heart valves
- Previous infective endocarditis
- Complex cyanotic congenital heart disease
- Transposition of great arteries
- Tetralogy of Fallot
- Surgically constructed systemic pulmonary shunts or conduits
- Mitral valve prolapse

Moderate risk
- Aquired valvular heart disease, for example, rheumatic heart disease
- Aortic stenosis
- Aortic regurgitation
- Mirtal regurgitation
- Ventricular septal defect and other structural cardiac defects
- Bicuspid aortic valve
- Primum atrial septal defect
- Patent ductus arteriosus
- Aortic root replacement
- Coarctation of aorta
- Atrial septal aneurysm/patent foramen ovale
- Hypertrophic obstructive cardiomyopathy
- Subaortic membrane

Low risk (not requiring antibiotic prophylaxis)
- Pulmonary stenosis
- Surgically repaired VSD; PDA
- Surgically repaired ASD although prophylaxis is still required for 12 months postoperatively dependant on surgical method
- Post Fontan or Mustard procedure without residual defect/murmur
- Previous coronary artery bypass surgery
- Isolated secundum ASD
- Mitral valve prolapse without regurgitation
- Innocent heart murmurs
- Cardiac pacemakers
- Coronary artery stent implantation
- Six months after heart–lung transplantation

Table 16.3   Dento-gingival manipulative procedures that need antibiotic prophylaxis

Recommended for antibiotic prophylaxis	Not recommended for antibiotic prophylaxis
Examination procedures Periodontal probing	Dental examination with mirror and probe
Investigation procedures Sialography	Intraoral radiographs Extraoral radiographs
Preventive procedures Nil	Fissure sealants Fluoride treatments
Professional cleaning procedures Polishing teeth with a rubber cup Oral irrigation with water jet Light scaling Deep scaling Scaling teeth with hand instrument Scaling with ultrasonic instrument	Air polishing

Anaesthetic procedures
Intraligamental local anaesthesia

Infiltration local anaesthesia
Nerve block local anaesthesia
Oral airway for general anaesthesia
Nasal airway for general anaesthesia
Laryngeal mask airway for general anaesthesia

Conservation (Restoration) Procedures(δ)
Rubber dam placement
Matrix band and wedge placement
Gingival retraction cord placement

Drilling of teeth (without rubber dam)

Periodontal procedures
Root planing
Antibiotic fibres or strips placed subgingivally (α)
Gingivectomy
Periodontal surgery

Endodontic procedures
Root canal instrumentation beyond the root apex

Root canal instrumentation within canal
Pulpotomy of primary molar
Pulpotomy of permanent tooth (β)

Avulsed tooth reimplantation (γ)

Orthodontic procedures
Tooth separation
Expose or expose and bond of tooth or teeth

Alginate impressions
Band placement and cementation
Band removal
Adjustment of fixed appliances

Surgical procedures
Extraction of a single tooth
Extraction of multiple teeth
Mucoperiosteal flap to gain access to tooth or lesion
Dental implants (as for mucoperiosteal flat)

Incision and drainage of an abscess
Biopsy

Dental implants transmucosal fixture (as for biopsy)

Postsurgical procedures
None

Suture removal
Removal of surgical packs (as for suture removal)

Other Events (Daily or Physiological Events)
Antibiotic prophylaxis not recommended as it is impractical despite
presence of bacteraemia following some of these events. This is
largely because of the significant risk of development of bacteria
resistant to the antibiotics used

Toothbrushing

Exfoliation of primary teeth

(α) No data but the procedure is very similar to that of gingival retraction cord placement.

(β) No data but the procedure is similar to pulpotomy of a primary molar.

(γ) The avulsed tooth can be quickly washed and reimplanted immediately by a parent or other responsible person and the antibiotic prophylaxis administered when the child attends the dental surgery provided this is within 2 h of the reimplantation. This is because antibiotic prophylaxis is still successful if administered after the bacteraemic episode.

(δ) It is common for a course of dental treatment to take place over several visits to the dentist. For patients at high or moderate risk of developing infective endorcarditis as much treatment as possible should be carried out at each visit. The antibiotic should be changed at alternate visits for example, Amoxicillin–Clindamycin–Amoxicillin, and so on. For young children the sequence would be Amoxicillin–Azithromycin–Amoxicillin, and so on. If penicillin or penicillin-related antibiotics are used as one of the antibiotics then a period of 1 month must be allowed between visits. Dentists can help further by planning dental care to minimize the number of times that patients are exposed to antibiotics by carrying out as much treatment as is feasible at each visit.

In an emergency when treatment needs to be carried out urgently the dental surgeon should make an assessment as to whether or not the patient is significantly at risk from infective endocarditis. If the answer is affirmative, the patient's clinical records should then be marked appropriately and consideration given to the risk of bacteraemia associated with the dental procedures to be carried out on the patient. If there is a risk of a significant bacteraemia then antibiotic prophylaxis should be given.

Table 16.4 Dental treatment under local anaesthesia (or procedures without local anaesthesia)

Clinical Situation	Drug	Regimen
Class I. high risk of developing infective endocarditis and class II. moderate risk of developing infective endocarditis		
Patients *not* allergic to penicillin or patients who must *not* have receive more than a single dose or course of penicillin in the previous month	Amoxicillin	**Adults** 　Oral amoxicillin 3 g administered 1 h before the procedure **Children** 　<5 years: oral amoxicillin 750 mg administered 1 h before the procedure 　5–10 years: oral amoxicillin 1.5 g administered 1 h before the procedure 　>10 years use adult dose
Patients *allergic* to penicillin or who have had more than a single dose or course of penicillin (or other β lactam antibiotic) within the last month	Clindamycin	**Adults** 　Oral clindamycin 600 mg administered 1 h before the procedure **Children** 　<5 years: oral clindamycin 150 mg administered 1 h before the procedure 　5–10 years oral clindamycin 300 mg administered 1 h before the procedure 　>10 years use adult dose
The oral suspension of Clindamycin is no longer available in the United Kingdom. If children are unwilling or unable to swallow tablets or capsules or patients are suffering with dysphagia, then azithromycin is a suitable alternative	Azithromycin (as a suspension)	**Adults** 　500 mg administered 1 h before the procedure **Children** 　<5 years: oral azithromycin 200 mg administered 1 h before the procedure 　5–10 years: oral azithromycin 300 mg administered 1 h before the procedure 　>10 years use adult dose of 500 mg 1 h before the procedure
Class III. low risk of developing infective endocarditis No antimicrobial prophylaxis required.		

Special considerations:

Multiple visits for treatment using local (or no) anaesthesia

For a care plan that will require several visits then a period of 1 month should elapse before the second dose of the same antibiotic. If treatment is planned to extend over more than two visits then amoxicillin should be used on one visit and clindamycin (or clarithromycin) for the next visit. This alternating sequence can be continued until treatment is complete and the time interval between different types of antibiotics does *not* need to exceed 1 month.

For those at highest risk, for example, patients with prosthetic heart valves of previous infective endocarditis

Adults	Intravenous amoxicillin 2 g administered 30 min before the procedure *plus* intravenous gentamicin, 1.5 mg/kg within the same time period. *Followed postoperatively by* intravenous administered amoxicillin 1 g *or* oral amoxicillin 1 g, 6 h post-procedure.
Children	<5 years as for <10 years <10 years intravenous amoxicillin 1 g 30 min administered before the procedure *plus* intravenous gentamicin, 1.5 mg/kg administered within the same time period. *Followed postoperatively by* oral amoxicillin at 6 h post-procedure.

For Patients Allergic to Penicillin,

Adults	Intravenous vancomycin 1 g infused over the 2 h before the procedure *plus* intravenous gentamicin, 1.5 mg/kg administered within the same time period.
Children	<5 years as for <10 years <10 years intravenous vancomycin, 20 mg/kg infused over the 2 h before the procedure *plus* intravenous gentamicin, 1.5 mg/kg administered within the same time period. >10 years, use the adult dose.
Adults and Children	Intravenous teicoplanin 6 mg/kg *plus* intravenous amikacin 15 mg/kg immediately before the procedure.

Table 16.5 Dental treatment under general anaesthesia (GA), intravenous sedation, or patients unable to take oral medications

Clinical Situation	Drug	Regimen
Patients *not* allergic to penicillin or patients who have *not* received more than a single dose or course of penicillin in the previous month	Amoxicillin or ampicillin	**Adults** IV amoxicillin 2 g administered upon attainment of GA and immediately before the dental procedure
		Children <5: years IV amoxicillin 500 mg administered upon attainment of GA and immediately before the procedure 5–10 years: IV amoxicillin 1 g administered upon attainment of GA and immediately before the procedure >10: years use adult dose 2 g administered immediately before the procedure
Patients allergic to penicillin or who have had more than a single dose or course of penicillin (or other β lactam antibiotic) within the last month	Clindamycin	**Adults** IV clindamycin 300 mg infused over at least 10 min upon attainment of GA and commenced before the start of the dental surgery. This is followed by oral or IV clindamycin 150 mg 6 h later
		Children <5 years: IV clindamycin 75 mg infused over at least 10 min upon attainment of GA and commenced before the start of the dental procedure 5–10 years: IV clindamycin 150 mg infused over at least 10 min upon attainment of GA and commenced before the start of the dental procedure >10 years: use adult dose

and they differ from the current BNF (2004). Readers are advised to read the latest editions of the BNF and to read the remainder of this section in that context.

There is a three-step approach to the use and choice of antibiotic prophylaxis.

1. Assessment of cardiac risk (Table 16.2)
   - Antibiotic prophylaxis is required only in moderate or high risk.
2. Assessment of the risk of significant bacteraemia associated with the dento-gingival manipulative procedure (Table 16.3)
   - If the detail of the planned dental procedure involves a dento-gingival manipulative procedure that will cause a significant bacteraemia then antibiotic prophylaxis is needed.
3. Assessment of antibiotic prophylaxis regimen: choice, dosage, and mode of administration (Tables 16.4 and 16.5)

   - The choice of regimen is determined by the use of anaesthesia and analgesia.
   - For multiple visits of treatment under local anaesthesia a period of 1 month should elapse before a second dose of the same antibiotic is given. Alternating the sequence of antibiotic between visits (e.g. penicillin then clindamycin) can be used to overcome this need to wait 1 month before the next visit.
   - The need for general anaesthesia or intravenous sedation requires a modification of the drug regimen particularly in regard to dosage.
   - Those patients with highest risk of infective endocarditis, for example, prosthetic heart valves or previous infective endocarditis. (1) Not allergic also require gentamycin and postoperative amoxicillin; (2) Penicillin allergic— require vancomycin and gentamycin.

Children who have had corrective surgery for a patent ductus arteriosus and those who have received a heart–lung transplant are considered to have normal hearts and only require prophylactic antibiotics for the initial 6 months following surgery. Those who had an atrial septal defect corrected using a catheter-based procedure require prophylactic antibiotics for 12 months following surgery. *If in doubt, contact the child's cardiologist!*

> **Key Points**
>
> Antibiotic prophylaxis considerations:
> - Assessment of cardiac risk,
> - Assessment of the risk of significant bacteraemia associated with the dento-gingival manipulative procedure,
> - Assessment of antibiotic prophylaxis regimen: choice, dosage, and mode of administration.

16.3 DISORDERS OF THE BLOOD

16.3.1 Bleeding disorders

The blood is in a dynamic equilibrium between fluidity and coagulation, but the haemostatic mechanism is more complex than just alterations in this equilibrium. It involves local reactions of the blood vessels, platelet activities, and the interaction of specific coagulation factors that circulate in the blood. In early childhood many of the bleeding disorders have a genetic background but with increasing age more become iatrogenic—usually due to anticoagulant medication. Patients who have had cardiac surgery for some congenital abnormality, those who have had a recent myocardial infarction, and those who have had cerebrovascular accidents may all be receiving long-term anticoagulant therapy. Table 16.6 gives a classification of bleeding disorders based on disorders of coagulation, bleeding problems due to decreased numbers of platelets, and disorders of bleeding where there are normal numbers of platelets. Many of these conditions are very rare and will not be considered further.

Haemophilia

Haemophilia A is an X-linked, recessively inherited condition caused by a deficiency of factor VIII. The degree of severity is very varied but tends to be consistent within the same family. Children with over 25% of normal levels of circulating factor VIII may lead normal lives, those with between 1% and 5% are moderately to severely affected by minor trauma, etc., while those with under 1% have multiple bleeds into joints (haemarthroses) and may be severely physically handicapped as a result. Obviously, prevention of trauma to those who have this condition is extremely important, but

Table 16.6 Classification of bleeding disorders

1.	Coagulation defects		
	(a) Inherited:	(i)	haemophilia A: factor VIII deficiency; (ii) haemophilia B: factor IX deficiency (Christmas disease)
	(b) Acquired:	(i)	liver disease; (ii) vitamin deficiency; (iii) anticoagulant drugs (heparin, warfarin); (iv) disseminated intravascular coagulation (DIC)
2.	Thrombocytopenic purpuras		
	(a) Primary:	(i)	idiopathic thrombocytopenic purpura (ITP); (ii) pancytopenia, Fanconi syndrome
	(b) Secondary:	(i)	systemic disease—leukaemia; (ii) drug induced; (iii) physical agents—radiation
3.	Non-thrombocytopenic purpuras		
	(a) Vascular wall alteration:	(i)	scurvy; (ii) infections; (iii) allergy
	(b) Disorders of platelet function:	(i)	inherited: von Willebrand's disease; (ii) drugs: aspirin, non-steroidal anti-inflammatories, alcohol, penicillin; (iii) allergy; (iv) autoimmune disease; (v) uraemia

the availability of factor VIII concentrates has revolutionized the quality of life of haemophiliacs. Unfortunately, some of these blood replacement products have been contaminated in the past with hepatitis and human immunodeficiency virus (HIV) and, therefore, cross-infection control is a high priority. It was found that a number of patients who were thought to be haemophiliacs did not respond to replacement with factor VIII (antihaemophiliac globulin) but were deficient in another factor—factor IX. This is known as Christmas disease or haemophilia B. This is also transmitted as an X-linked recessive trait with a wide range of clinical severity, but female carriers of this condition also have a tendency to bleed.

Key Points

Factor VIII level:

- >25%—mild;
- 1–5%—moderate to severe;
- <1%—severe.

Von Willebrand's disease

This is a dominantly inherited, complex, and variable condition characterized by a vascular abnormality of large irregular capillaries, defective platelets that do not adhere to each other, and decreased levels of factor VIII. Common clinical manifestations are nose bleeds and spontaneous gingival haemorrhage. Von Willebrand's disease is the most common inherited bleeding disorder affecting, ~1 in every 1000 individuals in the United States and the United Kingdom.

Thrombocytopenia

This is caused by a reduction in the numbers of circulating platelets in the bloodstream.

Normal levels are between 150 and $400 \times 10^9/l$. The platelet count should be at least $50 \times 10^9/l$ before surgery is attempted. Clinical signs are petechial haemorrhages into the skin and mucous membranes with haematemesis (blood in the vomit), haematuria (blood in the urine), and melaena (blood in the faeces).

In children the usual causes of thrombocytopenia are idiopathic, an acute immune response usually following an upper respiratory tract infection, leukaemic infiltration of the bone marrow, or following the administration of various drugs.

Key Points

- Genetic coagulation disorders:
  —haemophilia A (factor VIII)—80%
  —haemophilia B (factor IX)—13%
  —factor XI—6%
- Bleeding disorders:
  —haemophilia A—1 : 20,000
  —von Willebrand's disease—1 : 1000

16.3.2 Dental management of bleeding disorders

A good history is the best screening device, but a bleeding tendency may only become manifest after a surgical procedure or trauma. Effective communication with the child's physician or haematologist is important, not only to establish the aetiology of any bleeding tendency but also to liaise over any necessary medical treatment that is required to replace reduced levels of clotting factors. The cornerstone of dental care is prevention and regular review so that if disease does occur it can be treated at an early stage. Local anaesthetic infiltrations or intraligamentous injections are unlikely to cause problems if given carefully. Regional anaesthesia, such as an inferior dental block, is contraindicated as bleeding in the pterygomandibular region which may result in asphyxia. Pulp treatment of primary molar teeth may be required to avoid extractions. Most primary teeth exfoliate spontaneously with little haemorrhage; however, occasionally when they are very mobile, the soft tissues develop an inflammatory hyperplastic response and bleeding may be a problem. In these situations extraction may be necessary with the appropriate haematological replacement therapy. However, if dental extractions or surgery do become necessary then the patients are usually best managed in the hospital situation.

Haemophilia

Adequate replacement and careful monitoring of factor VIII and factor IX levels are required. This is usually done with fresh-frozen plasma or freeze-dried concentrate. Patients with mild to moderate haemophilia A can often be managed on an out-patient basis using replacement therapy or DDAVP (1 desamino-8, darginine vasopressin; also known as desmopressin) which stimulates the release of factor VIII. Antifibrinolytic agents such as EACA (epsilon-aminocaproic acid), and tranexamic acid are also given to prevent lysis of the clot. They also significantly reduce the requirement for replacement of factor VIII. Medications containing non-steroidal, anti-inflammatory drugs (NSAIDs) or aspirin should not be given (aspirin should not be given anyway to a child under 16 years because of the risk of developing Reye's syndrome).

Von Willebrand's disease

Factor VIII concentrates are not usually effective, but DDAVP is used in combination with EACA or tranexamic acid. Patients with more severe types of von Willebrand's disease will require fresh-frozen plasma or a cryoprecipitate replacement.

Thrombocytopenia

The platelet count should be at least $50 \times 10^9/l$ before surgery is attempted and continuous infusion of platelets may be required. In children with the idiopathic form of this condition, prednisolone (4 mg/kg per day for 1 week, given orally) will increase the platelet count to over $50 \times 10^9/l$ within 48 h in about 90% of cases. The necessary treatment can then be carried out.

16.3.3 Blood dyscrasias

There are several relatively common disorders of the red and white blood cells that may influence dental care in the child. Many of these conditions also give rise to abnormal bleeding but, in addition, may lead to delayed healing, infection, or mucosal ulceration. An outline classification is given in Table 16.7.

Table 16.7   Classification of blood dyscrasias

1.	Red blood cell disorders		
	(a) Anaemia:	(i)	iron deficiency; (ii) glucose 6-phosphate dehydrogenase deficiency (G-6-GD); (iii) sickle cell; (iv) thalassaemia
	(b) Polycythaemia		
2.	White blood cell disorders		
	(a) Leucocytosis:	(i)	infectious mononucleosis (glandular fever); (ii) neoplasia
	(b) Leucopenia:	(i)	neutropenia—congenital and drug induced
	(c) Leukaemias:	(i)	acute lymphocytic (ALL); (ii) acute myeloid (AML); (iii) chronic
	(d) Lymphomas:	(i)	Hodgkin's; (ii) non-Hodgkin's; (iii) Burkitt's

Red blood cell disorders: anaemia

When there is a reduction in the red blood cell volume or haemoglobin concentration, the oxygen carrying capacity of the blood is lowered. Anaemia is not a specific disease but a symptom of an underlying disorder. Children with anaemia may be very pale (examine the nail-beds, conjunctiva, and oral mucous membranes). They may also be tired, listless, and breathless.

IRON-DEFICIENCY ANAEMIA

This may result from chronic blood loss, possibly as a result of haemorrhagic disorders, but in children it is more commonly due to dietary deficiency or malabsorption. Vitamin B12 and folic acid are also needed for the maturation of red blood cells in the bone marrow.

GLUCOSE 6-PHOSPHATE DEHYDROGENASE (G-6-PD) DEFICIENCY

This enzyme is needed in the hexose monophosphate shunt pathway. In deficiency the accumulation of oxidants in the red blood cells causes their haemolysis and may result in jaundice, palpitations, dyspnoea, and dizziness. Drugs such as aspirin, phenacetin, and ascorbic acid, as well as infections, may precipitate haemolysis. As the gene for G-6-PD is located on the X-chromosome it is inherited as a sex-linked condition. There are many variants of the condition and it is common in certain ethnic groups; for example, type A is found in 11% of American black people and G-6-PD MED is relatively common in ethnic groups of Mediterranean origin.

SICKLE-CELL ANAEMIA

This is an inherited autosomal-recessive disorder that results in the substitution of a single amino acid in the haemoglobin chain. Sickle-cell *trait* is the heterozygous state in which the affected individual carries one gene for haemoglobin S. Approximately, 10% of American Black children and up to 25% of Central African Black children carry the trait. Sickle-cell *anaemia* is the homozygous state, with affected genes from both parents. The red blood cells containing haemoglobin S have a life of only 30–60 days and become clumped together under certain conditions, thus blocking small blood vessels and leading to pain and necrosis. Affected children may be pale, tired, weak, and breathless. They may complain of painful joints and swelling of the hands and feet. There tends to be a failure to thrive and growth retardation with an increased susceptibility to infection. Later problems include renal function impairment and retinal and conjunctival damage.

THALASSAEMIA

This is another inherited disorder of haemoglobin synthesis and may occur as a heterozygous trait or homozygous thalassaemia major. It occurs particularly in Mediterranean countries and in the Middle-Eastern Arab countries. It results, like sickle-cell anaemia, in a severe progressive haemolytic anaemia. Regular blood transfusions are necessary to maintain the haemoglobin level above 10 g/dl. If treatment is inadequate then hypertrophy of erythropoietic tissue occurs and this results in massive expansion of the marrow of the facial and skull bones producing maxillary hyperplasia and protrusion of the middle third of the face.

Dental management of anaemia

All anaemic children have a greater tendency to bleed after invasive dental procedures.

Therefore, any signs or symptoms suggestive of anaemia should be investigated. The haemoglobin level and haematocrit are simple tests used for screening, and a white blood cell and platelet count should also be obtained. If these reveal any abnormalities then further, more complex, tests may need to be undertaken. Ideally, the underlying defect should be corrected before embarking on a course of routine dental care.

A family history of conditions such as sickle-cell anaemia and thalassaemia is significant and all Black patients should be tested routinely for sickle-cell disease prior to a general anaesthetic. Sickle-cell crises occur due to inadequate oxygenation and, if possible, general anaesthetics should be avoided in preference to the use of local anaesthesia.

Key Points

Sickle-cell disease:

• All Black patients should be screened prior to general anaesthesia.

White blood cell disorders: leukaemia

Leukaemia is a malignant proliferation of white blood cells. It is the most common form of childhood cancer, accounting for about one-third of new cases of cancer diagnosed each year. Acute lymphocytic leukaemia accounts for 75% of cases with a peak incidence at 4 years of age. The general clinical features of all types of leukaemia are similar as all involve a severe disruption of bone marrow functions. Specific clinical and laboratory features differ, however, and there are considerable differences in response to therapy and long-term prognosis.

Acute leukaemia has a sudden onset but the initial symptoms are usually non-specific with anorexia, irritability, and lethargy. Progressive failure of the bone marrow leads to pallor, bleeding, and fever, which are usually the symptoms that lead to diagnostic investigation. The bleeding tendency is often shown in the oral mucosa (Fig. 16.4) and there may also be infective lesions of the mouth and throat. The dental practitioner may, therefore, be the first to diagnose the condition (Fig. 16.5). Bone pain and arthralgia are also important presenting complaints in about one-quarter of children. On initial haematological examination most patients will have anaemia and thrombocytopenia. A significant proportion will have white blood cell counts of less than 3000/mm³ and about 20% will have counts greater than 50,000/mm³. The diagnosis of leukaemia can be suspected on seeing blast cells on the blood smear confirmed on bone marrow biopsy, which will show replacement by leukaemic lymphoblasts. The treatment varies with the clinical risk features; children under 2 years and over 10 years with an initial white blood cell count of over 100,000/mm³ and central nervous system involvement (leukaemic cells in the cerebrospinal fluid) have the worst prognosis.

The basic treatment components are:

1. *Induction of remission*. To remove abnormal cells from the blood and bone marrow. Drugs used: vincristine and prednisone.
2. *Prophylactic treatment to central nervous system*. Drugs used: intrathecal methotrexate plus irradiation of central nervous system.
3. *Consolidation*. Drugs used: cytosine arabinoside plus asparaginase.
4. *Maintenance*. Drugs used: methotrexate plus mercaptopurine for approximately 2 years.
5. *Relapse*. If relapse occurs then bone marrow transplantation can be considered.

On this regimen over 70% of children now survive and can be regarded as cured.

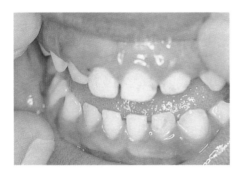

Fig. 16.4 This 3-year-old child was brought to the dental surgery with spontaneous bleeding from his gums. He had recently had several nosebleeds and had become very lethargic. His skin and mucosa were very pale. Haematological investigation showed acute lymphocytic leukaemia.

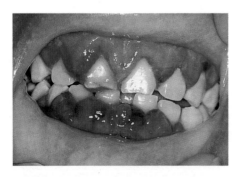

Fig. 16.5 Oral appearance of a patient with acute myeloid leukaemia, with infiltration of the gingivae and spontaneous bleeding. This oral presentation and type of leukaemia is less common than the lymphocytic type shown in Fig. 16.4. (Courtesy of Wolfe Publishing.).

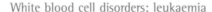

Key Points

Childhood leukaemia:

- 75% is acute lymphocytic leukaemia;
- peak incidence at 4 years of age;
- dentists can help early diagnosis, alerted by mucosal haemorrhage, and mouth and throat infections.

Dental management of leukaemia

In common with other medically compromising conditions, children with leukaemia are categorized as having a high risk of dental caries. Therefore, prevention is essential. Unless there is a dental emergency no elective operative dental treatment should be carried out until the child is in remission. The drug regimen used to induce remission has numerous side-effects, including nausea and vomiting, reversible alopecia (hair loss), neuropathy, and, most importantly from a dental point of view, oral ulceration (mucositis). It can be extremely difficult to carry out normal mouth care for children at this stage and many have difficulty with toothbrushing due to acute nausea. Swabbing the mouth with chlorhexidine mouthwash and the routine use of antifungal agents are essential. Local anaesthesia preparations such as 5% lignocaine (lidocaine) ointment, 20% flavoured benzocaine, or benzydamine hydrochloride (Difflam) applied before mealtimes can help to reduce the pain from ulceration or mucositis. The use of antibiotic paste or pastilles and ice chips can also be helpful. Once the leukaemia is in remission, and after consultation with the child's physician, routine dental care can be undertaken with the following adjustments:

1. If invasive procedures are planned then current haematological information is required to assess bleeding risks.
2. Prophylactic antibiotic therapy to prevent postoperative infection should be considered. This is given if the functional neutrophil count is depressed.
3. Children who are immunosuppressed are also at risk of fungal and viral infections. Fungal infections should be treated aggressively with amphotericin B, nystatin, or fluconazole, and herpetic infections with topical and/or systemic acyclovir.
4. Regional block anaesthesia may be contraindicated due to the risk of deep haemorrhage.
6. Oral preventive care is important. A typical protocol might include:

   While in hospital (paediatric dentistry specialist):
   - Relief of mucositis: Difflam mouthwash, topical anaesthesia, antibiotic pastilles, ice chips.
   - Elimination of bacterial plaque: chlorhexidine mouthwash 0.12%; povidone iodine topical application.
   - Nystatin 500,000 units 'swish and swallow'.
   - Topical fluoride therapy.
   - Manual plaque removal: toothbrushing instruction if platelet count is greater than 20×10^9/l; 'foam on a stick' with chlorhexidine if platelet count is less than 20×10^9/l.

   At home (primary care provider):
   - Oral surveillance.
   - Topical fluoride therapy.
   - Fissure sealants.
   - Diet advice.
   - Toothbrushing instruction.
   - Prescription of antifungals if required.

Key Points
- Oral side-effects of chemotherapy:
  —mucositis, oral ulceration;
  —infection (leucopenia);
  —haemorrhage (thrombocytopenia).
- Oral prophylaxis during chemotherapy:
  —oral hygiene;
  —pain relief for mucositis;
  —fluorides;
  —chlorhexidine;
  —antifungals.

16.4 RESPIRATORY DISORDERS

There are age-related disease patterns as far as the respiratory system is concerned; these patterns are also affected by sex, race, season of the year, geography, and environmental and socio-economic conditions. For example, the relatively short eustachian tube in infants and young children allows easy access to ascending infections from the pharynx. Cystic fibrosis largely affects Caucasians, whereas lung infections and infarctions associated with sickle-cell disease occur almost exclusively in Black children. Seasonal variation in the incidence of respiratory tract infections and asthma are quite marked and certain infections have a well-defined geographical distribution. The frequency of bronchitis may not be very different between socio-economic groups, but the severity may reflect differences in nutritional status and perhaps the availability of medical care.

16.4.1 Asthma

Asthma is a diffuse obstructive lung disease that causes breathlessness, coughing, and wheezing. It is associated with hyperreactivity of the airways to a variety of stimuli and a high degree of reversibility of the obstructive process. Asthma is a leading cause of chronic illness in childhood. Prevalence data are conflicting, but at least 10% of children will, at some time, have signs and symptoms compatible with a diagnosis of asthma. There is mounting recent evidence to suggest that the prevalence is increasing. Before puberty approximately twice as many boys as girls will suffer from asthma, thereafter, the sex incidence is similar. About half the children who are affected will be virtually free of symptoms by the time they become adults. The aetiology is poorly understood but it is a complex disorder involving immunological, infectious, biochemical, genetic, and psychological factors. Acute episodes of coughing and wheezing are often precipitated by exposure to allergens and irritants, such as cold air or noxious fumes and emotional stress. Drug therapy is now the mainstay of treatment both prophylactically and during acute exacerbations.

Dental management of asthma

Dental treatment itself can cause emotional stress, which may precipitate an attack. Routine dental care with local anaesthesia is not usually a problem; if in doubt, invite the child to take a puff of their inhaler before commencing. Steroid inhalers for asthma do not generally cause adrenal suppression and insufficiency. However, there is recent evidence that some of the newer generation of steroid inhalers may cause suppression. If in doubt contact the child's physician.

General anaesthesia for severe asthmatics usually requires in-patient hospital admission.

Recently, a study has been published linking dental erosion with asthma. This may be due to an increased likelihood of gastro-oesophageal reflux in people with asthma or to acidic long-term medication or to the increased consumption of erosive beverages due to 'drying' of the oral mucosa by inhalers.

> **Key Points**
>
> Of relevence to the dental management of asthma:
>
> - Erosion due to
>   —reflux;
>   —increase consumption of acidic beverages.
> - General anaesthesia may require in-patient admission.
> - The new generation of steroid inhalers may cause adrenal suppression.

16.4.2 Cystic fibrosis

Cystic fibrosis is an autosomal-recessive multisystem disorder predominantly of the exocrine glands. Thick viscid mucus is produced, particularly in the lungs, which leads to chronic obstruction and infection of the airways and to malabsorption. It is the most common genetic condition in Caucasians, with approximately 5% of the population being carriers and 1 in 2000 of live births affected. The abnormal gene has been located on the long arm of chromosome 7.

The clinical manifestations of the condition are variable and some patients remain asymptomatic for long periods. Coughing is the most constant symptom of pulmonary involvement and this may lead to recurrent respiratory infections and bronchiolitis. Sufferers often undergo regular physiotherapy to clear chest secretions. Lung disease progresses leading to exercise intolerance and shortness of breath (Fig. 16.6). More than 85% of affected children show evidence of malabsorption due to exocrine pancreatic insufficiency. Symptoms include frequent, bulky, greasy stools and a failure to thrive despite a large food intake.

Dental management of cystic fibrosis

There are reports of decreased caries prevalence attributable not only to the long term use of antibiotics and pancreatic enzyme supplements but also to increased

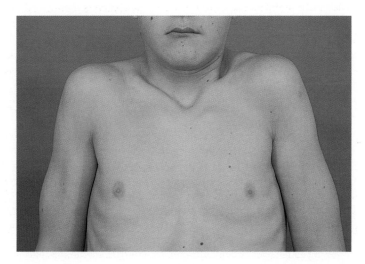

Fig. 16.6 This boy has cystic fibrosis and shows a 'barrel chest' deformity due to respiratory infections. Coincidentally, he also has a deformity of the clavicles. (Courtesy of Wolfe Publishing.)

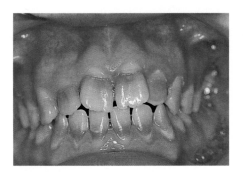

Fig. 16.7 Tetracycline was administered over a prolonged period to this patient who has cystic fibrosis. This has resulted in its incorporation into the mineral matrix with marked discoloration—alternative antibiotics are now used. Recent improvements in the management of people with cystic fibrosis have meant that an increasing number are not maintained on long-term antibiotic prophylaxis.

salivary buffering. Nevertheless, these children suffer from delayed dental development; more commonly have enamel opacities and are more prone to calculus. Moreover, they need to have a very high calorific intake and may have frequent refined carbohydrate snacks. As such, children with cystic fibrosis are an important priority group for dental health education and care. General anaesthetics should be avoided in view of the pulmonary involvement. A significant proportion of affected children also have cirrhosis of the liver, with resultant clotting defects and a liability to haemorrhage following surgical procedures. Children with cystic fibrosis sometimes still may be prescribed tetracycline to prevent chest infections, as a result of the development of multiple antibiotic sensitivities, even though it causes intrinsic dental staining (Fig. 16.7).

16.5 CONVULSIVE DISORDERS

16.5.1 Febrile convulsions

Convulsions are common; about 5% of children have had one or more convulsions and accurate diagnosis of the aetiology is very important. The vast majority of these are febrile convulsions and are associated with illnesses that cause high fever late in infancy such as otitis media. The seizures are usually tonic–clonic with loss of consciousness followed by sustained muscle contractions. Respiration may be impaired, which may lead to cyanosis. The teeth are often firmly clenched with possible tongue and lip-biting. There may also be a loss of bladder and bowel control. This tonic phase is followed by the clonic phase of intermittent muscular contraction. The duration is always less than 15 min. These convulsions usually occur early in the illness during the period of rapid temperature rise and may be the first indication that the child is ill. It is most important to eliminate the possibility of central nervous system infection; therefore examination of the cerebrospinal fluid is essential if there is persistent drowsiness following the attack.

16.5.2 Epilepsy

It may be difficult to differentiate these simple febrile convulsions from epilepsy but it is essential that this diagnosis is made as the therapy, prognosis, and implications differ enormously. Table 16.8 gives a list of conditions that are commonly associated with recurrent seizures. Epilepsy is not a disease in itself but a term applied to recurrent seizures, either of unknown origin (idiopathic epilepsy) or due to congenital or acquired brain lesions (secondary epilepsy). It affects about 0.5–2% of the population.

Table 16.8 Conditions commonly associated with seizures

Febrile convulsions
Idiopathic epilepsy: often genetic predisposition
Secondary epilepsy
  Cerebral neoplasms
  Cerebral vascular disorders, for example, subdural haemorrhage, especially seen in child abuse
  Cerebral malformation, for example, Down syndrome, hydrocephalus
  Neurocutaneous syndromes, for example, tuberous sclerosis, neurofibromatosis, Sturge–Weber disease
  Nutritional disorders, for example, pyridoxine deficiency, lead encephalopathy, drug intoxication
  Metabolic disorders, for example, hypoglycaemia, renal failure, phenylketonuria
  Atrophic cerebral lesions, for example, post-anoxic, post-traumatic, and postinfectious
  Degenerative cerebral disease, for example, Batten's disease
  Central nervous system infection, for example, meningitis, encephalitis, brain abscess

Medical management usually consists of long-term anticonvulsant drug therapy. The choice of drug depends on the seizure type, but the dosage needs to control the seizures with minimal side effects. New generation anti-epileptic drugs have become available, for example, Lamotrigine, Gabapentin, Oxcarbazepine, Tiagabine, and Topiramate but even these are not without problems, for example, hyperexcitability, dizziness, depression, weight loss, and abdominal problems. The most familiar anti-epileptic drugs are Sodium Valproate, Phenytion, and Carbamazepine.

Dental management of epilepsy

If possible, any liquid anti-epileptic medication should be sugar-free (Fig. 16.8). Sodium Valproate is not associated with gingival enlargement and like Carbamazepine, Lamotrigine, and Oxcarbazepine is available as a sugar-free liquid. Phenytoin results in gingival enlargement in about half of patients. The child with good control of seizures needs a minimum of restrictions, although the possibility of an attack occurring in the dental chair should be considered. A very high standard of oral hygiene is required to minimize the development of gingival enlargement and gingival surgery should never be contemplated unless the oral hygiene is good. Trauma to anterior teeth is often encountered in people with epilepsy who may have frequent, unpredictable falls. Reimplantation of avulsed teeth is usually contraindicated in those with severe learning difficulties. If prostheses are required then they should be well retained with clasps and unlikely to break or be inhaled during subsequent attacks.

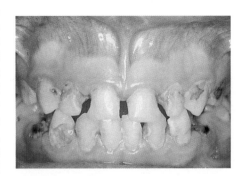

Fig. 16.8 This 3-year-old child with epilepsy has rampant caries of the primary dentition, with a somewhat unusual distribution of approximal lesions in both upper and lower incisors as well as molars. The child had been on long-term, sucrose-based medication but has now changed to the sugar-free sodium valproate liquid. (Courtesy of Wolfe Publishing.)

Key Points

Epilepsy:

- 0.5–1% of the population;
- gingival enlargement with phenytoin;
- check that any liquid medication is sugar-free.

16.6 METABOLIC AND ENDOCRINE DISORDERS

16.6.1 Diabetes mellitus

Diabetes is the most common endocrine/metabolic disorder of childhood and is due to the deficiency of insulin and abnormal metabolism of carbohydrate, protein, and fat. Type I diabetes mellitus is insulin-dependent (IDDM) and usually of juvenile onset. It is age-related with peaks of presentation between 5 and 7 years and at puberty. The prevalence of diabetes in school-age children is approximately 2 per 1000. Although there is a genetic predisposition, there may well be a triggering effect from viral infections in the aetiology of diabetes. The clinical manifestations are polydipsia (increased thirst), polyuria (increased urination), polyphagia (increased appetite), and weight loss. There may be an insidious onset of lethargy, weakness, and weight loss. The diagnosis is dependent on the demonstration of hyperglycaemia in association with glucosuria. The aims of treatment are to control the symptoms, prevent acute metabolic crises of hypo- and hyperglycaemia, and to maintain normal growth and body weight, with an active life-style. If there is good control of blood sugar levels with insulin therapy and nutritional management, then diabetic complications are minimized. One of the major hazards of insulin treatment is the development of hypoglycaemia. It is usually of rapid onset (unlike hyperglycaemia) with sweating, palpitations, apprehension, and trembling. This progresses to mental confusion, drowsiness, and coma. Hypoglycaemia in a diabetic child indicates too much insulin relative to food intake and energy expenditure. For an acute episode a carbohydrate-containing snack or drink should be given. Another problem, particularly in adolescents, is the psychological adjustment to the condition; the rebellious teenage years may lead to non-compliance with insulin therapy and nutritional management. Many of these problems can be averted by suitable education and counselling.

Dental management of diabetes

The well-controlled diabetic child with no serious complications can have any dental treatment but should receive preventive care as a priority. Uncontrolled diabetes can result in varied problems, which mainly relate to fluid imbalance, an altered response to infection, possible increased glucose concentrations in saliva, and microvascular changes. There may be decreased salivary flow, and an increased incidence of dental caries has been reported in uncontrolled young diabetics. There is also well-documented evidence of increased periodontal problems and susceptibility to infections, particularly with *Candida* sp. Dental appointments should be arranged at times when the blood sugar levels are well controlled; usually a good time is in the morning immediately following their insulin injection and a normal breakfast. General anaesthetics are a problem because of the pre-anaesthetic fasting that is required, and so these are normally carried out on an in-patient basis to enable the insulin and carbohydrate balance to be stabilized intravenously.

16.6.2 Adrenal insufficiency

There are a number of syndromes associated with adrenal insufficiency, such as Addison's disease and Cushing's syndrome. However, problems in the dental management of patients with steroid insufficiency are more likely to occur in children who are being prescribed steroid therapy for other medical conditions; for example, in the suppression of inflammatory and allergic disorders, acute leukaemia, and to prevent acute transplant rejection. In children, the risks of taking corticosteroids are greater than in adults and they should only be used when specifically indicated, in minimal dosage, and for the shortest possible time. If a child has adrenal insufficiency and/or is receiving steroid therapy, then any infection or stress may precipitate an adrenal crisis. For routine restorative treatment no additional steroid supplementation is usually necessary. However, if extractions under local anaesthesia or more extensive procedures are planned and/or if the patient is particularly apprehensive, then the oral steroid dosage should be increased. General anaesthesia should not be carried out on an out-patient basis. Consultation with the child's physician is necessary before prescribing steroids, and anaesthetists must be aware of such medication in order to avoid a precipitous fall in blood pressure during anaesthesia or in the immediate postoperative period.

16.6.3 Other disorders

Many other metabolic and endocrine disorders occur in children but these are rare events.

16.6.3.1 Thyroid disease

Thyroid disease may present in early adolescence, although it is generally more common in adults. Dental management should present no problems if the thyrotoxic patient is medically well controlled; however, liaison with the physicians is important.

16.6.3.2 Renal disorders

Nephrotic syndrome is a condition where protein leaks from the blood into urine via the glomeruli of the kidney resulting in hypoproteinaemia and generalized oedema. Left untreated, sufferers would die of infections but fortunately the majority respond to treatment using corticosteroids, usually prednisolone.

The kidney undergoes a complex developmental and migratory process leading to a high frequency of congenital anomalies, such as polycystic disease and unilocular cysts. Acute pyelonephritis is more common when there is a congenital abnormality present and so, even though it is simply treated with antibiotics, children often undergo further medical investigations to rule out congenital abnormality. Therefore, children with renal problems are likely to be, or have been, under specialist medical care. From a dental viewpoint, children with reduced renal function, or more importantly, progressive renal failure need extra consideration when prescribing drugs. Such children may: fail to excrete a drug or its metabolites, be more sensitive to the drug's effect; be less tolerant of side effects; and same drugs may even be less effective. Examples of drugs where caution should be exercised by the dentist include: midazolam and other benzodiazepines, chloral hydrate, NSAIDs, Fluconazole and co-trimoxazde. The BNF should always be consulted.

16.7 NEOPLASTIC DISORDERS

There are approximately 1200 new cases of childhood cancer each year in the United Kingdom. Child cancer patients largely reflect the child population in general and as such, represent a cross-section of the population. Cancer causes more childhood deaths between the ages of 1 and 15 years than any other disease, but is still considerably behind trauma as the most common reason for mortality. The incidence of malignant tumours in children under 15 years of age in developed countries is estimated to be in the region of 1 in 10,000 children per year but the mortality rate is high, at between 30% and 40%. Although leukaemia is the most common form of childhood cancer, tumours of the central nervous system and neural crest cells and lymphomas also form a significant proportion (Table 16.9). Prognosis varies with the type of tumour, the stage at which it was diagnosed, and upon the adequacy of treatment. Major advances have been made in the treatment of childhood malignancy in the last few decades, largely as a result of advances in chemotherapy and bone-marrow transplantation.

Dental management of children with cancer

The children may have untreated caries and, since many are under 5 years of age, and may not have had a previous dental examination. The oral side-effects of cancer treatment are shown in Table 16.10 but can be categorized into (1) immediate and (2) long term. The immediate problems include mucositis (oral ulceration) and exacerbations of common oral diseases that may become life threatening and are usually managed by paediatric dentistry specialists in liaison with their medical colleagues. Child cancer survivors later present with long-term problems relating to: - growth; puberty, and reproduction; cardiac; thyroid; cognitive deficit; and social function. Oral and dental development can also be impeded and specialist advice might again be required. Despite this, the introduction of a shared care arrangement between the primary dental practitioner and the paediatric specialist when the child is in remission is vital to ensure continued preventive therapy and good oral health while at the same time 'normalizing' care.

Table 16.9 The major types of childhood cancer

Leukaemia	48%
Central nervous system	16%
Lymphoma	8%
Neuroblastoma	7%
Nephroblastoma	5%
Others	16%

Key Points

- Children with cancer need the combined care of primary and specialist dental services;
- There are immediate and long-term effects of cancer treatment;
- Disease prevention is vital.

Table 16.10   Summary of oral problems associated with cancer therapy

Mucositis
  Acute inflammation of the mucosa
  White/ yellow fibrous slough, often with ulceration
  Painful to eat/ speak/ swallow
  Portal for microbial entry

Blood changes
  Spontaneous gingival/ mucosal bleeding
  Crusting of lips

Immunosuppression
  Non-vital primary teeth can become a medical emergency
  Acute herpetic gingivo stomatitis and candida can rapidly progress to systemic
    involvement in children

Changes in saliva
  Saliva becomes thick, viscous, and acidic
  Acute ascending sialadenitis can occur as a complication
  Loss/alteration of taste (may be difficult to persuade the child to eat so enticed by
    sugary snacks)
  Dysphagia (difficulty in swallowing)

Changes in oral flora
  Increase in cariogenic organisms
  Increased susceptibility to candidal infection
  Rapid progression of periodontal disease

Dental pain and trismus
  Leukaemic infiltration of dental pulp tissue or direct infiltration of jaws
  Jaw pain and trismus as a direct complication of drug therapy or fibrosis following
    radiotherapy

16.8 ORGAN TRANSPLANTATION

Kidney, heart, bone marrow, liver, and pancreas transplantation are now routine procedures. Most liver transplants in children occur because of biliary atresia. Bone marrow transplants are the treatment of choice for children with aplastic anaemia, those who fail conventional therapy for leukaemia, and for some immune deficiency disorders. Although children with end-stage renal disease can be kept alive by haemodialysis, their quality of life is considerably improved by kidney transplantation. Children who require organ transplantation are considered to be at a high caries risk and so prevention is important.

16.8.1 Pretransplant treatment planning

Any candidate for organ transplantation should be referred for specialist dental evaluation. Whenever possible, active dental disease should be treated before the transplant procedure and any teeth with doubtful prognoses extracted. This may present difficulties as many pretransplant patients can be seriously ill and have various associated medical problems. Moreover, some children will be placed on a high carbohydrate (cariogenic) diet, for example, 'maxijul', to 'build-them-up' in preparation for surgery and so the dental team will need to adopt a pragmatic approach to advice relating to sugar intake and frequency during this time, since the child's medical well being must take priority. Children undergoing bone marrow transplantation are prone to infection, bleeding, and delayed healing due to leucopenia and thrombocytopenia. However, the majority of children awaiting liver transplantation due to biliary atresia are of a very young age and have not experienced dental caries, though their teeth may have intrinsic green staining due to biliverdin deposition in the developing dental tissues. This is a time when intensive oral hygiene instruction and preventive advice and therapy are of paramount importance in helping to minimize later potential oral problems. Before any invasive dental procedures are undertaken, consultation with the child's physician is vital in order to establish the extent of the organ dysfunction and its repercussions. Prophylactic antibiotics will probably be required in patients with cardiac problems and depressed white blood cell counts. Any significant alterations in bleeding times and/or coagulation status must be checked. There are also certain drugs that should be avoided inpatients with end-stage liver or kidney disease.

16.8.2 Immediate post-transplant period

Drugs prescribed to prevent graft rejection have several side-effects. Azathioprine results in leucopenia, thrombocytopenia, and anaemia; hence, children in this immediate post-transplant phase may be even more prone to infections and haemorrhage than before. Cyclosporin (*Neoral*) and Tacrolimus are largely replacing azathioprine but these may cause severe kidney and liver changes leading to hypertension and bleeding problems. Cyclosporin is also associated with gingival enlargement. Steroids are prescribed at this time with the risk of adrenal suppression. Full supportive dental care is required and children complain of nausea and may develop severe oral ulceration. Routine oral hygiene procedures can become difficult but the use of chlorhexidine as a mouthwash, spray, or on a disposable sponge, together with local anaesthetic preparations is helpful.

16.8.3 Stable post-transplant period

Once healing has occurred and any acute graft rejection been brought under control then routine dental treatment can be undertaken. Reinforcement of all preventive advice and liaison with the child's dietitian may be helpful as many patients are still on high carbohydrate supplementation. Steroid therapy is discontinued in children with liver transplants after 3 months but may be continued for longer periods than this in those with other organ transplants. Antifungal prophylaxis is usually given in the first few months after transplantation to prevent oral candidal infections. Dental problems, apart from oral ulceration and those associated with immunosuppression and bleeding tendencies, include delayed eruption and exfoliation of primary teeth and ectopic eruption of permanent teeth. These are related to the gingival overgrowth associated with cyclosporin and nifedipine medication (Fig. 16.9).

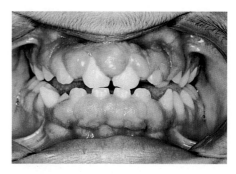

Fig. 16.9 These grossly hyperplastic gingivae are associated with cyclosporin and nifedipine medication in this 11-year-old boy who has had a kidney transplant. This combination of drugs is required to prevent rejection and to control his blood pressure.

Key Points

Transplant immunosuppression:

- leucopenia;
- thrombocytopenia;
- gingival enlargement.

16.9 SUMMARY

In all children who are medically compromised the dental team can not only play a vital part in the overall medical management but also in helping these children and their parents adjust to normal life following recovery. Oral care is extremely important in enhancing the quality of life by reducing the morbidity and mortality of oral conditions, and by allowing the child to eat without pain and so gain optimal nutrient intake. Preventive care should be the cornerstone of any oral care programme. Since many children travel long distances to regional and supra-regional units, shared care between the hospital paediatric dentistry specialist and the primary care provider can facilitate the child's reintegration into their local community and avoid lost schooling.

1. An increasing number of children with complex medical problems now survive due to improvements in medical care, and present difficulties in oral management.

2. An accurate, detailed medical history must be obtained for all children before any dental treatment is undertaken.

3. An aggressive preventive regimen is required for all children with significant medical problems; this must encompass dietary counselling, suitable fluoride therapy, fissure sealant applications, and oral hygiene instruction.

4. Congenital heart disease is more common in children than acquired conditions. Many of these malformations require prophylactic antibiotics prior to carrying out any invasive dental procedures.

5. Children with bleeding disorders, such as haemophilia, thrombocytopenic purpura, and Von Willebrand's disease, must be haematologically investigated prior to dental treatment. Haematological replacement therapy may be required before operative treatment.

6. Children with anaemia, whether from iron deficiency or from such inherited conditions as sickle-cell anaemia or thalassaemia, represent general anaesthetic risks in particular.

7. Leukaemia is the most common form of childhood cancer and the first disseminated cancer to respond completely to chemotherapy in a significant number of children. Dental management of affected children needs to consider their haematological status as well as their immunocompromised condition.

8. Asthma is a leading cause of chronic illness in childhood; severe asthmatics may be on systemic steroid therapy, which has implications for dental care.

9. Convulsions are common in children, occurring in approximately 5%, but many of these are associated with episodes of high fever in the child and not with epilepsy.

10. Diabetes mellitus is the most common endocrine/metabolic disorder of childhood; if there is good control of blood sugar levels with insulin therapy and nutritional management, then diabetic complications are minimized and dental care should be routine.

11. Organ transplantation in children is now being increasingly undertaken; there are many side effects of drug control of immunosuppression that affect treatment planning and oral care.

12. The participation of the dental team in the overall management of children with medical problems can significantly help to enhance the quality of life; preventive care should be the cornerstone of dental management.

16.10 FURTHER READING

Behrman, R. E. and Vaughan, V. C. (2003). *Nelson textbook of pediatrics* (17th edn). W. B. Saunders, Philadelphia, P A. (*The standard paediatric 'bible'; a huge amount of information about all types of medical problems in children.*)

Gorlin, R. J., Cohen, M. M., and Levin, L. S. (2001). *Syndromes of the head and neck* (4th edn). Oxford University Press, Oxford. (*The authoritative publication on this subject with erudite lists of references.*)

Grundy, M. C., Shaw, L., and Hamilton, D. V. (1993). *An illustrated guide to dental care of the medically compromised patient.* Wolfe, London. (*Basic information on a wider range of subjects than can be covered in the present chapter and with practical information on dental care.*)

Little, J. W. and Falace, D. A. (2002). *Dental management of the medically compromised patient* (6th edn). Mosby Year Book, St Louis, MO. (*Comprehensive information but with very helpful summaries on potential problems related to dental care.*)

Scully, C. and Cawson, R. A. (2004). *Medical problems in dentistry.* Churchill Livingstone, Edinburgh. (5th edn). (*The most comprehensive account of how to cope with medical problems.*)

17

Childhood impairment and disability

17 Childhood impairment and disability

J. H. Nunn

17.1 INTRODUCTION

An impairment becomes a disability for a child only if he or she is unable to carry out the normal activities of his or her peer group. For example, a child who has broken an arm is temporarily 'disabled' by not being able to eat and write in the normal way. However, for some children impairment is a permanent feature in their lives, although it may become a disability only if they are unable to take part in everyday activities, such as communicating with others, climbing stairs, and toothbrushing. One definition that helps to clarify which children are 'disabled', for the purposes of providing dental care, is as follows: 'dentally disabled' refers to patients who have some gross condition or deficit in their oral cavities, which necessitates special dental treatment for example, a cleft of the lip and palate. By contrast, children who are 'disabled for dentistry' are those who have a physical and/or intellectual or emotional condition that may prevent them from being treated in a routine manner.

There are a number of reasons why children with disabilities merit special consideration for dental care:

1. The oral health of some children with disabilities is different from that of their normal peers, for example, the greater prevalence of periodontal disease in people with Down syndrome and of toothwear in those with cerebral palsy.

2. The prevention of dental disease in disabled children needs to be a higher priority than for so-called normal peers because dental disease, its sequelae, or its treatment, may be life-threatening, for example, the risk of infective endocarditis from oral organisms in children with congenital heart defects (Fig. 17.1).

3. Treatment planning and the provision of dental care may need to be modified in view of the patient's capabilities, likely future co-operation, and home care, for example, the feasibility of providing a resin-bonded bridge for a teenager with cerebral palsy, poorly controlled epilepsy, and inadequate home oral care.

In the light of these considerations, do such children need special dental care? Most of the studies which have been undertaken on disabled children have indicated that the majority can in fact be treated in a dental surgery in the normal way, together with the rest of their family.

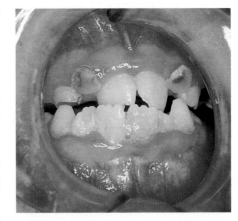

Fig. 17.1 A 13-year-old boy with Down syndrome and gross caries, who was prevented from going on a combined heart and lung as well as a renal transplant register because of his dental disease.

Key Points
The need for special dental care arises because of:
- differences in dental disease prevalence;
- dental disease/treatment may be life-threatening;
- the modifications required to treatment plans;
- the need for special facilities;
- treatment may be time-consuming.

This normality is desirable, provided the disabled person actually receives good dental care. The evidence from many studies is that, although the overall caries experience is similar between disabled children and their so-called normal contemporaries, the type of treatment they have experienced is different: disabled children have similar levels of untreated decay, but more missing teeth and fewer restored teeth. A minority of children with complex disabilities need special facilities, usually only available in dental or general hospitals, or from specialized community dental clinics. What *is* needed by all patients with disabilities is a very aggressive approach to the prevention of dental disease. Because of the potential for dental disease, or its treatment, to disable an impaired child, priority must be given to preventive dental care for such individuals from a very young age.

Children with a significant degree of impairment are termed 'children with special educational needs' or 'children with learning difficulties'. These terms, used synonymously, encompass a wide variety of impairments, but three main areas—intellectual, physical, and sensory impairments—predominate and will now be considered in more detail. It is important to stress, however, that impairment does not always present as a discrete entity; in any population of affected children, at least a quarter of the group will be multiply impaired, making it difficult to assign a 'label' to that child's impairment. Medical compromise, considered in more detail in Chapter 16, may also be imposed on these impairments. The way in which some of these present to a dentist are given below, together with the dental management issues relevant to each. Many of the issues raised are, of course, common to a number of impairments.

17.2 INTELLECTUAL IMPAIRMENT

The causes of intellectual impairment are numerous and for many children a cause for their disability may never be identified. Approximately, 25 per 1000 of the child population are affected, and the majority, as with other impairments, will be males. Children with intellectual impairment can be divided broadly into those who are either mentally retarded or have a learning difficulty. These are broad groups, often without a well-defined aetiology or consistent presenting features, but there are two distinct subgroups where the cause is known and the features are well described, namely Down and Fragile X syndromes. Intellectual impairment may be present in some children with cerebral palsy and those who have suffered birth anoxia, and severe infections, for example, meningitis and rubella. Intellectual impairment is also a feature of autism, microcephaly, and metabolic disorders (e.g. phenyl-ketonuria), and may also be acquired after significant trauma. Not every condition will have specific dental features like Down syndrome, but an understanding of the underlying impairment will help the dentist plan treatment more effectively.

Mental retardation, pervasive developmental disorders (autism and schizophrenia), learning disabilities, dyslexia, attention-deficit disorders, and hyperactivity are all controversial categories whose definition and processes of assessment are not universally agreed.

Key Points

Classification of children with impairments

- intellectually impaired—mentally retarded, learning difficulties;
- physically impaired—developmental, degenerative;
- sensory impairment;
- medically compromised;
- combination of impairments.

Mental retardation

This is sometimes called mental handicap, mental subnormality, or mental deficiency. It is a general category characterized by low intelligence, failure of adaptation, and early age of onset. Low general intelligence is the main characteristic. Affected children are slow in their general mental development and they may have difficulties in attention, perception, memory, and thinking. They may be stronger in some skills than others, for example, music and computing, but generally they are of low intellectual attainment. Children with low intelligence are not called mentally retarded unless they also have some problem in adaptation. That is, they are unlikely to be able to live independently and will always depend inappropriately on others as a source of income and support for daily living. According to IQ levels, five levels are traditionally described. The simplicity of the classification is somewhat illusory with great individual differences among people with mental retardation.

> **Key Points**
> Intellectual impairment may occur in:
> - cerebral palsy;
> - birth anoxia;
> - severe infections;
> - autism;
> - microcephaly;
> - metabolic disorders;
> - major trauma;
> - some syndromes.

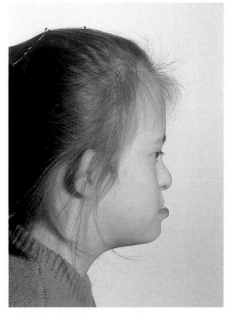

Fig. 17.2 Lateral view of a Down syndrome child, to show mid-face hypoplasia.

Down syndrome

Down syndrome is a chromosomal disorder, trisomy 21, with distinct clinical features. The prevalence is approximately 1 in 600 births but there is variation with maternal age, so that at 40 years of age the incidence is about 1 in 40 births. However, the numbers seen in any one country will vary depending on the prevailing attitude towards prenatal screening and termination. The general physical features associated with Down syndrome are a greater predisposition to cardiac defects, leukaemia of the myeloid type, infective hepatitis infection (especially in institutionalized males), although most children will have been vaccinated against viral forms. Coeliac disease as well as thyroid disorders are also clinical features of this condition. Increasingly, a form of early dementia, entitled disintegrative disorder is being recognized in adolescents with Down syndrome. The features seen are of a progressive loss of skills, both cognitive and physical and have obvious relevance in dentistry because of the impact on personal oral care.

Varying degrees of mental retardation occur, and upper respiratory tract infections and an inability to withstand infections generally are common. Physically, predominant features are a rounded, small face with an under-developed mid-face (Fig 17.2), especially of the nasal bridge, an upward slant of the eyes with prominent epicanthic folds, squints, cataracts, and Brushfield spots on the iris. The hands of children with Down syndrome are stubby with a pronounced transverse palmar crease. Intraorally the tongue is large, protruding, and sometimes heavily fissured (Fig 17.3). The palate may be high vaulted and narrow. There is usually a delay in the exfoliation of primary teeth and in the eruption of permanent teeth, while some teeth may be congenitally missing. Teeth that erupt are often microdont and/or hypoplastic (Fig. 17.4). There is a high prevalence of periodontal disease in the anterior alveolar segments, especially in the mandible. This is probably due to

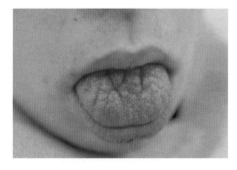

Fig 17.3 The protruberant, fissured tongue of an adolescent with Down syndrome.

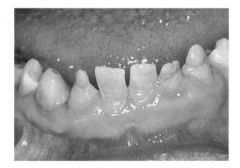

Fig 17.4 A Down syndrome patient with marked dental hypoplasia, conical teeth, and hypodontia.

impaired phagocyte function in neutrophils and monocytes, combined with poor oral hygiene. Other factors implicated in the pathophysiology of the extensive inflammation seen in Down syndrome patients are enhanced PGE_2 production and increased activity of plasminogen activators, and thus collagenase activity.

> **Key Points**
>
> Oral and dental features in Down syndrome:
> - mid-face hypoplasia;
> - large, fissured tongue;
> - narrow, high-vaulted palate;
> - delay in exfoliation/eruption;
> - congenitally absent teeth;
> - microdont/hypoplastic teeth;

Fragile X syndrome

Next to Down syndrome this is the most common cause of mental retardation. This disorder is largely under-diagnosed; and people who have been classified as having 'mental handicap of unknown origin', especially if they are male, probably have Fragile X syndrome. The condition is of particular significance because a high proportion of affected individuals have congenital heart defects, usually mitral valve prolapse, that may require antibiotic prophylaxis. Although males are predominantly affected, milder versions of the disability may be seen in females.

Pervasive developmental disorders

This group encompasses autism and childhood schizophrenia. The former is characterized by its early onset, usually before 30 months of age, whereas childhood schizophrenia presents later. They are conditions that represent profound adaptive problems in thinking, language, and social relationships. Autism in particular has the distinctive feature of restricted and stereotypical behaviour patterns. Most children score below normal on IQ testing and thus experience significant developmental delay. The more severely delayed children seem oblivious to their parents or carers, express themselves minimally, show a low level of interest in exploring objects, avoid sounds, and engage in ritualistic behaviour. Children with Asperger's syndrome display some of the features of autism but may also possess a level of skill in some areas well above the average for their peers.

These features need to be taken into consideration when attempting dental care, and underlines the particular importance of acclimatization and familiarity of routine (rituals) as part of that process.

The causes of autism are unknown but are thought to be prenatal and not social in origin. Much interest was generated in a possible link with MMR vaccine as a possible aetiological factor but this evidence has since been discredited. A major malformation in the cerebellum has recently been implicated as a possible causative factor. The prevalence of autism ranges from 0.03% to 0.1% with fluctuations that may point to an environmental cause.

Learning difficulties

Learning difficulty is associated with dyslexia, minimal brain damage, attention-deficit disorder, and hyperactivity. All these categories are controversial, mainly because they have been overextended.

Historically, a child with a learning difficulty has been defined as one whose performance in one academic area is more than 2 years behind the child's ability.

Thus the impairment is restricted in its range and there is a discrepancy between academic performance and tested general ability. In these two ways a learning difficulty differs from mental retardation because the latter is characterized by *general* delay and academic performance is usually at the level expected from ability. In practice, learning difficulty has been used to characterize any child with a learning problem who cannot be labeled mentally retarded, no matter how broad the range of impairment or the discrepancy from the tested ability level. This overextension of the definition has not only increased the apparent prevalence of learning disability but has also made the whole area rather confusing.

In general, the prevalence of learning difficulties is estimated on average to be about 4.5%. There is overlap between learning difficulties and other problems, for example, higher levels of classroom behavioural problems and an increased risk of delinquency. In part, this accounts for the greater predominance of males in groups with intellectual impairment as they are more likely than females to be disruptive at school and thus be referred for assessment by educational psychologists.

Dyslexia

This widely discussed form of learning disability is a specific problem with cognition. The broadest definition of dyslexia includes those children whose reading skills are delayed for any reason, and it is usually associated with a number of cognitive deficits. Prevalence varies from 3% to 16% depending on the breadth of the definition and the country. For example, prevalence rates are higher in the United States than they are in Italy, perhaps due to the complexity of the English language as compared with Italian!

Minimal brain damage

This category of impairment is used to describe the child who has minor neurological signs, which are often transitory. They are not reliable predictors of future behavioural and educational problems.

Attention disorder and hyperactivity

These disorders are often confused with one another. Children who cannot sit still are thought to be inattentive to their lessons in school. A child who does not pay attention often: fails to finish activities; acts prematurely or redundantly; infrequently reacts to requests and questions; has difficulties with tasks that require fine discrimination, sustained vigilance, or complex organization; and improves markedly when supervised intensively. A child who is hyperactive: engages in excessive standing up, walking, running, and climbing; does not remain seated for long during tasks; frequently makes redundant movements; shifts excessively from one activity to another; and/or often starts talking, asking, or making requests. This elevated activity level expresses itself differently at different ages. Inattentive, hyperactive children are disturbing to their parents, other children, and to professionals like teachers, doctors, and dentists. They are often judged to be behaviourally disturbed. The variation in definition, age, sex, source of the data, and cultural factors produces prevalence estimates of up to 35%. However, most estimates are under 9% for boys and even less for girls.

Emotional and behavioural disorders

There are many manifestations of emotional disorder: fear, anxiety, shyness, aggressive, destructive or chronically disobedient behaviour, theft, associating with bad companions, and truancy. When parents or teachers believe that these problems interfere with the child's socialization, they are often referred for professional help. In considering the prevalence of emotional or behavioural disorders, account has to be taken of the very common, seemingly identical, behaviour of normal children. Eating disorders, which may be of concern to dentists because of self injurious behaviour as well as dental erosion, are important in the preschool period and, in different ways, in adolescence.

17.2.1 General considerations

Access to care

Segregated special education and institutions, especially in rural areas, were characteristic of services for disabled children until after the Second World War. During the 1950s there was a move towards *normalizing* the lives of 'handicapped' children. This movement set about making major changes in the lives of affected children and adults but cannot yet be considered as completely successful. The move to normalization came about largely for ideological, legal, and probably in some countries for financial reasons.

The philosophy of this movement, which originated in Sweden, centered on the idea that an impaired person should live in an environment as near normal as possible. This involved residing in home-like residences and attending schools, work places, and recreational programmes that were part of the community. On the basis of this ideology, many mildly impaired people were moved out of long-stay institutions into community homes. This movement was fostered by the belief that institutionalization retarded emotional and cognitive growth. De-institutionalization would also reduce the state's expense in maintaining impaired people, and the onus would be shifted to parents, private charities, and local authorities. Contemporary concepts within this movement are embodied in social role valorization—that is, the concept of social devaluation of which social exclusion, for whatever reason, is just one aspect.

While most people would agree with the principle of normalization, inadequate funding has produced a less than satisfactory alternative in community care and disastrous consequences for some mentally ill people and those with whom they interact. While many children and adults with impairments were resident in long-stay institutions the provision of dental services was relatively efficient. With the move to normalization, children were often returned to parents/guardians or housed by social services in homes in the local community, thereby placing an additional burden on these families or carers to organize dental care.

Alongside this programme has been the move to integrate as many children as possible into mainstream education. This may mean that these children are not as readily identifiable as was the case when they attended 'special schools' and thus may miss out on the opportunity to receive the prioritized dental care they need. For teenagers, it has become apparent that some managers of the adult training centres that they attend feel that, as part of normalization, their clients should receive 'normal' dental care, that is, from a general dental practitioner. This would be desirable, provided general dental practitioners were happy to provide this service. The evidence to date is that this is not generally the case. In the meantime, teenagers and young adults could lose out by not continuing to receive the special dental services that the publically funded service has been able to offer, simply because it is felt by their advocates that this runs contrary to the philosophy of 'normalization'.

Consent for dental care

A treatment plan for a child (less than 16 years of age in most jurisdictions) requires the consent of a parent before embarking upon active treatment. This is often by implied consent; that is, the parent brings the child to the surgery and the child sits in the chair, the implication being that the parent has consented to treatment. This is no different to the scenario with an impaired child. The United Nations Convention on the Child requires that children's rights are protected and in this context, cognizance taken of the child's views on whether they wish treatment to be carried out. As with any patient, best interests must be protected. Difficulty arises in adolescents with an intellectual impairment who are over the age of consent. In this situation parents or carers are unable to give a valid consent on their charge's behalf. That is, an adult cannot consent for treatment on behalf of another adult. Dentists would be well advised to obtain a second opinion on their treatment plan before embarking on dental care for an impaired young person who is judged to be incapable of giving their own valid, that is, informed, consent. This is particularly the case where dental care under general anaesthesia is being contemplated. It is prudent, also, to discuss the proposed treatment plan and to obtain the agreement for the care that is being suggested from those who have an interest in the patient.

There will be occasions when it will not be possible to easily undertake an examination for a child or adolescent with a profound learning disability. In those circumstances, a decision has to be made as to whether some form of physical intervention, previously termed restraint, may need to be used. The clinician must decide, on the basis of a number of factors, what is the best way forward. At all times, as part of the dentist's duty of care, she or he must act in the patient's best interest in reaching a decision as to whether to use some form of physical intervention. This decision must be taken in the light of a number of factors, modified after Schuman and Bebau and incorporated into the British Society of Disability and Oral Health's Policy Document on Physical Interventions (www.bsdh.org) as follows:

Key Points

Physical interventions

- Minimum to be effective.
- Clearly documented —type/reason.
- Only employed by trained staff.
- Beneficial for individual to complete treatment.
- Not seen as punishment/for convenience.
- Not likely to cause physical trauma.
- Not likely to cause more than minimal psychological trauma.
- A means of avoiding more severe restraint (e.g. GA).
- To control involuntary movements.
- To avoid injury to self, others.
- Agreed with others close to patient.

17.2.2 Oral health

Dental caries

In the absence of targeted preventive and treatment programmes, children with impairments fare less well than their normal peers. While overall disease experience as measured using the dmf/DMF index (decayed, missing, filled primary/permanent teeth) is similar, for the child with impairments there is often more untreated decay, more missing, and fewer filled teeth. Early studies point to a reduced prevalence of dental caries in children with Down syndrome, but this feature may be attributable more to the later eruption of teeth relative to a control group of unaffected children so that the teeth are 'at risk' in the mouth for a shorter period. The relative microdontia/spacing seen in young people with Down syndrome may also be a contributory factor in this supposed reduction in dental disease prevalence.

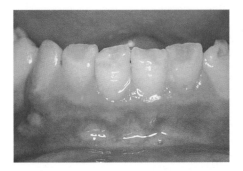

Fig. 17.5 Chronological hypoplasia in a child with coeliac disease.

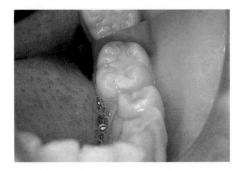

Fig. 17.6 Glass ionomer cement fissure sealant.

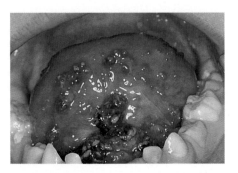

Fig. 17.7 Fluoride varnish on primary molars in a child with a mixed lymph/haemangioma and a learning disability.

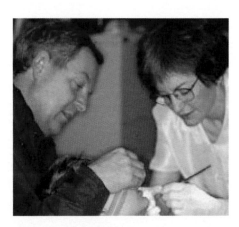

Fig. 17.8 A parent of a boy with crebral palsy assisting in the delivery of nitrous oxide sedation for routine scaling.

Periodontal disease

The periodontal status of children who are intellectually impaired may be compromised by their inability to comprehend and thus comply with oral hygiene measures. In these children periodontal disease is more prevalent, possibly as a result of an altered immune state (Chapter 11.). Almost universally, plaque and gingivitis indices scores are higher in children with impairments.

Malocclusion

There are no studies that deal specifically with the problems of malocclusion in intellectually impaired children. However, in published data on general dental health, the number of orthodontic anomalies is frequently higher because many remain untreated. In Down syndrome the relative mid-face hypoplasia contributes to the pseudoskeletal class III relationship and this, in combination with the narrow, high-vaulted palate produces buccal cross-bites (Fig. 17.2).

Other oral defects

One feature of note is the prevalence of enamel defects often caused by the aetiological agent that produced the impairment. It is possible that dentists could play a part not only in the diagnosis of some disabilities, for example, coeliac disease (Fig. 17.5), but also in the timing of the insult that led to the impairment. Teeth provide a good chronological record of the timing of severe systemic upsets (Chapter 13).

17.2.3 Operative procedures

Children who are intellectually impaired may be able to co-operate for dental treatment, but their ability to accept specific procedures such as the use of local anaesthetic and high speed instruments will depend on their degree of understanding and level of maturity. Isolation may be difficult due to a large tongue and poor control of movement, and in these situations it may be necessary to compromise on the treatment approach. In fissure sealing it may be more practicable to use a glass ionomer cement, protected by occlusal adjustment wax or a gloved finger during the setting phase, rather than to struggle with all the stages of applying a conventional resin sealant (Fig. 17.6). Human clinical trials are now underway in both the United Kingdom and the United States to investigate the use of intraoral fluoride-releasing devices. These are small diameter glass beads that are attached by composite resin, to the buccal surface of a tooth (Chapter 6). The device dissolves slowly in saliva, releasing fluoride as it does so. Those currently on trial have continued to elevate salivary fluoride levels for up to 2 years. Whether the released fluoride is equitably distributed around the mouth is not yet known. The placement, and retention *in situ*, of the glass beads in such children may be a challenge.

Duraphat fluoride varnish (5% sodium fluoride = 22,600 p.p.m. fluoride, Colgate) is an almost ideal preventive agent for children with poor tolerance of dental procedures. The amber-coloured polyurethane-based material is applied to the tooth surfaces, preferably dry, although the varnish is water tolerant, and the resulting adherent film slowly releases fluoride (Fig. 17.7). The exercise should be repeated up to four times a year depending on caries risk. A reduction of caries in permanent teeth of between 30% and 62% has been reported using Duraphat ™ varnish.

Recourse to one or other forms of conscious sedation may be indicated for a child with impairments who finds it difficult to co-operate for dental care. However, a degree of compliance is necessary in order to retain the nasal hood for the delivery of nitrous oxide/oxygen for inhalation sedation(Fig. 17.8) as it is for the insertion of a cannula for intravenous sedation. However, IV sedation is not usually indicated for children although the drug used most commonly in the United Kingdom, Midazolam, can be given orally although again, the outcome may not be predictable.

For some patients general anaesthesia will be necessary to provide adequate dental care (Fig. 17.9). This facility is not widely available and often means

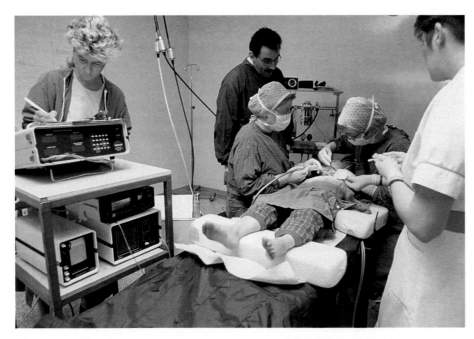

Fig. 17.9 Dental treatment under day-stay general anaesthesia for a child with impairments.

considerable disruption for the family because of the distance involved in travelling to specialist centres. Additionally, the child may be unsettled by the whole process of being starved, looked after by strange personnel, being anaesthetized, and then waking up with a sore throat and perhaps a mouth full of blood. There is evidence that this experience is only in the short-term memory as many parents comment on how much better their child is in terms of behaviour, sleeping patterns, and eating after the immediate postoperative period.

Treatment planning for dental care under general anaesthesia has to be more radical. The opportunity to reduce a 'high' restoration or to review a doubtful tooth is not necessarily available without recourse to another general anaesthetic. Radiography is an important aid in theatre, especially for the patient who is totally unco-operative in the dental chair. It is particularly important for detecting otherwise hidden pathology and for early enamel lesions. The latter cannot normally be left in the hope that they will remineralize by preventive means. Similarly, the chances of restoration failure can be reduced by the use of pulpotomy techniques and preformed metal crowns. Most forms of treatment can be carried out under general anaesthesia provided there is sufficient operating time and the patient's general condition permits it.

Success is dependent upon careful pre-anaesthetic assessment by dentist and anaesthetist. Appropriate perioperative care in theatre, for example, steroid or antibiotic cover, and the back-up of in-patient facilities where medically or socially indicated, are vital to a successful outcome. Patients with Down syndrome may have altlanto-axial joint instability and will need extra care in moving from trolley to theatre table as well as during the recovery phase.

Key Points

Pre-anaesthetic assessment—important features:
- accurate medical history;
- previous anaesthetic history;
- significant airway difficulties;
- need for premedication;
- transport arrangements;
- home care.

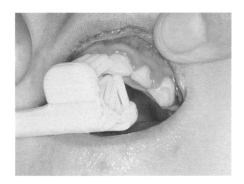

Fig. 17.10 A 'superbrush' in use in a child with cerebral palsy.

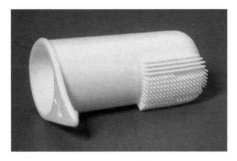

Fig. 17.11 An infadent brush for use with a patient who is uncooperative for oral hygiene measures.

17.2.4 Home care

Oral hygiene

There is little to be gained in embarking on elaborate treatment plans including advanced restorative work when it will not be maintained by regular oral hygiene measures at home.

Parents or carers need specific advice and practical help in the best way to care for their child's mouth. Great reliance is thus placed on the parent or carer who must be actively involved in oral hygiene instruction and given positive suggestions for modifications to the standard techniques. Examples include advice on the way to position a child (a bean bag can be helpful), in order to clean their mouth more efficiently and less traumatically. Another aid is the use of a prop such as a toothbrush handle to gain access to tooth surfaces on the other side of the mouth. Modification of existing, often very narrow-handled toothbrushes or the use of specially modified brush heads can be helpful (Fig. 17.10). Carers may be concerned about being bitten when they attempt to clean a child's mouth, in situations when toothbrushing is a battle. In these circumstances, use of an infadent brush (Fig. 17.11), with bristles incorporated onto the end of a plastic-type material that fits over the end of a finger, similar to a finger-stall, can overcome these problems and ensure adequate tooth cleaning.

For some children, the mechanical removal of plaque can be more readily accomplished using a powered toothbrush. Once the child has become accustomed to the sensation, results can be better than by conventional toothbrushing. Chemical agents are effective in reducing plaque in the short term, but not enough is known about the effects of their long-term usage. Many children find the taste of 0.2% chlorhexidine gluconate, either as a gel or solution, unpalatable and parents or carers are unhappy about the extrinsic brown staining. Many patients with impairments may be unable to use a mouthwash correctly and either swallow or spit out anything distasteful. An alternative technique is to opt for chairside application of chlorhexidene as a varnish. Originally intended for treating dentine hypersensitivity, application of the varnish has been shown to reduce the incidence of both gingival signs and dental caries.

Some schools for children with special educational needs provide toothbrushes for their pupils during their learning of personal hygiene skills. However, supervising staff may be unaware of the best method of mouth cleaning, which may be more dependent on their own perceptions of oral health and the perceived difficulty than any other factor (Fig. 17.12).

Toothbrushing can be taught in the same way as other skills, but it requires time for the individual as well as commitment on the part of the regular carer to ensure that all areas of the mouth are being cleaned each time. However, many disabled children are intolerant not only of toothbrushing but also of toothpaste and they may gag when toothpaste, which they cannot swallow because of poor reflexes, is introduced into the mouth. Toothpaste also obscures the view for the carer during toothbrushing and they cannot always be sure that the tooth surfaces are clean. In these circumstances, where toothpaste is unacceptable to the child, parents or carers should attempt to clean around the mouth with a piece of gauze moistened in a 0.2% chlorhexidine gluconate solution or a toothbrush dipped in fluoride mouthrinse (0.05% sodium fluoride if used on a daily basis). Alternatively, chlorhexidine in gel form or fluoride toothpaste can be rubbed as vigorously as possible around the tooth surfaces using a finger. Since chlorhexidene is inactivated by the traditional foaming agents in toothpastes, the former should be used at a different time of the day to the latter.

Children who are tube-fed for some or all of their nutrient intake still need oral care. They will frequently accumulate significant quantities of calculus, which, if detached might be inhaled. Regular mouth cleaning and the use of a 'tartar control' toothpaste are necessary (Fig. 17.13).

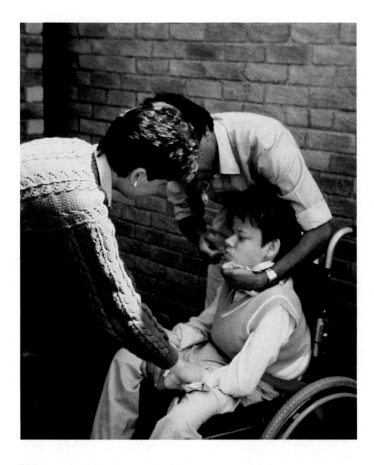

Fig. 17.12 Staff in a special school brushing the teeth of a child with an impairment.

Diet

More severely impaired children may have well-regulated eating times and a reduced likelihood of snacking. The food consumed may be semi-solid or even liquidized, but those foods which are easily reduced to this form are often dentally undesirable. In these circumstances the dentist should offer advice on limiting the number of intakes of food, provided it conforms to the child's general nutritional and dietary needs.

For some children establishing a normal eating routine while 'growing up' becomes a battlefield and impaired children are no exception to this. It is often easier for parents to 'give in' to a child and allow them to eat a limited variety of unsuitable foods frequently. This will be justified by parents saying they are desperate to get the child to eat something, and so biscuits, and other snacks high in non-milk extrinsic sugars, become the norm. This pattern is further endorsed in some children with impairments where weight gain is paramount and the dental implications are secondary, if indeed they are even considered. Drinks can also be a difficult area, particularly the use of sweetened bottles for an extended period in a child's life. It is not uncommon for children of 2 years of age or older still to be using a bottle containing milk, often for naps, last thing at night before going to bed and even during the night. This is an extremely difficult habit to break, but the most successful approach has been to advise the parent gradually to dilute the contents with water over a period of weeks, until eventually the child is drinking water only. This not only eliminates the undesirable habit but also gives the parent of the child, who is able to be toilet trained, some prospect of getting the child dry and out of nappies overnight.

For a number of children with impairments, the use of sweetened medication has led to an increase in dental caries (Fig. 17.14). In the past this has arisen because of a lack of sugars-free alternatives. However, with the pharmaceutical industry's greater awareness it is often only due to ignorance among the medical profession that such outmoded prescribing continues. Some children will be taking medication

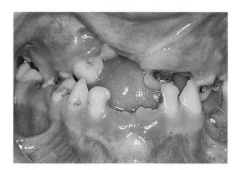

Fig. 17.13 Loose calculus deposits in a child with chromosome 4p-syndrome.

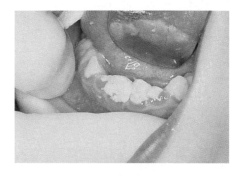

Fig. 17.14 The dental effects of frequent medication in a child with a cleft of the lip and palate.

as dispersible tablets or in an effervescent form, some of which, with chronic use, may predispose to dental erosion.

Another consideration is spoiling. For any parent the birth of a child who is impaired in some way, is a shock. Months of eager anticipation are followed by disbelief, anger, denial, frustration, and guilt. Parents have to grieve for the normal child they will never have, before coming to terms with their new responsibilities. Parents continue to feel guilty; maybe their child has an impairment because of something they have done, or something they should not have done. Either way, they may attempt to assuage that guilt by spoiling the child. This may take the form of easy to eat sweet foods, which are thought to be pleasurable and are welcomed by the child with a poor appetite, thus compounding the problem of poor eating. Poor eating habits resulting in oral disease need to be tackled together with the paediatrician and dietician, as well as the parents or caregivers.

> **Key Points**
> General dietary advice:
> - Restrict sweet foods/drinks to mealtimes.
> - Limit sweetened foods/drinks to three times a day.
> - Keep food and drinks clear of bedtime by about an hour.
> - Remember that carbonated drinks, and some medicines are erosive to teeth.
> - Ask for sugars-free medicines.

Fluorides

Many special milk formulas and food supplements, as well as containing non-milk extrinsic sugars to boost the child's calorie intake, in some cases also have quite substantial amounts of fluoride. It is wise therefore to check the diet carefully before advocating the use of fluoride supplements for such children. Where dental caries is potentially a real problem and in the absence of any other form of systemic fluorides, then the daily fluoride supplement regimen of 0.25 mg from 6 months of age, followed by an increase to 0.5 mg at 3 years of age, and then 1.0 mg from 6 to 16 years of age is to be advocated. Once the concentration of fluoride in the local water supply is known from the water company, fluoride supplements can be prescribed by the general dental practitioner if indicated, either as drops for the younger child or tablets for the preschool child. It is likely that some children with impairments will never cope with fluoride tablets and have to remain on drops. As long as the parent is given written instructions to overrule the prescribing schedule given for younger children on the label of the bottle, there is no reason why older children should not be prescribed fluoride drops.

The dentist should also advise on the appropriate fluoride toothpaste to be used in conjunction with fluoride supplementation or water fluoridation. Each case should be considered individually taking into account the relative risks and benefits that may occur. Paramount is consideration of the risk of developing dental caries versus the potential for enamel opacities in the permanent dentition. As a guideline, if the risk of caries is minimal, and if the diet is reasonably well controlled and home oral care is generally good, then it is sensible to suggest the use of a pea-sized amount of toothpaste containing approximately 500–600 p.p.m. of fluoride for the child under 6 years of age, provided that toothpaste can be used successfully. Older children, in the same situation should use a toothpaste containing between 1000 and 1500 p.p.m. of fluoride, as the risk of enamel opacities on anterior teeth is non-existent and this formulation will provide optimal protection against caries. In the child where the development of dental disease would pose a real hazard to their general health, and where home care in terms of oral hygiene and diet is poorly controlled, it is advisable to confer maximum protection by recommending the use of a toothpaste containing 1000–1500 p.p.m. of fluoride, even during the preschool years.

Because of the inability of many disabled children to hold solutions in their mouths or to expectorate, fluoride mouthwashes are contraindicated; however, they can be used on a toothbrush (dipped) where toothpaste is not well tolerated, to mimic the amount of topical fluoride received from toothpaste.

Key Points

Fluoride advice:

- supplements to give optimal caries protection;
- fluoride mouthwash on a toothbrush instead of paste in cases of paste intolerance;
- low caries risk: 500–600 p.p.m. of fluoride paste (<6 years), 1000–1500 p.p.m. of fluoride paste (>6 years);
- high caries risk: 1000–1500 p.p.m. of fluoride paste (pea-sized amount) from the time of tooth eruption onwards.

17.3 PHYSICAL IMPAIRMENT—CEREBRAL PALSY

The common physical impairments the dentist will encounter are: *developmental* neuromuscular disorders, for example, cerebral palsy, spina bifida, scoliosis, and osteogenesis imperfecta; and *degenerative* neuromuscular disorders, for example, muscular dystrophy and juvenile forms of arthritis. Included in this general category of physical impairment are children with clefts of the lip and/or palate (Chapter 14), where there may well be an associated syndrome in up to 19% of cases.

17.3.1 General considerations

Cerebral palsy occurs in 1–2 children per 1000 of school age, a figure which has been relatively stable because of the improved quality of survival of premature babies. This is a group of non-progressive neuromuscular disorders caused by brain damage, which can be pre-, peri-, or postnatal in origin, and is classified according to the type of motor defect:

1. *Spasticity*—impaired ability to control voluntary movements. There is the appearance of severe muscle stiffness and the planned movement of an affected limb results in a hypotonic tendon reflex, especially with rapid movements. Spasticity occurs in about 50% of cases of cerebral palsy.

2. *Athetosis*—uncontrolled, slow twisting, and writhing movements, which are frequent and involuntary and occur in over 16% of cases.

3. *Rigidity*—resistance to passive movement, which may be overcome by sudden action. It is uncommon and the majority of these children are intellectually impaired.

4. *Ataxia*—disturbance of equilibrium as well as difficulty in grasping objects. It is also uncommon.

5. *Hypotonia*—all muscles are flaccid with decreased function.

6. *Mixed*—a combination of the above.

The last 25 years has seen a change in the proportion of the different subtypes. For example, with the decrease in kernicterus (neonatal jaundice), there has been a fall in the athetoid form, but the spastic form, associated with prematurity, has increased. An affected child may be monoplegic with only one limb affected

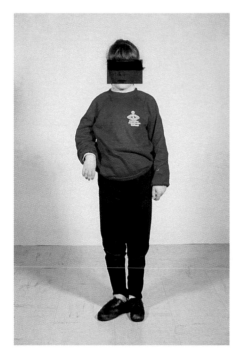

Fig. 17.15 Monoplegia of the right arm in a child with cerebral palsy and a congenital heart defect.

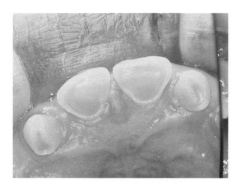

Fig. 17.16 Palatal erosion on maxillary incisors in a child with cerebral palsy.

(Fig. 17.15) or have all four limbs affected (quadriplegia). In addition, they may be disabled by other impairments such as convulsions, intellectual impairment, sensory disorders, emotional disorders, speech and communication defects, and a poorly developed swallowing and cough reflex.

17.3.2 Oral health

The oral and dental features that may be seen in children with cerebral palsy are:

(1) poor oral hygiene, increased periodontal disease, and drug-induced gingival enlargement;

(2) malocclusion (increased prevalence of skeletal class II with anterior open-bite);

(3) a tendency to bruxism;

(4) tongue thrust and mouth breathing;

(5) an increase in caries prevalence;

(6) increased prevalence of anterior trauma;

(7) enamel hypoplasia;

(8) heightened gag reflex and peri-oral sensitivity;

(9) drooling;

(10) decreased parotid flow rate.

Although not confined to children with cerebral palsy, gastric reflux is relatively common (Fig. 17.16). There may be an obvious aetiology, for example, a hiatus hernia, but quite often a cause for the erosion cannot be identified (Chapter 10).

17.3.3 Operative procedures

Children who are severely physically impaired will probably be brought to the dental surgery in a wheelchair or be carried. Care is required in the handling of such patients (see Section 17.4.1).

> **Key Points**
> Oral features in cerebral palsy:
> - gingival hyperplasia;
> - increased caries prevalence;
> - malocclusion;
> - dental trauma;
> - enamel hypoplasia;
> - heightened gag reflex;
> - dental erosion and abrasion (bruxism).

Altered gag and cough reflexes may complicate the delivery of dental care or the provision of prostheses, as well as adding to the patient's anxiety. Plentiful reassurance, efficient suction and skilled assistance are vital to success in these situations. Impaired ventilation may accompany scoliosis and becomes an even more important consideration if procedures involving a general anaesthetic are contemplated. Children who spend long periods in one position may be predisposed to pressure sores, therefore lengthy procedures in the dental chair without a break are best avoided.

Hypoplastic teeth can be very sensitive, particularly to extreme cold. Patients can experience acute discomfort during tooth preparation or ultrasonic scaling (even when the affected teeth are distant from the operating site), merely from the cold produced by high volume aspiration. The use of a desensitizing agent like Duraphat fluoride varnish or fissure sealing the symptomatic surface can be helpful if a restoration is not indicated. Hypoplastic enamel does not have the same ordered prism structure as normal enamel and, despite acid etching, may not provide optimum retention for conventional resins. In this situation, glass ionomer cements may be a more suitable alternative.

Some less severely disabled children will have little or no intellectual impairment but will have a degree of spasticity or rigidity. This may prevent them from co-operating fully with dental procedures, despite their willingness to do so, and they may be helped by nitrous oxide sedation (Chapter 4). Such sedation may also help diminish an exaggerated gag reflex.

17.3.4 Home care

Oral hygiene

Physical impairment may hinder oral hygiene procedures and for the child who has gingival enlargement the problem may be compounded. Most children require help with brushing until they are 7 years or older, but for the child with physical limitations this may be a permanent commitment on the part of carers. Limited or bizarre muscle movements prevent normal mouth clearing and food is often left impacted in the vault of the palate. This is readily removed with the end of a toothbrush handle or a spoon handle, but carers need to be aware of the potential for this, otherwise food residues may be left in the oral cavity for days. Powered toothbrushes may be helpful for a child with limited dexterity, not only because of the relative efficiency of cleaning but also because of the larger size of the handle of most of these brushes.

When normal limb movement is impaired or absent and/or normal speech is impossible, the mouth assumes an even greater importance as a means of holding mouthsticks to grasp pens or to operate a variety of equipment. It is vital the dentition is maintained to the highest standard as the successful use of such mouthsticks is reliant on having a good occlusal table for balanced contact (Fig. 17.17).

Children with cerebral palsy, especially where there is accompanying intellectual impairment, will on occasion adopt a habit of self-mutilation by chewing soft tissues around the mouth (Fig. 17.18). This can be triggered by teething, although often no cause may be found. It is distressing for the parents as the child is obviously in pain from the ulcerated areas and may refuse all food and drink, but there is little they can do to break the habit. It may be helpful to discuss the child's medication with their

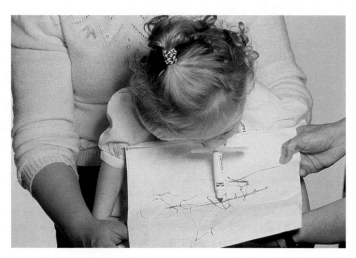

Fig. 17.17 A modified pen holder for a child with arthrogryphosis.

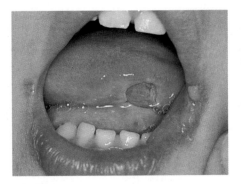

Fig. 17.18 Self-mutilation in a child with cerebral palsy.

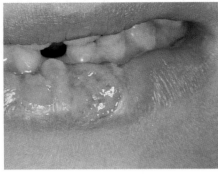
(a)

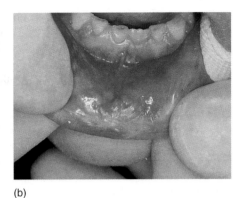
(b)

Fig. 17.19 (a) and (b) Traumatic self-mutilation in a boy with cerebral palsy—before and after the use of a composition 'splint' to protect the traumatized area.

physician as the prescription of a drug to reduce muscle tonus, which can be an exacerbating factor in this situation, could be considered.

There are a number of solutions to the problem depending on the cause and the severity of the condition. In a child who is erupting primary teeth it may be possible to fit an occlusal splint, provided that sufficient teeth are available for retention. Fabrication of the splint may necessitate a short general anaesthetic for impression-taking. Alternatively, addition of glass ionomer cement to the occlusal surfaces of the primary molars, to open the occlusion and prevent the teeth contacting the soft tissues, may be successful. If only anterior primary teeth are present then composition, moulded over the offending tooth surfaces as a temporary splint, may break the habit and allow healing (Fig. 17.19(a) and (b)). If the problem is more severe and a splint is not feasible, it is sensible to extract the primary teeth involved. In the permanent dentition, rounding-off the pointed or sharp tooth surfaces and/or fitting a splint is usually successful. During the acute phase the use of a topical analgesic such as 0.15% benzydamine hydrochloride (Difflam) in spray form increases mouth comfort prior to eating; and 0.2% chlorhexidine gluconate solution (Corsodyl) swabbed around the mouth or applied as a gel on a finger promotes more rapid healing by keeping the area clean. Ensuring that the child has plenty of fluids is of paramount importance as small, debilitated children rapidly become dehydrated.

The other area of concern to parents and carers is drooling. For some disabled children this can be excessive, although surgery to divert the submandibular flow more posteriorly may alleviate the problem. However, this is not always successful and carries the risk of increasing caries prevalence as a result of the greatly diminished salivary volume. The use of acrylic training plates that encourage the formation of an oral seal as well as promoting a more active swallowing mechanism so that saliva does not pool in an open mouth may be helpful (Fig. 17.20). Concurrent work with speech and language therapists will help with the necessary therapy that is fundamental to the success of such treatment. Anecdotal case reports support the use of these plates, but few studies have been published that give objective data on their success. However, one relatively non-interventional method of reducing saliva flow is the use of hyoscine hydrobromide, a drug which blocks parasympathetic transmission to the salivary glands. It is applied as a patch behind the ear and changed every three days.

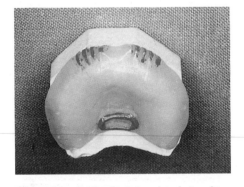

Fig. 17.20 A palatal training plate designed to improve lip and tongue posture.

Diet

Considerations on dietary aspects have been covered in the section on intellectual impairment (Section 17.2.4). Some children, because of a failure to thrive, will be fed through a gastrostomy site. If the child is exclusively fed via this route, they will tend to accumulate large deposits of calculus. These need to be removed from surfaces adjacent to the gingival margins in particular. This can be difficult unless there is good cooperation from the patient; an impaired airway makes the safe removal of such deposits hazardous, with the risk of inhalation of calculus. The gastrostomy site can be useful also for sedative drugs, especially bitter intravenous sedation drugs that might otherwise not be tolerated orally. However, such sedation procedures need to be carried out in specialist units.

17.4 PHYSICAL IMPAIRMENT—SPINA BIFIDA

Spina bifida occurs as a result of non-fusion of one or more posterior vertebral arches, with or without protrusion of some or all of the contents of the spinal canal. It may be accompanied by hydrocephalus in up to 95% of cases. It is estimated that in 50–60% of affected children the defect is inherited and that environmental agents may be responsible for the remainder. In the United Kingdom the incidence is 2.5 per 1000 births and, unlike other malformations, is commoner in females. A quarter of children will also have epilepsy and about a third will have some degree of intellectual impairment.

17.4.1 General considerations

Children with spina bifida will, unless the defect is slight, spend much of their time confined to a wheelchair (Fig. 17.21) and be incontinent. Urinary tract infections are common and the child may be on frequent courses of antibiotics. Hydrocephalus, unless arrested, is treated by the insertion of a shunt (fitted with a Spitz–Holter valve) to drain fluid from the ventricles into either the superior vena cava or more usually the peritoneum. It is important to protect the venous shunt from blockage, which may arise from a bacteraemia of oral origin, otherwise intracranial pressure will increase, causing convulsions. Although opinion is divided on the necessity to cover invasive dental procedures in children who have a shunt, those erring on the side of caution will use the same prophylaxis regimen as in cardiac disease (Chapter 16). However, there is no indication for antibiotic prophylaxis if the shunt is a ventriculo-peritoneal one.

Children who are confined to a wheelchair for much of the time will need to be treated either in their chair or transferred carefully to the dental chair. There are commercially available chair adaptations to accommodate a patient in their wheelchair (Fig 17.22). These are helpful if the child is too heavy to transfer easily to the dental chair or if the procedure is more easily accomplished for the operator and patient in this position. Shaped body supports, which are essentially modifications of a bean bag, are also available for use in the dental chair for any patient with a physical disability who cannot otherwise be comfortably accommodated. These supports contain a material that allows them to mould to the body shape of the patient and be remoulded for subsequent patients (Fig. 17.23).

17.4.2 Oral health and operative procedures

There is little in the dental literature to suggest that the oral/dental health of children with spina bifida is different from other children with impairments. The same principles of treatment apply to these children as to others who are impaired, namely aggressive prevention and early intervention with a radical approach if dental treatment under general anaesthesia is required.

17.4.3 Home care

The issues relevant to spina bifida have been covered in the appropriate sections under intellectual and physical impairment.

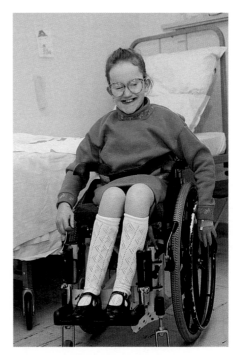

Fig. 17.21 A girl with spina bifida—wheelchair-aided.

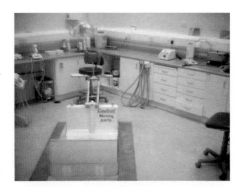

Fig. 17.22 A customized floor insert to accommodate a patient's wheelchair (courtesy of Dr Alistair Boles, National Rehabilitation Hospital, Ireland).

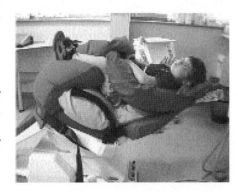

Fig. 17.23 Dental chair with moulded cushion supports (courtesy of Dr Bitte Ahlborg, Mun-H-Center, Sweden).

17.5 PHYSICAL IMPAIRMENT—MUSCULAR DYSTROPHY

Muscular dystrophy is a group of muscle diseases which present as progressive atrophy and weakness of skeletal muscles with resultant disability and deformity. The muscle fibres degenerate and are replaced by fatty and fibrous tissue. The disease is eventually fatal as a result of recurrent respiratory infections. Prevalence rates in children are of the order of 4 per 100,000 children.

17.5.1 General considerations

The child with muscular dystrophy will initially be mobile but as the disease progresses, they will become reliant on a wheelchair to move around. A respirator will be necessary in the later stages of the disease and patients are then confined to home or to residential care. There are a number of variants of the disease with different signs and symptoms. Males are exclusively affected in the Duchenne-type, while facial musculature is always affected in the fascioscapulohumeral-type, but rarely in other forms.

17.5.2 Oral health

The oral/dental effects of the disease are numerous and include:
- weakness of the facial muscles;
- poor oral hygiene secondary to the general inability to provide oral self-care;
- increased dental decay;
- increased potential for periodontal disease;
- malocclusion secondary to decreased facial muscle tone while retaining tongue function;
- decreased protective reflexes and reduced ability to swallow or clear secretions from the oropharynx, thus increasing the potential for aspiration.

17.5.3 Operative procedures

Consideration needs to be given to wheelchair transfer techniques and padding as well as the length of appointments (see above). The use of sedation and general anaesthesia may need to be avoided due to the decrease in respiratory function and the risk of post-anaesthetic complications. Frequent recall is important, with applications of topical fluorides and antiplaque agents (0.2% chlorhexidine gluconate). There are no contraindications to dental treatment, with the exception of orthodontics because of the changing muscle forces. As a consequence of tooth movement seen as part of the disease, and the likely development of anterior or posterior open-bites, prosthetic appliances may become non-functional.

17.5.4 Home care

Appropriate support and training needs to be given to the parent or carer so that in the later stages of the disease, when contact with dental services may be difficult, adequate plaque control can be maintained. Dental treatment may need to be provided within the home environment, although this will usually be at the stage when the patient has reached adulthood. It is important that every effort is made to optimize oral function and facial appearance and thereby encourage a positive self-image.

17.6 OTHER MUSCULOSKELETAL IMPAIRMENTS

There are a variety of other defects, some degenerative and some developmental, which also affect children; however, these are relatively rare and unlikely to be encountered regularly in practice—for example, osteogenesis imperfecta, juvenile arthritis, and multiple sclerosis. When patients present with such disabilities there may be significant oral signs, for example, in rheumatoid arthritis there is an increased incidence of Sjögren's syndrome (autoimmune) and anaemia (secondary to anti-inflammatory and steroid medication). Aggressive prevention is vital to prevent dental disease.

17.7 BLINDNESS AND VISUAL IMPAIRMENT

Visual impairments vary from total blindness to sight limitations of size, colour, distance, and shape. The prevalence is in the order of 3 per 1000 children.

17.7.1 Oral health

The oral and dental health of children with a visual impairment is no different from the normal population and with good home care this can be maintained. In the United Kingdom many children are educated in boarding schools and their supervision, with regard to personal hygiene and diet (restraint from between-meal snacking), often means that their oral health is good.

17.7.2 Operative procedures

Consideration should be given to the design and format of written material available for use by patients who may be visually impaired, for example, instructions for the wearing of orthodontic appliances and diet history sheets. Highly stylized type should be avoided and a mix of upper and lower case should be used. Letters should be at least one-eighth of an inch high (about 3 mm; 14 point) and be on uncoated (non-glare) paper. The best contrast for ease of reading is black type on white or off-white paper.

It is important to assist the visually impaired person according to their individual needs. Patients with a sight defect object to being forcefully guided around by a nurse or dentist who is enthusiastic to help. Many sight-impaired patients will have an increased sensitivity to bright lights and perhaps touch. The operating light should therefore be used with caution and the latter should be utilized to enhance the patients' perception of what is being done; for example, being allowed to feel the instruments and the dental chair.

It is not unusual for people to shout at those with a visual impairment. Sight-impaired children are not usually deaf as well and should therefore be addressed in a normal voice. It is important to the patient, and not only those with visual impairments, that conversation is addressed to them and not to the person with them—the so-called 'Does he take sugar?' approach. Because vision is impaired and the sense of touch may be heightened, it can be startling suddenly to feel a cold mirror in your mouth without warning. A 'tell-feel-then-do' approach is important for these children who may be unnerved by contact without forewarning. With these considerations in mind, there are no areas of dental treatment that are unsuitable for the child with a visual impairment, provided that they, or their parent or carer, can maintain an adequate standard of oral hygiene. Insertion of orthodontic appliances may initially be difficult and techniques like flossing take time to master.

17.8 DEAFNESS AND HEARING IMPAIRMENT

Loss of hearing is an impairment acquired by many with increasing age. However, some children are born with either a partial or total loss of hearing and this can occur in isolation or in combination with other impairments, for example, rubella syndrome (auditory, visual, intellectual, and cardiac defects). The prevalence is 3 per 1000 children.

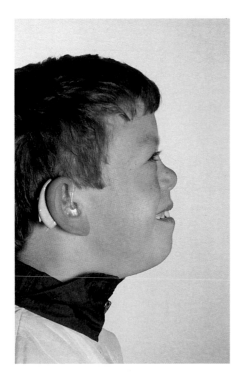

Fig. 17.24 A child with William's syndrome wearing hearing aids.

17.8.1 General considerations

Patients who have hearing impairment may be fearful, or even hostile, because they feel they are not going to understand what is being asked of them. The child may not hear what has been said but pretends they have done so to avoid embarrassment. In this situation visual aids assume an even greater importance. It is important for optimizing hearing that all extraneous background noise is removed when communicating with the hearing-impaired child. Piped music in the surgery, noise from the reception area, as well as internal noises from aspirators and scavenging systems should be reduced or eliminated.

Many deaf or hearing-impaired children will wear aids (Fig. 17.24) to enable them to pick up more sounds, and older children may have become skilled not only in lip-reading but also in signing. However, there is now a trend towards discouraging the use of signing and to positively encourage a child to acquire some speech, utilizing any residual vocal potential.

17.8.2 Oral health

There is a paucity of data concerning the oral health of children with hearing impairment. As with visually impaired children, residence away from home in special boarding schools sometimes means that eating patterns are more desirable dentally, with less opportunity for between-meal snacking compared to day pupils. Supervision of oral hygiene measures can also be better in children living in institutions and is reflected in their oral hygiene scores, but this is very variable. Like many other impaired children, hearing-impaired patients are initially wary of powered toothbrushes because of the sensation they produce intraorally. But, although these brushes have not been shown to be better in terms of plaque removal than a well-manipulated manual brush, in children particularly, the novelty aspect may be a motivating factor to use this type of brush to greater benefit.

17.8.3 Operative procedures

For those children who can lip-read it is necessary to sit well in front of the child, with good lighting to the operator's face. Both dentist and assistant should move their lips clearly during speech and avoid the temptation to shout. Masks are therefore to be put to one side and bearded operators should ensure that facial hair does not obscure clear visualization of lip movement! A comment as to the best hearing side should be inserted in the patient's notes so that staff are aware of this at each visit.

Children wearing hearing devices may be disturbed by the high-pitched noise produced by handpieces and ultrasonic scalers. This may make them less co-operative and less amenable to treatment. Similarly, the conduction of vibrations from the handpiece and burs via bone is more disturbing for the hearing-impaired child. After initial communications are complete it may be advisable to suggest that the hearing device is removed or turned off and only re-inserted on completion of the dental treatment in time for final instructions. Very young children often have difficulty keeping the aids in place simply because of the size of the immature pinnae. This is especially so when lying supine in the dental chair.

17.9 SUMMARY

1. Children with impairments present the dental team with the challenge of adapting familiar skills to new situations.
2. To meet this challenge effectively we need to re-examine some of the stereotypes of impairment we carry in our own minds.

3. An impairment becomes a disability by virtue of other people's attitudes, the things we do or do not do, the facilities we do not offer, as well as the physical barriers the environment interposes.

4. Oral and dental health are little different between children with impairments and others. What is different is the type of treatment provided, with more missing teeth and fewer filled teeth in populations with impairments.

5. Some children have specific oral conditions as a result of their impairment, for example, periodontal disease in Down syndrome.

6. A degree of common-sense, a willingness to be flexible, as well as a working familiarity with the commoner medical conditions and their implications for oral and dental health, are most of what a general dental practitioner requires to provide dental care for the child with impairments in his or her community.

17.10 FURTHER READING

Nunn, J. H. (2000). *Disability and oral care*. FDI World Dental Press Ltd., London. (*A comprehensive coverage of aspects of oral and dental care for people with disabilities.*)

Nunn, J. H. (2003). Preventing childhood impairment. In *The prevention of oral disease* (4th edn). (eds. J. J. Murray, J. H. Nunn, and J. G. Steele), pp. 200–16. Oxford Medical Publications, Oxford. (*A more comprehensive review of preventive aspects of oral/dental care.*)

Shuman, S. K., Bebeau, M. J. (1994). Ethical issues in nursing home care: practice guidelines for difficult situations. Spec Care Dent, **16**, 170–7. (*Covers criteria for the safe use of physical intervention.*)

Index